Fluoride in Dentistry

FLUORIDE IN DENTISTRY

2nd edition

Edited by

Ole Fejerskov • Jan Ekstrand • Brian A. Burt

Munksgaard

Fluoride in Dentistry

2nd edition, 1st printing

Copyright © 1996 Munksgaard, Copenhagen

All rights reserved

Cover: Tegnestuen Munksgaard

Drawings, composition and typesetting: Tegneren Jens ApS, Vejle

Reproduction: Boisen Print, Grindsted

Printed in Denmark by: Fr. Martin, Christiansfeld

ISBN 87-16-11282-2

PREFACE

From the time it was first added to the drinking water of Grand Rapids, Michigan, in January 1945, the benefits of fluoride have become truly global in their scope. Over the last generation, the extent and severity of dental caries in the economically developed world has declined to an extent that was unimaginable in the days when many of today's dental practitioners attended dental school, and most indicators are that this trend is still in progress. Fluoride, in the different ways it is used today, is universally agreed to have been the principal influence in this major public health phenomenon. It has profoundly affected the way dentistry is practiced today, and it has led to extensive changes in the curricula of dental schools.

Despite extensive research with both unerupted and erupted teeth, however, there are still some fundamental aspects of fluoride's action on dental tissues which are not yet fully understood. Research continues into the mechanisms by which fluoride affects the initial mineralization of the teeth, as well as the ways in which it inhibits demineralization and promotes the reprecipitation of minerals at the tooth surface. Practical delivery methods continue to be developed, and the challenge of bringing fluoride's benefits to the economically developing world continues to be studied. In some countries, the use of fluoride is so pervasive that increases in the prevalence and severity of dental fluorosis have been reported. To deal with this issue, refinement in the amounts and timing of the mass provision of fluoride is still needed.

When the first English edition of this book appered in 1988, it was already clear that the principal action of fluoride in reducing caries was by its effect on the demineralization and subsequent remineralization of enamel during caries initiation and progression. This action has been confirmed by a solid body of research evidence since then. The aim of this second edition has thus been to collate the most pertinent recent research on fluoride, with special emphasis on making its benefits applicable in everyday dental practice.

This second edition has been thoroughly revised and expanded by including contributions from a broad spectrum of experts in various fields of fluoride research, most of them active teachers and researchers in academic institutions in Europe and North America. It is presented in four sections to enable the reader to gain easy access to its wealth of information. The first section covers the occurrence and distribution of fluoride in the environment, and the methods of chemical analysis employed to determine fluoride content. The second section presents physiological and toxicological aspects of fluorides with emphasis on their effect on humans. The third section focuses on the nature of dental caries and the effect of fluoride in the oral environment. To complete the picture, the fourth section covers the major clinical and public health uses of fluoride today.

This book is intended to help dental students and graduate students receive the most up-to-date knowledge about fluoride as a cornerstone of preventive dentistry today. Dental practitioners, dental hygienists and public health administrators will also benefit from the information in this book. The multiplicity of authors gives the book a heterogeneity of style which, we hope, readers will find refreshing. The world of fluoride research moves rapidly, and while extraordinary progress has been made in reducing the scourge of dental caries, much still remains to be done. We hope this book will serve to help us all reach that goal.

January 1996

Ole Fejerskov, Jan Ekstrand, Brian A. Burt

CONTENTS

Section III FLUORIDE AND THE ORAL ENVIRONMENT – THE EFFECT ON THE CARIES PROCESS

9

LIST OF CONTRIBUTORS

Dr. Vibeke Baelum
Royal Dental College
Faculty of Health Sciences
Aarhus University
Aarhus C
Denmark

Professor David W. Banting
Faculty of Dentistry
University of Western Ontario
London, Ontario
Canada

Professor George H.W. Bowden
Faculty of Dentistry
University of Manitoba
Winnipeg, Manitoba
Canada

Professor Brian A. Burt
School of Public Health
The University of Michigan
Ann Arbor, Michigan
USA

Professor Brian H. Clarkson
School of Dentistry
The University of Michigan
Ann Arbor, Michigan
USA

Dr. Pamela DenBesten
School of Dentistry
University of California,
San Francisco, California
USA

Professor Jan Ekstrand
Karolinska Institutet
School of Dentistry
Huddinge
Sverige

Dr. Erik Fink Eriksen
Aarhus County Hospital
Aarhus C
Denmark

Professor John D.B. Featherstone
School of Dentistry
University of California,
San Francisco, California
USA

Professor Ole Fejerskov
Royal Dental College
Faculty of Health Sciences
Aarhus University
Aarhus C
Denmark

Professor Emeritus Samuel J. Fomon
Department of Pediatrics
University of Iowa
Iowa City, Iowa
USA

Professor Ian R. Hamilton
Faculty of Dentistry
University of Manitoba
Winnipeg, Manitoba
Canada

Dr. Herschel S. Horowitz
Consultant, Dental Research & Public Health
6307 Herkos Court
Bethesda, Maryland
USA

Professor Amid I. Ismail
Faculty of Dentistry
Dalhousie University
Halifax, Nova Scotia
Canada

Dr. Jennifer Kirkham,
School of Dentistry
The University of Leeds
Leeds
England

Professor Emeritus Thomas M. Marthaler
Dental Institute
University of Zürich
Zürich
Switzerland

Professor Flemming Melsen
Aarhus County Hospital
Aarhus C
Denmark

Professor Leif Mosekilde
Aarhus County Hospital
Aarhus C
Denmark

Professor Emeritus Aaron S. Posner
2 Longview Drive
Scarsdale, New York
USA

Dr. Alan Richards
Royal Dental College
Faculty of Health Sciences
Aarhus University
Aarhus C
Denmark

Professor Colin Robinson
School of Dentisty
The University of Leeds
Leeds
England

Professor Gunnar Rölla
Faculty of Dentistry
University of Oslo
Oslo
Norway

Professor Frank A. Smith †
Medical Center
University of Rochester
Rochester, New York
USA

Professor Jacob M. (Bob) ten Cate
Academic Centre for Dentistry Amsterdam
(ACTA)
University of Amsterdam
Amsterdam
The Netherlands

Dr. Pothapragada Venkateswarlu
3M/Specialty Materials Divison
Saint Paul, Minnesota
USA

Dr. Gerald Lee Vogel
American Dental Association Health
Foundation
National Institute of Standards and
Technology
Gaithersburg, Maryland
USA

Professor John A. Weatherell
School of Dentistry
The University of Leeds
Leeds
England

Professor Gary M. Whitford
School of Dentistry
Medical College of Georgia
Augusta, Georgia
USA

Section I

General Aspects of Fluorides

CHAPTER 1

THE OCCURRENCE AND THE CHEMISTRY OF FLUORIDE

F.A. Smith • J. Ekstrand

Introduction – Chemistry – Fluoride in the lithosphere – Fluoride in the hydrosphere
Fluoride in the atmosphere – Fluoride in the biosphere

Introduction

When considered from the biological viewpoint, fluoride is usually classed with the trace elements. This is reasonable, inasmuch as fluoride can occur biologically in very small amounts, and concentrations in biological materials generally are in the parts per million (ppm) range or less. However, fluorides are present in the environment to a far greater extent than is implied by the term "trace" element. Fluoride is apparently ubiquitous and has been reported in the atmosphere of Venus, in meteorites, and in lunar samples. It ranks thirteenth among the elements in order of abundance in the earth's crust. In the combined state, fluoride constitutes about 0.065% by weight of the crust.[14]

The dispersion of fluoride in the environment is represented in Fig. 1-1. Fluoride enters the atmosphere by volcanic action and by the entrainment of soil and water particles due to wind action on these surfaces. It is returned to the earth's surface by deposition as dust or rain, snow and fog. Fluoride enters the hydrosphere by leaching from soils and minerals into ground water and by entry with surface waters. Fluoride enters vegetation by uptake from soil and water, by absorption of gaseous fluorides from the air, and by deposition of particulate fluorides from the atmosphere and from rain splash. It is returned to the soil through plant waste, or it may enter the food chain and be returned as animal or human waste.

Fluoride may enter these pathways directly or indirectly from various industrial processes such as grinding, drying and calcining of fluoride-containing minerals, acidulation of these minerals, metallurgic processes involving fluoride fluxes or melts, melting raw materials in glassmaking, kiln firing of brick and ceramic materials, and the use of fluoride-containing materials in cleaning, etching and electroplating. Principal industries with a potential for appreciable fluoride release include electric power generation at coal-burning stations, and the production of aluminum, steel, phosphate fertilizers, phosphoric acid, phosphorus and the manufacture of glass, ceramic and brick products.

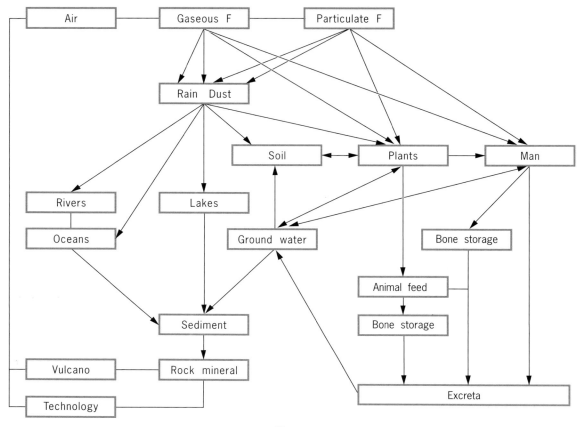

Fig. 1-1. Dispersion of fluoride in the environment.[25]

Chemistry

The chemistry of fluorine and fluorides has been reviewed in depth by Banks & Goldwhite and by Glemser.[21] Pertinent information from those reviews can be summarized as follows.

Because of the small radius of the fluorine atom, its effective surface charge is greater than that of any other element. As a consequence, fluorine is the most electronegative and reactive of all the elements. It reacts promptly with its surroundings and is rarely found in the free or elemental state. Indeed, at appropriate temperatures fluorine directly attacks all elements except oxygen and nitrogen. The standard potential of the fluorine-fluoride ion electrode is +2.8v. No other redox potential approaches this value, meaning that elemental fluorine cannot be produced by chemical oxidation of fluoride ions or by electrolysis of solutions containing any negative ion other than fluoride. This latter condition underlies both the first isolation of fluorine in 1886 by Moissan and the modern day large-scale production of fluorine; in both instances fluorine was or is released by the electrolysis of a mixture of molten potassium fluoride and anhydrous hydrogen fluoride. Fluorine is exclusively monovalent, which is not true for the other halogens. The common states for the fluorine atom in combination are the ionic form F^- and the electrovalent or covalent form. Metallic fluorides are usually ionic in nature, with melting and boiling points usually higher than the other corresponding halides. Most of the ionic fluorides are readily soluble in water, although the fluorides of lithium, aluminum, strontium, barium, magnesium, calcium and manganese are only slightly soluble. Covalent compounds are formed with nonmetals, e.g. silicon tetrafluoride and sulfur hexafluoride. Covalent fluorides often have much lower melting and boiling points than do the corresponding chlorides and bromides. Many of the covalent non-metal fluorides are extremely stable.

Fluoride in the lithosphere

Because of its extreme reactivity, fluorine rarely occurs in nature in its elemental form, but is found most frequently as inorganic fluoride. It concentrates in the last stages of crystallizing magmas and in the residual solutions and vapors. Thus, concentrations are increased in siliceous rocks, alkalic rocks, in geothermal waters and hot springs, and in volcanic fumaroles and gases. About 150 fluoride-containing minerals are known, of which fluorspar (fluorite, CaF_2, 49% F), fluorapatite ($Ca_{10}F_2(PO_4)6$, 3.4% F) and cryolite (Na_3AlF_6, 54% F) are the most important. Fluorspar and fluorapatite are widespread and are mined in many countries. The once enormous deposits of cryolite in Greenland are now largely depleted. Fluorine replaces the hydroxyl group in hydroxy silicates, e.g. in topaz $[Al_2SiO_4(OH,F)]$, and in hydroxyapatites to form fluorapatite.

Fluoride concentrations in several rock types are listed in Table 1-1. In sedimentary rocks fluorides is usually found in fluorite, mica, amphiboles, apatite and clay minerals and is richest in shales; in igneous rock the granites are

Table 1-1

Fluoride concentrations in different rock types (concentrations in mg/kg ~ppm)

Igneous		Sedimentary	
felsic	735	shales	740
intermediate	500	sandstones	270
mafic	400	carbonates	330

Data from Fuge[19]

the richest.[20] Granites vary widely, however. Fuge & Andrews[20] have reported that the mean fluoride concentrations of granite rocks from different sites in England, Northern Ireland, Wales and Scotland ranged from 569 to 15,464 mg/kg; other igneous rocks from Wales and Scotland contained 429-913 ppm; sedimentary rocks from Wales, Scotland and England averaged 110-691 ppm; meta-igneous rocks from Land's End and from Wales averaged 1014 and 542 ppm, respectively. Finnish rapakivi granites have been reported to contain 2000-4000 ppm fluoride, whereas average granites in Finland contained 500-1000 ppm fluoride.[30] Fluoride concentrations of 1500-3200 ppm were found in young alkaline volcanic rocks in Tanzania (loc. cit.). Geologic sources of fluoride in the United Kingdom have been mapped by Fuge & Andrews,[20] in Finland by Lahermo et al.,[30] and in the United States by Shacklette et al.[38]

Fluoride in soils is derived primarily from the geologic parent material with only minor proportions coming from airborne sea spray.[30] In acid soils (pH < 6) fluoride is bound chiefly in complexes with aluminum and with iron. At pH > 6 the dominant species is the fluoride iron.[12,13] During weathering, fluorine-containing minerals may be rapidly broken down, particularly in acid soils.[20] Soil fluoride varies widely but generally ranges from 50 to 500

19

ppm. Samples of non-industrially contaminated soils from Germany, Greece, Finland, Japan, Morocco, New Zealand, Sweden, USA and USSR have been reported as containing from 30 to over 500 ppm of fluoride though soils near fluorite, and other types of mineralization may show enrichment up to more than 5000 ppm.[20] In normal circumstances there is a tendency for concentrations to increase with increasing sampling depth, due to leaching.[9,10] This is particularly true in acid soils. High calcium levels tend to block the downward migration, as do also clay minerals and aluminum.[20] It is the available or labile fluoride which is of special interest, because of the potential for damage to plant and animal life. In nonsaline soils, calcium is the principal agent for fixation of fluoride and the limited solubility usually leads to water-soluble fluoride concentrations of less than 1 ppm. In saline soils, the dominance of sodium and the resultant greater solubility of fluoride can result in water-soluble concentrations of several ppm.[10]

Volcanic activity can contribute large amounts of fluoride to surface soils by way of ash deposited on the nearby terrain. During the 1970 eruption of Mt. Hekla in Iceland, the ash deposited in the first days in southern and northern Iceland contained 2000 and 1400 ppm fluoride, respectively. A fortnight later it had dropped to 10% of the original amount and was only 1% of the original concentration 3 weeks later.[18]

Human activities are known to contribute to the fluoride burden in soils. The addition of fluoride-containing phosphate fertilizers and sewage sludges to agricultural soils have been reported to increase soil fluoride appreciably.[20] Increases in soil fluoride have been reported in the vicinity of a plant producing elemental phosphorus from phosphate rock containing calcium fluoride[40] and near aluminum production facilities.[23] However, soil fluoride was unchanged in samples taken downwind from a coal-fired electric power generating plant.[49]

Fluoride in the hydrosphere

Ground waters in the United States have been reported to contain up to 67 ppm F;[17,51] ground waters in the rapakivi granite area of Finland contain, on average, 1.0-2.0 ppm F.[30] Concentrations are affected by factors such as availability and solubility of fluoride-containing minerals, porosity of the rocks or soils through which the water passes, residence time, temperature, pH, and the presence of other elements, e.g. calcium, aluminum and iron, which may complex with fluoride. Most surface waters contain less than 0.1 ppm of fluoride, the concentrations being influenced by the contributing sources, and the amounts of runoff and precipitation. Most US rivers contain less than 0.5 ppm fluoride, though higher concentrations have been noted.[16,17,41] Swedish rivers have been reported to contain 0.09-0.60 ppm, French rivers 0.08-0.25 ppm and rivers in Spain, Quebec Province in Canada, the UK, Japan and Finland 0.03-1.0 ppm F. Most of the fluoride exists as free fluoride ion, but complexed fluoride increases with increasing salinity, reaching 50-60% in sea water.

Surface water fluoride can be increased by the discharge of industrial wastes and municipal sewage into the streams. Evaluations of the fluoride status of several French rivers polluted by effluents from facilities producing aluminum of phosphate fertilizers showed fluoride concentrations to be increased near the point of entry of the effluent into the stream, but to be normal again at points further downstream.[29] Municipal water fluoridation programs have been shown not to increase environmental fluoride concentrations to toxic levels.[34]

Sea water contains 1.2-1.4 ppm fluoride (c. 0.07 mM)[7,19,22], depending on the chlorinity. In the Baltic Sea, concentrations ranged from 0.14 ppm with a chlorinity of 1.10% (Ajos, Gulf of Bothnia) to 0.69 ppm in water with a chlorinity of 8.83% (Helsingør, The Kattegat).[2] Concentrations may be enhanced locally by undersea volcanic activity. Fluoride exists in sea water in the ionic form and in fluoride complexes; MgF^+ constituting nearly half of these. Fluoride is lost from the seas by incorporation by life forms into carbonates and phosphates and by ejection or surface spray into the atmosphere. The airborne fluoride is returned by way of rain- and snowfall, and via the rivers when these events occur over land. Carpenter is of the opinion that the principal source of oceanic fluoride is the input from rivers.[7]

Hot waters associated with volcanic activity have been reported to contain elevated fluoride concentrations.[32] Acid spring waters located close to volcanic activity may contain 5000-6000 ppm fluoride. Geothermal waters in Yellowstone National Park, in the USA, contain up to 24 ppm fluoride and are responsible for the typical fluorotic damage to the bones and teeth of deer, elk and bison foraging in this region.[39]

Rain samples collected in areas of minimal or no local fluoride pollution were found to contain 2-20 parts per billion (ppb).[3] Anthropogenic sources of fluoride may appreciable increase fluoride in rain samples. Fluoride in snow cover may serve as a convenient way to monitor environmental pollution control programs. For example, snow samples collected in the vicinity of aluminum smelters in Quebec, Canada prior to the installation of control measures contained an average of 0.925 ppm fluoride; 6 years later, after installation of control measures to reduce the emissions of gaseous and particulate fluorides, the average fluoride concentration in snow had been reduced to 0.097 ppm. Natural background concentration in the area was 0.05 ppm.[35]

Fluoride in the atmosphere

Fluorides are found in the air of rural communities as well as that over cities. The sources are varied and include effluvia from volcanoes, dust generated by the weathering of fluoride-containing soils and outcroppings of fluoride-containing minerals, ocean spray, smoke from burning coal and releases from a variety of industrial processes.

An in-depth air monitoring study in Great Britain[31] showed that concentrations of water-soluble fluoride in total suspended airborne particles collected at 11 sites varied from place to place, ranging from 0.01 to 0.07 mg/m^3 at the six primary sites and from 0.05 to 0.17 mg/m^3 at five secondary sites. The variations appeared to reflect local sources, and were little affected by the heating or the nonheating season. Fluoride constituted 0.04-0.13% by weight of samples from all sites in both seasons. The major component was sulfate, at 6.9-25.7% by weight.

Similar concentrations of water-soluble fluorides in particulate matter were found in an earlier survey done in the US.[46] In this investigation more than 88% of all urban samples showed concentrations < 0.05 mg/m^3, the minimum detectable concentration. Only 0.2% of the urban samples exceeded 1.00 mg/m^3; the maximum concentration found was 1.89 mg/m^3. These urban samples were characterized as center-city business-commercial and were not taken at industrial locations. More than 98% of samples from non-urban sites showed < 0.05 mg/m^3; 0.1% contained > 0.10 mg/m^3 (maximum, 0.16 mg/m^3). Over 90% of all urban and non-urban samples did not contain detectable fluoride. Similar background concentrations of airborne fluoride (< 0.1 mg/m^3) have been reported by others.[11,26,36,48]

Ambient airborne fluoride concentrations have been measured in the vicinity of industrial operations. Most frequently, these have measured total fluoride. In some instances, gaseous and particulate fluoride have been determined separately and have demonstrated that the gaseous components represent less than half of the total fluoride. The common gaseous components are HF and SiF_4. Treshow[47] is

Table 1-2
Airborne fluoride concentrations near industrial facilities

Facility	Airborne fluoride, mg/m^3	Country	Reference
Aluminum, phosphates	3.0	The Netherlands	5
Aluminum	ca. 0.60	Canada	15
Aluminum	0.54	Norway	42, 43
Aluminum	0.63	Norway	28
Phosphate mining	12.6 (0.5 km downwind)	US	8
Sugerphosphate	2.0	Belgium	36
Manufacture fluorides	0.2	Spain	48
Manufacture fluorides, steel, glass (Rotherham)	1-6 gaseous 0-1 particulate	England	26
Industrial cities	0.1-1.0	Great Britain	9
Stoke-on-Trent	1.9 (winter) 2.8 (summer)	England	4,33
Rhine-Rhur region	0.2-0.4	Germany	6
Duisburg	1.3	Germany	37

quoted by Haidouti et al.[23] as stating that gaseous compounds account for more than half of airborne fluorides around industrial sites. Some of these data are listed in Table 1-2. These concentrations should not be accepted in an absolute sense, however. Concentrations in such surveys are influenced by many factors, the cyclic nature of some observations, season of the year, and local meteorologic conditions. Nevertheless, concentrations associated with industrial activities usually are distinctly different from those encountered in rural or nonurban localities.

Other sources of airborne fluorides include the domestic use of coal as a fuel and volcanic activity. Coals have been reported to contain up to approximately 500 ppm fluoride, though most contain less than this.[41] Davison et al.[11]

found a mean concentration of 0.28 mg F/m^3 in air samples collected in urban coal-burning areas vs. a mean of 0.05 mg F/m^3 in rural areas. Yixin et al.[52] found 21 and 3.6 mg F/m^3, respectively, in the air of kitchens and bedrooms of homes burning coal as a fuel in the Pingxiang region of China; in homes burning wood for heating and cooking, the corresponding airborne concentrations were 1.2 and 0.9 mg/m^3. Symonds et al.[45] determined that hydrogen fluoride is the predominant species of fluorine in volcanic gases. The authors estimated the annual global volcanic emission of fluoride to be 0.06-6 Tg. Less than 10% of this is released in large, infrequent explosive emissions that project fluoride to the stratosphere; the remainder is vented to the troposphere by small explosive eruptions and passive degassing.

Fluoride in the biosphere

As summarized by Weinstein[50] the normal accumulation of soil fluoride in plants is small. Leaves generally contain 2-20 ppm. There is little relationship between fluoride concentrations in soils and plants; fluoride added to soil as a contaminant in fertilizer has little effect on fluoride in the crop, although plants grown in acidic soils tend to have higher fluoride concentrations than do those grown in calcareous soils. The uptake of fluoride varies among plant species, being influenced by age of the leaf, soil, use of fertilizers, irrigation and other factors.

A few species of plants are known to accumulate several hundred parts per million of fluoride, for example, tea (*Camillea sinensis*) and other members of the genus *Camillia*.[10]

Industrial air pollution is thought not to add enough fluoride to soils to significantly affect the soil-derived fluoride in plants. However, vegetation grown in the vicinity of industrial facilities may show elevated fluoride concentrations as a result of the absorption of particulate and gaseous fluorides impinging on leafy surfaces. Concentrations decrease with increasing distance from the source. For example, leaves of white birch were sampled 0.7-18.7 km from a plant producing elemental phosphorus from fluoride-containing phosphate rock. At the end of the growing season, leaves taken at 0.7 km contained 357 ppm fluoride; concentrations decreased with increasing distance from the source to 7 ppm at 18.7 km. Airborne fluoride also decreased at the end of the growing season from 4.34 mg/m^3 at 0.7 km to 0.15 $\mu g/m^3$ at 18.7 km.[40] Fluoride accumulations in the foliage of wild raspberry plants 1.4 km from this source and at a control site were 403 and 8 ppm respectively, while foliage samples of wild blueberry were 216 and 9 ppm respectively.[43] Investigations into the effects of fluoride emissions on the natural vegetation surrounding an aluminum reduction plant in Greece have been reported by Haidouti *et al.*[23] Three response zones in the area ranging out to 15 km from the source were identified, using the effects seen in *Olea europea var. oleaster* as a criterion. In the zone nearest to the source, the *Olea* leaves showed a necrosis associated with 200-400 ppm fluoride. In the next zone *Olea* leaves showed a chlorosis associated with 100-200 ppm fluoride. In the outermost zone there were no visible signs of injury and the leaves contained < 100 ppm fluoride.

Fluorosis has been reported in livestock in Morocco where grass, forage, straw and barley have been contaminated by gaseous and particulate fluoride emissions from phosphate mining and processing facilities. The fluorosis endemic in human populations in the same regions is thought to originate from the inhalation of fluoride-bearing dusts.[24,27]

Background literature

Fluorides – effects on vegetation, animals and humans. Shupe JL, Peterson HB, Leone NC, eds. Salt Lake City: Paragon Press, 1983.

Environmental Protection Agency. Reviews of the Environmental Effects of Pollutants: 1X. Fluoride. Report Number EPA-600/1-78-050. Prepared for Health Effects Research Laboratory, US Environmental Protection Agency, Cincinnati, Ohio, by Oak Ridge National Laboratory, Tennessee.

Koritnig S. Fluorine. Chapter 9. In: Wadepohl KH, ed. Handbook of Geochemistry. Berlin: Springer-Verlag, 1977.

Smith FA, Hodge HC. Airborne fluorides and man: Part I. Crit Rev Enviro Control 1978; 8: 293-371.

Literature cited

1. Banks RE, Goldwhite H. Fluorine chemistry. In: Smith FA, ed. Handbook of experimental pharmacology, vol. XX/1, Pharmacology of fluorides. New York: Springer-Verlag, 1966: 1-52.

2. Barbaro A, Francescon A, Polo B. Fluoride distribution along chlorinity gradients in Baltic Sea waters. Finn Marine Res 1981; No. 248: 129-36.

3. Barnard WR, Nordstrom DK. Fluoride in precipitation – II. Implications for geochemical cycling of fluorine. Atmos Environ 1982; 16: 105-11.

4. Bennet AJ, Barratt RS. Some observations on atmospheric fluoride concentrations in Stoke-on-Trent. Roy Sci Health J 1980; 100: 86-94.

5. Biersteker K, Zielhuis RL, Backer Dirks O, van Leeuwen P, vanRaay A. Fluoride excretion in the urine of school children living close to an aluminum refinery in The Netherlands. Environ Res 1977; 13: 129-34.

6. Buck M, Ixfield H, Ellermann K. Die Veränderung der Imissionsbelastung in den letzten 15 Jahren in Rhein-Ruhr-Gebiet. Staub-Reinhalt Luft 1982; 42: 51-8.

7. Carpenter R. Factors controlling the marine geochemistry of fluorine. Geochin Cosmochim Acta 1969; 33: 1153-67.

8. Chamblee JW, Arey F, Powell JW, Heckel E. Fluoride in the ambient air over the Pamlico estuary in North Carolina. J Air Pollut Control Assoc 1980; 30: 397-400.

9. Davison AW. Pathways of fluoride transfer in terrestrial ecosystems. In: Coughtry PJ, Martin MH, Unsworth MH, eds. Pollutant transport and fate in ecosystems. Special Publication Numbers 6 of the British Ecological Society. Oxford: Blackwell Scientific Publications, 1987: 193-210.

10. Davison AW. Uptake, transport and accumulation of soil and airborne fluorides by vegetation. In: Shupe JL, Peterson HB, Leone NC, eds. Fluorides – Effects on vegetation, animals and humans. Salt Lake City: Paragon Press, 1983: 61-82.

11. Davison AW, Rand AW, Betts WE. Measurement of atmospheric fluoride concentrations in urban areas. Environ Pollut 1973; 5: 23-33.

12. Elrashidi MA, Lindsay WL. Solubility of aluminum fluoride, fluorite and fluorophlogopite minerals in soils. Soil Sci Soc Am J 1986; 50: 594-8.

13. Elrashidi MA, Lindsay WL. Chemical equilibria of fluorine in soils: a theoretical development. Soil Sci 1986; 141: 274-84.

14. Environmental Protection Agency. Reviews of the Environmental Effects of Pollutants: IX. Fluoride. Report Number EPA-600/1-78-050 prepared for Health Effects Research Laboratory, US Environmental Protection Agency, Cincinnati, Ohio, by Oak Ridge National Laboratory, Tennessee.

15. Ernst P, Thomas D, Becklake MR. Respiratory survey of North American Indian children living in proximity to an aluminum smelter. Am Rev Respir Dis 1986; 133: 307-12.

16. Fleischer M, Robinson WO. Some problems of geochemistry of fluorine. In: Shaw DM, ed. Studies in analytical geochemistry. The Royal Society of Canada, Special Publications, No. 6. Toronto, Canada: University of Toronto Press, 1963; 58-75.

17. Fleischer M, Forbes RM, Harriss RC, Krook L, Kubota J. Fluorine. In: Geochemistry and the environment, Vol. 1. The relation of selected trace elements to health and disease. Report of workshop Feb. 7-12, 1972 under auspices of Subcommittee on the Geochemical Environment in Relation to Health and Disease, US National Committee for Geochemistry, Div. Earth Sci, Nat Res Council. Washington, DC: Natl Acad Sci 1974: 22-5.

18. Fridriksson S. Fluoride problems following volcanic eruptions. In: Shupe JL, Peterson HB, Leone NC, eds. Fluorides – effects on vegetation, animals and humans. Salt Lake City: Paragon Press, 1983: 339-44.

19. Fuge R. Sources of halogens in the environment, influences on human and animal health. Environ Geochem and Health 1988; 10: 51-61.

20. Fuge R, Anderews MJ. Fluorine in the UK environment. Environ Geochem Health 1988; 10: 96-104.

21. Glemser O. Inorganic fluorine chemistry, 1900-1945. J Fluorine Chem 1986; 33: 45-69.

22. Gomez M, Corvillo MAP, Rica CC. Determination of fluoride in drinking water and sea water by aluminum monofluoride molecular absorption spectrometry using an electrothermal graphite furnace. Analyst 1988; 113: 1109-12.

23. Haidouti C, Chronopoulos A, Chronopoulos J. Effects of fluoride emissions from industry on the fluoride concentration of soils and vegetation. Biochem Systematics Ecol 1993; 21: 195-208.

24. Haikel Y, Voegel JC, Frank RM. Fluoride content of water, dust, soils and cereals in the endemic dental fluorosis area of Khouribga (Morocco). Archs Oral Biol 1986; 31: 279-86.

25. Hodge HC, Smith FA. Chapter 7. Fluorides. In: Lee DHK, ed. Fogarty Intl Cent Proc No. 9, Metallic contaminants and human health. Washington, DC: Am Chem Soc 1972: 163-87.

26. Horner JM. Pollution by fluorine compounds. J Roy Soc Health 1989; 4: 147-50.

27. Kessabi M, Assimi B. The effects of fluoride on animals and plants in the south Safi zone. Sci Total Environ 1984; 38: 63-8.

28. Kongerud J, Grønnesby JK, Magnus P. Respiratory symptoms and lung function of aluminum potroom workers. Scand J Work Environ Health 1990; 16: 270-7.

29. Kudo A, Garrec JP, Plebin R. Fluoride distribution and transport along rivers in the French Alps. Ecotoxicol Environ Safety 1987; 13: 263-73.

30. Lahermo P, Sandström H, Malisa E. The occurrence and geochemistry of fluorides in natural waters in Finland and East Africa with reference to their geomedical implications. J Geochem Exploration 1991; 41: 65-79.

31. Lee RE Jr, Caldwell J, Akland GG, Fanchauser R. The distribution and transport of airborne particulate matter and inorganic components in Great Britain. Atmos Environ 1974; 8: 1095-109.

32. Mahon WA. Fluorine in the natural thermal waters of New Zealand. J Sci 1964; 7: 3-28.

33. Martin AE, Jones CM. Some medical considerations regarding atmospheric fluorides. HSMHA Health Rep 1971; 86: 752-8.

34. Osterman JW. Evaluating the impact of municipal water fluoridation on the aquatic environment. Am J Public Health 1990; 80: 1230-5.

35. Ouellet M. Reduction of airborne fluoride emissions from Canadian aluminum smelters as revealed by snow chemistry. Sci Total Environ 1987; 66: 65-72.

36. Rondia D, Sartor F, Dans JM. Impregnation par le fluor atmosphérique d'une population habitant au voisinage d'une usine d'engrais phosphates. Arch B Med Soc, Hyg, Med Tr Med Leg 1987; 45: 269-87.

37. Schneider W. Daueruntersuchungen zum Fluorproblem in einem industriellen Ballungsgebiet. Staub-Reinhalt Luft 1968; 28: 13-8.

38. Shacklette HT, Boerngen JG, Keith JR. Selenium, fluorine, and arsenic in superficial materials of the conterminous United States. Geol Survey Circular 692. Reston, VA: US Geological Survey Center 1974.

39. Shupe JL, Olson AE, Peterson HB, Lou JB. Fluoride toxicosis in wild ungulates. J Am Vet Med Assoc 1984; 185: 1295-300.

40. Sidhu SS. Fluoride levels in air, vegetation and soil in the vicinity of a phosphorus plant. J Air Pollu Cont Assoc 1979; 29: 1069-72.

41. Smith FA, Hodge HC. Airborne fluorides and man: Part I. Crit Rev Environ Control 1978; 8: 293-371.

42. Söyseth V, Kongerud J. Prevalence of respiratory disorders among aluminum potroom workers in relation to exposure to fluoride. Br J Ind Med 1992; 49: 125-30.

43. Söyseth V, Kongerud J, Ekstrand J, Boe J. Relation between exposure to fluoride and responsiveness in aluminium potroom workers with work-related asthma-like symtoms. Thorax 1994; 49: 984-9.

44. Staniforth RJ, Sidhu SS. Effects of atmospheric fluorides on foliage, flower, fruit, and seed production in wild raspberry and blueberry. Can J Bot 1984; 62: 2827-34.

45. Symonds RB, Rose WI, Reed MH. Contribution of Cl^- and F^- bearing gases to the atmosphere by volcanoes. Nature 1988; 334: 415-8.

46. Thompson RJ, McMullen TB, Morgan JB. Fluoride concentrations in the ambient air. J Air Pollut Control Assoc 1971; 21: 484-7.

47. Treshow M. Symptomatology of fluoride injury on vegetation. In: Handbook of effect assessment: vegetation damage, vol. 7, University Park, PA: Pennsylvania State Univ Center for Air Environment Studies 1969: 1-41.

48. Villar E, Bonet A, Diaz-Caneja N, Fernandez E, Fernandez PL, Quindos LS, Soto J. A study of the impact of industrial fluoride emissions on a rural environment. J Air Pollut Control Assoc 1989; 39: 1098-100.

49. Wangen LE, Williams MD. Elemental deposition downwind of a coal-fired power plant. Water, Air, Soil Pollut 1978; 10: 33-44.

50. Weinstein LH. Effects of fluorides on plants and plant communities: an overview. In: Shupe JL, Peterson HB, Leone NC, eds. Fluorides – effects on vegetation, animals and humans. Salt Lake City: Paragon Press, 1983: 53-9.

51. Worl RG, Van Alstine RE, Shawe DR. United States mineral resources. Fluorine. US Geol Survey Prof Paper 820, 1973; 223-35.

52. Yixin C, Meiqi, Zhaolong H, Xiaomao X, Yongquan L, Yuandong X, Jing Z, Yong F, Xiwen X, Fengshen X. Air pollution-type fluorosis in the region of Pingxiang. Jiangxi, Peoples Republic of China. Arch Environ Health 1991; 48: 246-9.

CHAPTER 2

FLUORIDE ANALYTICAL METHODS

P. Venkateswarlu • G. Vogel

Introduction – Forms of fluorine in biological materials – Methodology
Analysis of inorganic fluoride, total fluorine and organic fluorine
Special aspects of analysis of samples from the oral environment – Conclusion

Introduction

The emergence of fluoridation of public water supplies as a safe and economic mass caries-control measure was based on epidemiologic studies and on the concurrent elucidation of the transport and metabolism of fluoride, the mechanism of action of fluoride compounds, their biological effects, and the environmental aspects of fluorides. The success of these studies depended, among other things, on the development of sound fluoride analytical methods. This involved fluorine analysis of water, soil, minerals, vegetation, foods and a host of other biological materials such as bone, teeth (enamel, dentin, cementum), body fluids (urine, blood, saliva) and soft tissues (kidney, liver, muscle).

Forms of fluorine in biological materials

Based on the work of Taves[45] and Venkateswarlu et al.,[69] it is now clearly established that human and animal blood sera contain two normal forms of fluorine:

- A fraction that is diffusible as hydrogen fluoride (HF) or as a fluorosilane from an acid medium or readily adsorbable at neutral pH onto calcium hydroxyapatite (presumably through formation of calcium fluorapatite) and

- Another fraction that is not so diffusible or adsorbable.

These two fractions have been found to be *inorganic fluoride* and *organic fluorine,* respectively. In the latter fraction, fluorine is covalently bound within an organic molecule. Inorganic fluoride bound to organic molecules (proteins) or to organic sediments in saliva should not be confused with organic fluorine (covalent fluorine). Recognition of the two fractions of fluorine calls for determination of both inorganic fluoride and organic fluorine in biologic materials. However, depending on the goals of the investigation, either one or both of the fractions may be determined.

Inorganic fluoride in biological samples could be in different forms: (a) ionic fluoride, to which the fluoride ion electrode responds, and (b) nonionic fluoride, to which the electrode does not respond. The former is represented by

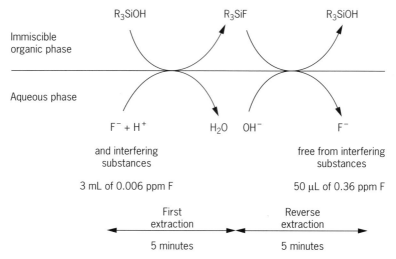

Fig. 2-1. Schematic representation of the principles of the reverse-extraction technique for isolation of fluoride. "R" stands for acyl- or aryl-groups.

free (uncomplexed) fluoride ions in solution. The latter is represented by inorganic fluoride, which is complexed as (i) fluoride bound to protons as in HF at low pH, (ii) fluoride bound to metal ions (Ca^{2+}, Mg^{2+}, Fe^{3+}, Al^{3+}, etc.), (iii) fluoride that is adsorbed or complexed by mineral/organic sediments, as in saliva, (iv) apatitic fluoride, which is inorganic fluoride incorporated into the apatite lattice of bones and teeth, and (v) nonapatitic fluoride, calcium fluoride or calcium fluoride-like fluoride formed on tooth enamel following topical application of fluoride. All these forms of fluoride can be separated and analyzed by appropriate methods.

Methodology

Ideally, the results of analysis are corroborated by at least two analytical methods, which differ widely with regard to pretreatment of the sample, separation and concentration of F and the final mode of F analysis. These requirements are met by a judicious blending of alter-native approaches. Some of the more common approaches are indicated below. Detailed descriptions of these and more alternative approaches are provided in a more comprehensive review by Venkateswarlu.[59]

Pretreatment of samples

The goal is to release fluoride ions from other matrices in the sample (inorganic or organic) that might complex or bind the fluoride ions and to get rid of organic matter that may interfere in the analysis. Attainment of this goal may call for open ashing, fusion,[30,33] or confined combustion procedures such as the use of oxygen flask,[35] oxygen bomb,[57] pyrohydrolysis,[22,24,53] and oxyhydrogen flame.[80] In these procedures organic fluorine (covalent fluorine), when present, is also converted into inorganic fluoride. The conversion of organic fluorine into inorganic fluoride can also be accomplished at room temperature (in the absence of oxygen) by the use of sodium biphenyl reagent, which cleaves the C-F covalent bonds and releases fluoride ions.[60]

Separation and concentration of fluoride ions

Diffusion of fluoride
The classic Willard-Winter distillation,[81] which has provided a wealth of information through the mid-decades of this century, has largely been replaced by simpler techniques such as diffusion, originally developed by Singer & Armstrong[37,38] and rendered more rapid by Taves[46] through the use of hexamethyldisiloxane. These diffusions are normally carried out in Conway diffusion cells, which require application of grease for sealing along the edges of the cells. Recently, diffusion has been accomplished by Venkateswarlu[63] in 5-mL stoppered test tubes without the need for grease. These diffusion techniques require from 6-48 h for quantitative diffusion of fluoride, depending on the nature of the sample.[47]

Reverse extraction of fluoride
A more rapid procedure, requiring minutes instead of several hours for separation of fluoride from interferences and with a tremendous increase in the concentration of fluoride, as well as a lower fluoride concentration blank, is the reverse extraction technique developed by Venkateswarlu.[55] The fluoride from a large sample is extracted as a fluorosilane (free from interfering substances) into an organic layer and then back-extracted as fluoride ions into a few microliters of an aqueous phase (Fig. 2-1).

Adsorption of fluoride
Adsorption provides yet another rapid means to concentrate fluoride from a variety of samples. It involves boiling the test solution (e.g. water or urine) at neutral pH with magnesium oxide[67,68] or calcium phosphate.[66,69,70] The fluoride adsorption is complete in a matter of minutes. The fluoride so adsorbed is readily separated by centrifugation. Because of the coagulation and viscosity problems in the case of serum and saliva samples, such samples are handled slightly differently. The samples are diluted, and the adsorption on calcium phosphate is carried out at 35-40 °C for 1 hour.

Strong acid conditions are employed in the separation and concentration of fluoride by the above diffusion and reverse extraction procedures. Fluoride measured with these techniques includes native inorganic fluoride plus additional inorganic fluoride released from acid-labile organic (covalent) fluorine compounds (if any) such as the circulating fluorometabolites following methoxyflurane anesthesia.[48] The calcium phosphate adsorption technique measures only the inorganic fluoride.[55] Normal human blood serum and saliva do not contain acid-labile organic fluorine compounds.

Final measurement of fluorine

Spectrophotometric and fluorometric methods
When the fluoride has been separated from interferences by appropriate procedures, it can be analyzed readily by spectrophotometry[19] or fluorometry.[44] There are many spectrophotometric and fluorometric methods, and they are included in the review by Venkateswarlu.[59] Used under the right circumstances, these methods are faster and more convenient than the fluoride electrode.

Fluoride electrode
One of the most significant advances in the determination of fluoride is the development of the fluoride ion specific electrode by Frant & Ross.[16] The fluoride electrode has tremendous tolerance for extraneous ions like sulfate, phosphate and organics, which invariably interfere in spectrophotometry and fluorometry.

The fluoride electrode responds to fluoride ion activity (free fluoride ions) and not to fluoride ions that are complexed by certain metal ions (iron, aluminum, magnesium). To measure total inorganic fluoride in such solutions, agents (ethylenediaminetetraacetic acid, 1,2-cy-

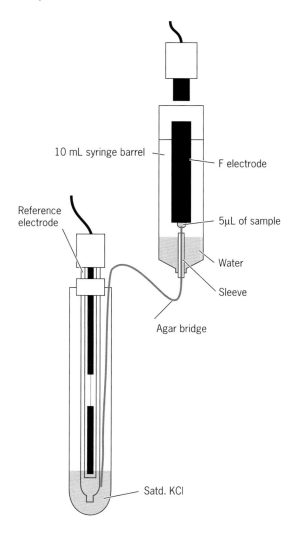

10 mL syringe barrel

F electrode

Reference electrode

5µL of sample

Water

Sleeve

Agar bridge

Satd. KCl

Fig. 2-2. Hanging-drop electrode assembly.

sponds to hydroxide ions, which interfere when the hydroxide concentration is more than 10 times the fluoride concentration. These facts require that the pH of the test solution be ideally maintained at about 5 to 6 for reliable measurements with the fluoride electrode. The fluoride ion activity also varies with the background ionic concentration, and it is necessary that the ionic strength and composition in sample and standard solutions be maintained essentially the same. These requirements are met by adding a total ionic strength adjustment buffer (TISAB, ATI Orion, Cambridge MA, or its equivalent) to the standards and samples prior to measurement with the fluoride electrode. TISAB also contains reagents to release fluoride from complexing metal ions and to provide the right pH.

Measurement of extremely low levels of fluoride (around 1 µmol/L) with the electrode requires extreme care in the maintenance of the fluoride electrode, adequate equilibration times and the use of an appropriate number of standards. It is possible to overcome these problems, however, and to obtain more reliable results with the electrode following concentration of fluoride in such samples by the diffusion, reverse-extraction or adsorption techniques described earlier. Gel-filled reference electrodes with high porosity junction can trap a significant amount of fluoride when exposed to a high fluoride concentration sample and then contaminate a subsequent low fluoride concentration sample, especially if the volume of the latter is small. Thus the correct choice of the reference electrode is important. It is always good practice first to screen rapidly fluoride standards and samples with the fluoride electrode and to arrange the standards and samples, interspersed, in the order of increasing fluoride concentration and then to take the final measurements in that order, starting with the lowest fluoride standard.

To measure fluoride in microliter volumes of samples (the reverse-extracts, blood serum,

clohexylenedinitrilotetraacetic acid, tartaric acid, citric acid, acetyl acetone, etc.) are used to complex the metal ions and release fluoride ions. HF is a weak acid and at low pH fluoride exists mostly as unionized HF, to which the fluoride electrode does not respond. At pH values above 5, fluoride is essentially completely ionized. However, the electrode also re-

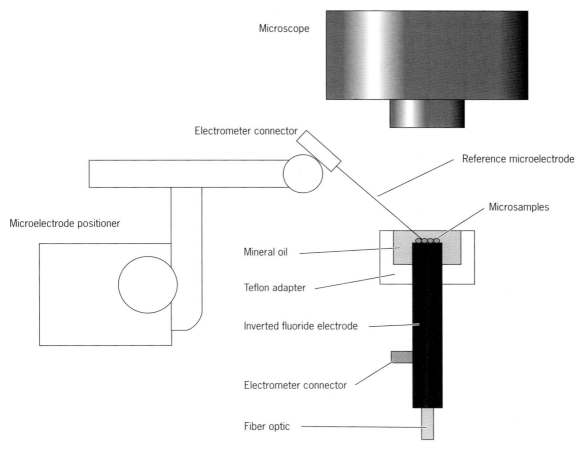

Fig. 2-3. Inverted under oil fluoride electrode assembly.

urine, milk, saliva), the hanging-drop fluoride electrode has been conceived by Venkateswarlu.[55,56] The use of Parafilm to cover the fluoride-sensing membrane of the electrode described in the original paper[55] has since been discontinued by the author to avert any possible cross contamination between successive samples. Also, a few millimeters of the agar bridge coming in contact with the sample can be snipped off with a sharp scalpel between reading high and low fluoride samples. Of the several modifications of the electrode available for the measurement of reduced volumes,[8,13,] the hanging-drop fluoride electrode (Fig. 2-2) is relatively easy to assemble. It has been successfully used in a wide variety of situations by Ophaug[29] and Venkateswarlu.[55,56, 57,60] The multiwell adapter method of Vogel et al.[72,74] is considerably more difficult to manufacture but has the advantage of allowing six samples to be equilibrated simultaneously with the surface of a fluoride electrode so that a single electrode can perform as six independent electrodes. However, the integrity of the seal of the adapter to the electrode surface can be a problem; defective sealing leads to cross contamination of samples. The technique of Hallsworth et al.[21] utilizing a ground sleeve junction to sandwich the sample between the fluoride electrode and the reference electrode is also popular with several investigators.

For measuring fluoride in nanoliter volumes of samples such as dental plaque fluid (available sample volumes are submicroliters), a significant breakthrough has been achieved by Vogel et al.,[75] who designed delicate instrumentation whereby micro-drops of samples placed under oil on an inverted fluoride electrode are monitored with a capillary microreference electrode (Fig. 2-3). As in the case of the multiwell adapter method numerous samples can be simultaneously brought to equilibrium with the fluoride electrode and measurements rapidly made simply by moving the reference electrode from sample to sample. The application of these microtechniques has been reviewed by Vogel et al.[74]

The fluoride electrode does not respond to covalently bound fluorine either in inorganic salts such as monofluorophosphate or in organic fluorine compounds. However, monofluorophosphate can be determined with the fluoride electrode after acid hydrolysis.[20] Monofluorophosphate and fluoride can also be separated and measured by ion chromatography.[25] In the case of organic fluorine compounds, the C-F covalent bonds must be cleaved to release fluoride ions if measurements are to be made with the electrode.[60]

There are some interesting developments in monitoring fluoride concentrations in solutions even at the low pH values of 1-2, when the most predominant form of fluoride would be HF and not F^-. The technique developed by Diggens & Ross[9] involves the use of a differential electrode cell containing two electrodes, the fluoride ion electrode and a pH electrode. This technique has been successfully used by Tyler & Comer[51] and Tyler & Poole[52] for fluoride analysis of enamel biopsy samples and saliva. They report that the differential cell responds

faster (2 minutes) than the single electrode (20 minutes).

Gas chromatography

Based on the first demonstration by Bock & Semmler[1] that fluoride could be analyzed by gas chromatography after conversion to volatile fluorosilanes, Fresen et al.[17] reported a gas chromatographic method for determination of fluoride in blood serum, urine and saliva (fluoride is converted to trimethylfluorosilane, b.p. 16.4 °C, by shaking the test sample plus acid with trimethylchlorosilane).

Aluminum monofluoride molecular absorption spectrometry (AlF MAS)

A very rapid method for measurement of nanogram amounts of inorganic fluoride, requiring no more than 2-3 minutes per sample, is the aluminum monofluoride molecular absorption technique developed by Tsunoda et al.[50] and adopted with certain modifications by others. [18,22,71] In this procedure the sample containing fluoride is mixed with an aluminum nitrate solution containing certain modifiers and fired to 2200 °C, at which temperature aluminum monofluoride (AlF) is formed in the gas phase. The concentration of AlF is determined by its absorption of light at 227.5 nm. This method, however, cannot distinguish between inorganic fluoride and organic fluorine and therefore should not be used to measure one form of fluorine in the presence of a significant amount of the other. This method has been successfully adapted by Venkateswarlu[62] for analysis of bone fluoride. Application of this rapid technique in fluoride analysis of enamel biopsy samples, saliva, etc., remains to be investigated.

Miscellaneous advanced instrumentation techniques

These include techniques such as secondary ion mass spectrometry (SIMS), proton-induced x-ray emission (PIXE), proton-induced gamma-ray emission (PIGE), electron probe microanalysis (EPM), and x-ray-induced photoelectron spectroscopy (XPS also called ESCA). Most of these techniques are for surface analysis of fluorine and are described in reviews by Duckworth & Gilbert[11] and Ten Bosch & Booij.[49]

Analysis of inorganic fluoride, total fluorine and organic fluorine

Inorganic fluoride

For the determination of inorganic fluoride in biological samples, ashing is avoided because ashing converts organic fluorine, if present, to inorganic fluoride. Analyses are, therefore, carried out on unashed samples, homogenates, digests or extracts of the samples. The fluoride ion electrode has been extensively used in these analyses.

Total fluorine

For a long time, total fluorine determination in biologic samples was carried out by diffusion of unashed samples, followed by colorimetric analysis.[38,39,79] This method was shown to give erroneous results in the case of normal body fluids and tissues, and foods as well, because (a) the diffusates contained interferences that masqueraded as fluoride released from the organic fluorine fraction,[41,58] and (b) it has been unequivocally demonstrated that the organic fluorine in normal blood serum is not available for diffusion.[58]

Total fluorine in biological materials has been determined after open ashing[40] or, more preferably, after combustion in the oxygen-bomb.[57] The two problems of (a) loss of fluoride or (b) contamination with extraneous fluoride encountered in the open ashing procedure are eliminated in the oxygen-bomb technique. However, oxygen-bomb combustion is cumbersome. For measuring organic fluorine in the blood of workers in fluorochemical manufacturing plants, this method has been es-

sentially replaced by the sodium biphenyl technique developed by Venkateswarlu.[60,66,71] The usefulness of the sodium biphenyl technique in determination of organic fluorine in normal human plasma needs to be explored.

The AlF MAS method has been claimed by Chiba et al.[5] to yield total fluorine values in the case of blood serum samples. However, it has been demonstrated by Venkateswarlu et al.[65,71] that significant losses of organic fluorine occur in this technique, depending on the volatility of the compounds involved. Thus, in order to obtain reliable results for total fluorine by this technique, it is best to convert all organic fluorine into inorganic fluoride, e.g. by using the sodium biphenyl technique, prior to injection of the samples into the furnace for analysis by AlF MAS.[66,71]

Organic fluorine

Organic fluorine is obtained by subtracting inorganic fluoride from total fluorine. Organic fluorine in a sample can be determined also by extracting it from the sample into a water-immiscible solvent and then applying the sodium biphenyl method[60] for analysis of the extract. Inorganic fluoride would remain in the aqueous phase.

Details of procedures for analysis of both inorganic and organic fluorine in diverse materials (water, plants, soils, foods, body fluids and tissues, etc.) are covered in earlier reviews by Venkateswarlu.[54,59,61,64] Fluoride analytical methods pertaining to less frequently analyzed tissues (hair, nails and skin) and the relevance of the results to determining the body burden of fluoride are critically reviewed by Ophaug.[28]

Special aspects of analysis of samples from the oral environment

The analysis of saliva, plaque, plaque fluid and tooth-bound fluoride often requires measurements of small biologically complex samples containing low levels of fluoride. The fluoride electrode, because of its low cost, high sensitivity, good specificity (considerable tolerance for interference), and relative ease of modification for reduced volumes, has been extensively employed in these analyses as described below.

Saliva

Whole uncentrifuged saliva is contaminated by soft tissue and plaque sediments that could be significant sources of fluoride.[43,83] Fluoride released from these sediments has been postulated as the reason why the fluoride concentration of the whole saliva is generally found to be higher than that in centrifuged saliva.[11] Since it is the soluble fluoride in saliva that is available for interaction with the teeth, the use of centrifuged saliva[27,73] is to be preferred.

When saliva is allowed to stand for long periods of time, the pH rises due to CO_2 loss, and as a result calcium phosphate mineral precipitation is favored. During this process, fluoride in the saliva appears to be partly removed, presumably through the formation of insoluble fluoridated apatites.[82] Although some investigators[12,52] have found that the original fluoride levels are recovered following addition of the TISAB, the immediate addition of the buffer would be a prudent precaution. However, if the samples contain very high levels of fluoride (i.e. following shortly after a fluoride rinse), TISAB addition may not be adequate to prevent precipitation of fluoridated apatites, especially if the samples are stored for extended periods (Vogel, unpublished results). Ideally, to overcome this precipitation problem, measured aliquots of saliva could be dispensed into suitable containers immediately following collection and fluoride separated by diffusion or reverse-extraction at any convenient time.

Salivary fluoride concentrations commonly encountered are often near the limit of sensitivity of the electrode, and these conditions impose stringent requirements, including extensive conditioning of the electrode, the use of numerous standards, and standardization of electrode equilibration times.[12,23,56] Again, concentration of fluoride by the extraction-concentration methods described earlier can be employed to increase the accuracy.[83]

Whole plaque

Although early studies by Jenkins & Edgar[23] suggested that a significant portion of plaque fluoride required strong acid digestion for recovery, recent studies by Ophaug et al.[29] showed that 85% of the fluoride was extractable in 5 min with 0.5 mol/L $HClO_4$ and 100% in 15 min. Even with the high levels of plaque fluoride found after a fluoride rinse, more than 90% of the fluoride was released by the 0.5 mol/L $HClO_4$ extraction. However, levels of fluoride higher than 50 μmol/L seem to promote precipitation of fluoridated apatites (after TISAB addition) due to the high concentration of calcium and phosphate in plaque so that it is important to extract into an adequate volume of acid.

As noted by Tatevossian,[43] many of the analyses of whole plaque fluoride are near the limit of the sensitivity of the fluoride electrode. This problem can be overcome by taking advantage of the concentration-extraction techniques described earlier and by employing any of the electrodes adapted for reduced volume measurements; for example, Sidi[36] has resorted to a microdiffusion technique. The use of these extraction techniques also obviates the possibility of fluoridated apatite precipitation noted above in the case of high fluoride samples.

Plaque fluid

Few measurements have been made of plaque fluid fluoride due to the difficulty of measuring the very small amounts of fluid that can be recovered from human dental plaque.[43] However, Vogel et al.[73,77] and Carey et al.[3] have recently employed the under-oil inverted fluoride electrode (Fig. 2-3) to obtain a profile of the oral distribution of plaque-fluid fluoride after a fluoride rinse.

Enamel biopsies

These techniques have been developed to determine the profile of fluoride concentration with depth in enamel under physiological conditions as well as after the topical application of fluoride. Although the instrumental methods noted above have recently been adapted for *in vitro* tooth biopsy, the most popular technique for *in vivo* studies on human enamel remains the method first introduced by Munksgaard & Bruun.[26] An area of enamel surface is delineated by covering it with an adhesive tape with a tiny perforation, and successive superficial enamel biopsies are obtained by a series of applications of microliter volumes of dilute acid to the exposed enamel. The amount of the tooth mineral in the samples is derived from phosphate or calcium analysis. This technique was adapted by Retief *et al.*[31] for similar studies in small experimental animals. Reduced volume fluoride electrodes described above are used with considerable advantage in these studies.[32,76] Sample areas of less than 2 mm diameter can be used so that several biopsies (i.e. before and after treatment) can be obtained from the same tooth,[42] and the increments in depth can be smaller than 3 μm. However, calculation of the depth with each biopsy relies on the assumption that the mineral dissolution is homogeneous and that the samples have the same fluoride profile.[10,11] Recently, Chow *et al.*[6] described a mathematical procedure that could be used to calculate fluoride at a standardized depth, thereby allowing more subtle differences between specimens to be detected.

Acid-etch biopsy cannot be used to sample porous tissue (e.g. carious enamel). In such cases, samples are obtained by microdrilling or by microabrasive techniques. Abrasive biopsy

of enamel was apparently first carried out by Brudevold *et al.*,[2] who described the analysis of enamel using a dental felt cone impregnated with abrasive. Sakkab *et al.*[34] describe the drill biopsy of enamel white spots with a carbide bur dressed to 500 μm, while Vogel *et al.*[74] described the analysis of carious regions of enamel thin sections with a 100 μm diameter diamond microdrill. More recently, Weatherell *et al.*[78] mounted small pieces of teeth on a Mikrokator before removing samples with an abrasive. This method has the advantage that the depth (ca. 1 μm) is directly measured by a gauge on the instrument.

In the above procedures, the total inorganic fluoride in the samples is measured. However, especially in studies on topical application of fluorides, two fractions of inorganic fluoride have been recognized: (a) apatitic fluoride and (b) nonapatitic fluoride, calcium fluoride or calcium fluoride-like fluoride. Because of its ready leachability it is labeled "labile" fluoride. It is also referred to as "alkali-soluble" fluoride because calcium fluoride can be extracted for analysis with 1 M KOH, although it can be extracted by water as well. The real role of KOH is in suppressing the dissolution of the apatitic fluoride,[4] whereby more accurate results of calcium fluoride analysis are ensured. Recently, Chow & Takagi[7] described a method in which the amount of labile fluoride can be measured under defined conditions; a constant composition method is used to measure the amount of fluoride released when teeth are exposed to an artificial saliva with a constant driving force for calcium fluoride dissolution.

Conclusion

A more complete understanding of the cariostatic effects of fluoride and the development of improved fluoride treatment methods rest in no small measure on the development of accurate and sensitive methods of fluoride analysis. Conversely, inaccurate and misleading analysis can hinder understanding and retard the devel-opment of promising therapies. It is hoped that the methods and guidelines described here will be useful in this regard.

Background literature

Caslavska V, Moreno EC, Brudevold F. Determina-tion of the calcium fluoride formed from in vitro exposure of human enamel to fluoride solutions. Arch Oral Biol 1975; 20: 333-9.

Ekstrand J. A micromethod for the determination of fluoride in blood plasma and saliva. Calcif Tissue Res 1977; 23: 225-8.

Munksgaard EC, Bruun C. Determination of fluoride in superficial enamel biopsies from human teeth by means of gas chromatography. Arch Oral Biol 1973; 8: 735-44.

Retief DH, Summerlin DJ, Harris BE, Bradley EL. An evaluation of three procedures for fluoride ana-lysis. Caries Res 1985; 21: 248-54.

Singer L, Ophaug R. Ionic and nonionic fluoride in plasma (or serum). In: CRC Critical Reviews in Clinical Laboratory Science. Boca Raton, FL: CRC Press, 1982: 111-40.

Tatevossian A. Fluoride in dental plaque and its ef-fects. J Dent Res 1990; 69 (Spec Iss): 645-52.

Taves DR. Separation of fluoride by rapid diffusion using hexamethyldisiloxane. Talanta 1968; 15: 969-74.

Ten Bosch JJ, Booij M. A quantitative comparison of methods measuring fluoride in solutions or ena-mel. J Dent Res 1992; 71 (Spec Iss): 945-8.

Venkateswarlu P. Reverse extraction technique for the determination of fluoride in biological ma-terials. Anal Chem 1974; 46: 878-82.

Venkateswarlu P. Determination of fluorine in biol-ogical materials. In: Glick D, ed. Methods of bio-chemical analysis. New York: Wiley-Interscience 1977: 93-201.

Venkateswarlu, P. Overview of analytical methods for fluorine in air, water, soil, vegetation, body fluids and tissues. In: Shupe JL, Peterson HB, Leone NC, eds. Fluorides: effects on vegetation, animals and humans. Salt Lake City: Paragon Press, 1983: 21-52.

Venkateswarlu P. Evaluation of analytical methods for fluorine in biological materials. J Dent Res 1990; 69 (Spec Iss): 514-21.

Venkateswarlu P. Determination of fluorine in biol-ogical materials. A review. Adv Dent Res 1994; 8: 87-91.

Vogel GL, Carey CM, Chow LC, Ekstrand J. Fluoride analysis in nanoliter- and microliter-size fluid samples. J Dent Res 1990; 69 (Spec Iss): 522-8.

Vogel GL, Chow LC, Brown WE. Amicroanalytical procedure for the determination of calcium, phos-phorus and fluoride in enamel biopsies. Caries Res 1983; 17: 23-31.

Literature cited

1. Bock R, Semmler HJ. Abtrennung und Bestim-mung des Fluorid-ions mit hilfesiliciumorgani-scher Verbindungen. Z Anal Chem 1967; 230: 161-84.

2. Brudevold F, McCann HG, Gron P. An enamel biopsy method for determination of fluoride in human teeth. Arch Oral Biol 1968; 13: 877-85.

3. Carey CM, Gregory TM, Rupp NW, Tatevossian A, Vogel GL. The driving forces in human dental plaque fluid for demineralization and remin-eralization of enamel mineral. In: Leach AS, ed. Factors Relating to Demineralization and Re-mineralization of the Teeth. Oxford: IRL Press Ltd. 1986: 163-73.

4. Caslavska V, Moreno EC, Brudevold F. Determi-nation of the calcium fluoride formed from in vitro exposure of human enamel to fluoride sol-utions. Arch Oral Biol 1975; 20: 333-9.

5. Chiba K, Tsunoda K, Haraguchi H, Fuwa K. Determination of fluorine in urine and blood serum by aluminum monofluoride absorption spectrometry and with a fluoride ion selective electrode. Anal Chem 1980; 52: 1582-5.

6. Chow LC, Beaudreau GM, Brown WE. Enamel fluoride profile construction from biopsy data. Caries Res 1985; 19: 103-12.

7. Chow LC, Takagi S. Deposition of fluoride on tooth surfaces by a two-solution mouth rinse in vitro. Caries Res 1991; 25: 397-401.

8. Deutsch D, Zarini S. Determination of subnanogram and nanogram amounts of fluoride by fluoride and calomel reference electrodes. Anal Chem 1977; 52: 1167-8.

9. Diggens AA, Ross JW. UK Patent Application GB 2064 131 A, 1981.

10. Dijkman AG, Arends J. Thickness of enamel layer removed by HClO4 etching. Caries Res 1982; 16: 129-37.

11. Duckworth RM, Gilbert RJ. Intraoral models to assess cariogenicity: evaluation of oral fluoride pH. J Dent Res 1992; 71 (Spec Iss): 934-44.

12. Duckworth RM, Morgan SN, Murray AM. Fluoride in saliva and plaque following use of fluoride-containing mouthwashes. J Dent Res 1987; 66: 1730-4.

13. Durst RA. Fluoride microelectrode – fabrication and characteristics. Anal Chem 1969; 41: 2089-90.

14. Durst RA, Taylor JK. Modification of the fluoride activity electrode. Anal Chem 1967; 39: 1483-5.

15. Ekstrand J. A micromethod for the determination of fluoride in blood plasma and saliva. Calcif Tissue Res 1977; 23: 225-8.

16. Frant MS, Ross JW. Electrode for sensing fluoride ion activity in solution. Science 1966; 154: 1553-5.

17. Fresen JA, Cox FH, Witter MJ. The determination of fluoride in biological materials by means of gas chromatography. Pharm Weekblad 1968; 103: 909-14.

18. Fujimori S, Itai K, Sakurai S, Tsunoda H. Microdetermination of total fluoride in serum by aluminum monofluoride molecular absorption spectrometry and its significance. Fluoride 1982; 17: 27-35.

19. Greenhalgh R, Riley JP. The determination of fluoride in natural waters, with particular reference to sea water. Anal Chim Acta 1961; 25: 179-88.

20. Gron P, Brudevold F, Aasenden R. Monofluorophosphate interaction with hydroxyapatite and intact enamel. Caries Res 1971; 202-14.

21. Hallsworth AS, Weatherell JA, Deutsch D. Determination of sub-nanogram amounts of fluoride with the fluoride electrode. Anal Chem 1976; 48: 1660-4.

22. Itai K, Tsunoda H. Determination of submicrogram quantities of fluoride by a rapid and highly sensitive method. In: Tsunoda H, Yu M, eds. Studies in Environmental Science 27. Fluoride Research, Amsterdam: Elsevier 1985: 25-9.

23. Jenkins GN, Edgar WM. Distribution and forms of F in saliva and plaque. Caries Res. 1977; ll Suppl. 1: 226-37.

24. Kakabadse GJ, Manohin B, Bather JM, Weller EC, Woodbridge P. Decomposition and determination of fluorine in biological materials. Nature 1971; 229: 626-7.

25. Lindahl CB. Fluoride and monofluorophosphate analysis. Caries Res 1983; 17 (Suppl. 1): 9-20.

26. Munksgaard EC, Bruun C. Determination of fluoride in superficial enamel biopsies from human teeth by means of gas chromatography. Arch Oral Biol 1973; 8: 735-44.

27. Oliveby A, Tweetman S, Ekstrand J. Diurnal fluoride concentration in whole saliva children living in a high- or low-fluoridated area. Caries Res 1990; 24: 44-7.

28. Ophaug RH. Reaction paper to "Microdetermination of fluorine in biological materials. A review." Adv Dent Res 1994; 8: 87-91.

29. Ophaug RH, Jenkins GN, Singer L, Krebsbach PH. Acid diffusion analysis of different forms of fluoride in human dental plaque. Arch Oral Biol 1987; 32: 459-62.

30. Remmert LF, Parks TD, Lawrence AL. Determination of fluorine in plant materials. Anal Chem 1953; 25: 450-53.

31. Retief DH, Navia JM, Lopez H. Microanalytical technique for the estimation of fluoride in rat molar enamel. Arch Oral Biol 1977; 22: 207-11.

32. Retief DH, Summerlin DJ, Harris BE, Bradley EL. An evaluation of three procedures for fluoride analysis. Caries Res 1985; 21: 248-54.

33. Rowley RJ, Grier JG, Parsons RI. Determination of fluoride in vegetation. Anal Chem 1953; 25: 1061-5.

37

34. Sakkab NY, Cilley WA, Haberman JP. Fluoride in deciduous teeth from an anticaries clinical study. J Dent Res 1984; 63: 1201-4.

35. Schoniger W. A rapid microanalytical determination of halogens in organic substances. Mikro Chim Acta 1955: 123-9.

36. Sidi AD. Effect of brushing with fluoride toothpastes on the fluoride, calcium, and inorganic phosphorus concentration in approximal plaque of young adults. Caries Res 1989; 23: 268-71.

37. Singer L, Armstrong WD. Determination of fluoride. Procedure based on diffusion of hydrogen fluoride. Anal Chem 1954; 26: 904-6.

38. Singer L, Armstrong WD. Determination of fluoride. Procedure based on diffusion of hydrogen fluoride. Anal Biochem 1965; 10: 495-500.

39. Singer L, Armstrong WD. Determination of fluoride in ultrafiltrates of sera. Biochem Med 1973; 8: 415-22.

40. Singer L, Ophaug RH. Determination of fluorine in blood plasma. Anal Chem 1977; 49: 38-40.

41. Singer L, Ophaug RH, Harland BF. Fluoride intake of young male adults in the United States. Am J Clin Nutr 1980; 33: 328-32.

42. Takagi S, Chow LC, Schreiber CT. Enhanced root fluoride uptake by monocalcium phosphate monohydrate gels. Caries Res 1990; 24: 18-22.

43. Tatevossian A. Fluoride in dental plaque and its effects. J Dent Res 1990; 69 (Spec. Iss.): 645-52.

44. Taves DR. Determination of submicromolar concentrations of fluoride in biological samples. Talanta 1968; 15: 1015-23.

45. Taves DR. Evidence that there are two forms of fluoride in human serum. Nature 1968; 217: 1050-1.

46. Taves DR. Separation of fluoride by rapid diffusion using hexamethyldisiloxane. Talanta 1968; 15: 969-74.

47. Taves DR, Forbes N, Silverman D, Hicks D. Inorganic fluoride concentrations of human and animal tissues. In: Shupe JL, Peterson JB, Leone NC, eds. Fluorides: Effects on vegetation, animals and humans. Salt Lake City: Paragon Press, 189-93.

48. Taves DR, Fry BW, Freeman RB, Giles AJ. Toxicity following methoxyflurane anesthesia. II Fluoride concentrations in nephrotoxicity. J Am Med Assoc 1970; 214: 91-5.

49. Ten Bosch JJ, Booij M. A quantitative comparison of methods measuring fluoride in solutions or enamel. J Dent Res 1992; 71 (Spec. Iss.): 945-8.

50. Tsunoda K, Fujiwara K, Fuwa K. Subnanogram fluorine determination by aluminum monofluoride molecular absorption spectrometry. Anal Chem 1977; 49: 2035-9.

51. Tyler JE, Comer JEA. Novel ion-selective electrode system for simultaneous determination of fluoride and calcium in acid solution. Analyst 1985; 110: 15-8.

52. Tyler JE, Poole DFG. The rapid measurement of fluoride concentration in stored human saliva by means of a differential electrode cell. Arch Oral Biol 1989; 4: 995-8.

53. Van Gogh H. The isolation and determination of micrograms fluorine in biological material. Pharm. Weekblad. 1966; 101: 881-98.

54. Venkateswarlu P. Overview of analytical methods for fluorine in air, water, soil, vegetation, body fluids and tissues. In: Shupe JL, Peterson HB, Leone NC, eds. Fluorides: Effects on vegetation, animals and humans. Salt Lake City: Paragon Press, 1983: 21-52.

55. Venkateswarlu P. Reverse extraction technique for the determination of fluoride in biological materials. Anal Chem 1974; 46: 878-82.

56. Venkateswarlu P. A micromethod for direct determination of fluoride in body fluids with the hanging drop fluoride electrode. Clinica Chim Acta 1975; 59: 277-82.

57. Venkateswarlu P. Determination of total fluorine in serum and other biological materials by oxygen-bomb and reverse extraction techniques. Anal Biochem 1975; 68: 512-21.

58. Venkateswarlu P. Fallacies in the determination of total fluorine in the diffusates of unashed sera and ultrafiltrates. Biochem Med 1975; 14: 368-77.

59. Venkateswarlu P. Determination of fluorine in biological materials. In: Glick D, ed. Methods of Biochemical Analysis. New York: Wiley-Interscience 1977; 24: 93-201.

60. Venkateswarlu P. Sodium biphenyl method for determination of covalently bound fluorine in organic compounds and biological materials. Anal Chem 1982; 4: 1132-7.

61. Venkateswarlu P. Evaluation of analytical methods for fluorine in biological materials. J Dent Res 1990; 69 (Spec. Iss.): 514-21.

62. Venkateswarlu P. Determination of fluoride in bone by aluminum monofluoride absorption spectrometry. Anal Chim Acta 1992; 262: 33-40.

63. Venkateswarlu P. Separation of fluoride from fluoroelastomers by diffusion in test tubes. Anal Chem 1992; 64: 346-9.

64. Venkateswarlu P. Determination of fluorine in biological materials. A review. Ad Dent Res 1994; 8: 80-6.

65. Venkateswarlu P, Blackwell JA, Jewell K, Kirsch GW. Direct determination of individual organic fluorine compounds by aluminum monofluoride molecular absorption spectrometry. J AOAC Int 1992; 75: 672-7.

66. Venkateswarlu P, LaCroix MA, Kirsch GW. Determination of organic (covalent) fluorine in blood serum by furnace molecular absorption spectrometry. Microchem J 1993; 48: 78-85.

67. Venkateswarlu P, Narayanarao D. Investigations on removal of fluoride from water. Factors governing the adsorption of fluoride by magnesium oxide. Ind J Med Res 1954; 42: 135-40.

68. Venkateswarlu P, Narayanarao D. Investigations on removal of fluoride from water. Rapid removal of fluoride with magnesium oxide. Ind J Med Res 1953; 41: 473-7.

69. Venkateswarlu P, Singer L, Armstrong WD. Determination of ionic (plus ionizable) fluoride in biological fluids. Procedure based on adsorption of fluoride ion on calcium phosphate. Anal Biochem 1971; 42: 350-9.

70. Venkateswarlu P, Sita P. A new approach to the determination of fluoride. Adsorption-diffusion technique. Anal Chem 1971; 43: 758-60.

71. Venkateswarlu P, Winter LD, Prokop RA, Hagen DF. Automated molecular absorption spectrometry for determination of fluoride in biological samples. Anal Chem 1983; 55: 2232-6.

72. Vogel GL, Brown WE. Microanalytical techniques with inverted solid state ion selective electrodes. II. Microliter volumes. Anal Chem 1980; 52: 377-9.

73. Vogel GL, Carey CM, Ekstrand J. Distribution of fluoride in saliva and plaque-fluid after a 0.048 mol/L NaF rinse. J Dent Res 1992; 71: 1553-7.

74. Vogel GL, Carey CM, Chow LC, Ekstrand J. Fluoride analysis in nanoliter- and microliter-size fluid samples. J Dent Res 1990; 69 (Spec Iss): 522-8.

75. Vogel GL, Chow LC, Brown WE. Microanalytical techniques with inverted solid-state ion electrodes. I. Nanoliter volumes. Anal Chem 1980; 52: 375-7.

76. Vogel GL, Chow LC, Brown WE. A microanalytical procedure for the determination of calcium, phosphorus and fluoride in enamel biopsies. Caries Res 1983; 17: 23-31.

77. Vogel GL, Mao Y, Carey CM, Chow LC, Takagi S. In vivo fluoride concentrations measured for two hours after a NaF or a novel two-solution rinse. J Dent Res 1992; 71: 448-52.

78. Weatherell JA, Robinson C, Strong M, Nakagaki H. Microsampling by abrasion. Caries Res 1985; 19: 97-102.

79. Wiatrowski E, Kramer L, Ossis D, Spencer H. Dietary fluoride intake of infants. Pediatrics 1975; 55: 517-22.

80. Wickbold R. Quantitative combustion of fluorine containing organic substances. Angew Chem 1954; 66: 173-4.

81. Willard HH, Winter OB. Volumetric method for determination of fluorine. Ind Eng Chem (Anal. Ed.) 1933; 5: 7-10.

82. Yao K, Gron P. Fluoride concentrations in duct saliva and in whole saliva. Caries Res 1970; 4: 321-31.

83. Zero D, Raubertas RF, Pedersen AM, Fu J, Featherstone JDB. Studies of fluoride retention by oral soft tissues after the application of home-use topical fluorides. J Dent Res 1992; 71: 1546-52.

This chapter was supported, in part, by USPHS Research Grant DE04385 to the American Dental Association Health Foundation from the National Institutes of Health – National Institute of Dental Research and is part of the dental research program conducted by the National Institute of Standards and Technology in cooperation with the American Dental Association Health Foundation.

Certain commercial materials and equipment are identified in this paper to specify the experimental procedure. In no instance does such identification imply recommendation or endorsement by the National Institute of Standards and Technology or the ADA Health Foundation or that the material or the equipment identified is necessarily the best available for the purpose.

CHAPTER 3

FLUORIDE INTAKE

S.J. Fomon • J. Ekstrand

Introduction
Fluoride concentrations of foods and beverages and fluoride intake from these sources
Fluoride exposure from dental products and miscellaneous sources
Fluoride supplements

Introduction

Water is the predominant source of fluoride for most individuals living in communities in which the fluoride concentration of the water supply is 0.7 mg/L or more. In some countries, such as the United States, where the water supply in many communities is fluoridated, individuals living in communities with low concentrations of fluoride in the drinking water may still obtain a substantial intake of fluoride from beverages and other foods commercially prepared in locations with fluoridated water. As will be discussed, a few foods are rich sources of fluoride. The use of fluoride-containing dentifrices and other fluoride-containing dental products adds appreciably to total fluoride intake. In this chapter we shall consider the fluoride content of foods and beverages, and the usual fluoride intake of individuals in various age groups. Because the fluoride content of their diet is extremely low in breast-fed infants and in infants fed undiluted milk from other mammals, but quite high in infants fed certain formulas, the fluoride intake of infants varies widely. Moreover, it has been shown that fluoride intake during infancy may be an over-riding factor in the development of enamel fluorosis of the permanent teeth.[28,62] Special attention will therefore be paid to the fluoride intake of infants.

Fluoride concentrations of foods and beverages and fluoride intake from these sources

Methods suitable for estimating concentrations of fluoride in water have been widely available for many years, but much of the data on fluoride concentrations in foods have in the past been obtained with a colorimetric method applied to diffusates of unashed samples of food. This method appears to overestimate fluoride concentration (see Chapter 2). Concentrations of fluoride in foods as presented in this chapter have been obtained by modern analytic methods.

The medical/dental significance of various intakes of fluoride may be considered in the context of estimates of intakes necessary to produce adverse effects. The adverse effects of excessive fluoride intake are entirely systemic in origin and cannot be produced after completion of enamel formation. They consist of enamel fluorosis, which may be cosmetically objectionable but, except in its most severe form, is of no other medical or dental significance. Dental fluorosis is of greatest concern with respect to the permanent teeth. For the permanent incisors and canines – the teeth of greatest cosmetic importance – enamel formation is generally complete by 7 years of age. Thus, although beneficial effects of fluoride intake may be realized by fluoride intake throughout the life span, concern about development of dental fluorosis applies primarily to the first 7 years of life.

Adults, adolescents and school-age children

The beverages and foods that account for most of the dietary fluoride intake of adults also account for most of the dietary fluoride intake of adolescents and school-age children. Age categories other than preschool children and infants will therefore be considered together.

Water and other non-dairy beverages

"Market basket" food collections in the United States have demonstrated that most of the fluoride intake of adults is obtained from water and other beverages. The percentage of dietary fluoride intake from these sources in market basket collections in 1965 was 60% in a community with fluoride content of the water 0.4 mg/L and 66 to 73% in three communities with 0.8-1.0 mg/L fluoride in the drinking water.[53] A large number of market basket collections made between 1975 and 1982 demonstrated that water and other beverages accounted for 66% of fluoride intake in communities with a fluoride content of the drinking water of less than 0.3 mg/L, and for 75-80% of fluoride intake in communities with greater fluoride concentrations of the water supply.[51]

Because of the increase in consumption of soft drinks in the USA and Canada over the past 30 years,[10,33,46] the proportion of fluoride

Table 3-1
Estimated fluoride intake from various food categories by adults in the united states*

Food category	Fluoride intake (% of total)
Water and non-dairy beverages	75
Grain and cereal products	7
Meat, fish and poultry	6
All other foods	12

* Simplified summary of "market basket" data of Singer et al.[51]

intake from this source is greater now than in the 1960s and 1970s. As indicated in Table 3-1, it seems likely that approximately 75% of dietary fluoride intake by adults in the USA is obtained from water and beverages.

Fluoride concentration of fruit-flavored and carbonated beverages in the USA and Canada is commonly 0.6-0.9 mg/L.[11,44,49] Schulz et al.[49] reported a range of fluoride concentrations from 0.55 to 1.05 mg/L, with a mean of 0.889 mg/L for 24 canned beverages and a mean of 0.875 mg/L for 39 bottled beverages.

The fluoride content of beer and other alcoholic beverages generally reflects the fluoride concentration of the water used in production of the beverage.[47] Tamacas et al.[57] reported that fluoride concentrations of a few beers produced "in areas where fluoride levels in the water were high" ranged up to 1 mg/L, but fluoride content of most beers was less than 0.2 mg/L.

The fluoride content of bottled waters used for drinking is quite variable. Water prepared by deionization, steam distillation, reverse osmosis or a combination of methods generally provides no more than 0.2 mg fluoride per liter, whereas various methods for filtering water have relatively little effect on the fluoride content.[2,38,42,58] Some brands of mineral water from France and other European countries contain 1.8-5.8 mg fluoride per liter.[2,9,37,38] Most of the brands with high fluoride content are naturally effervescent or carbonated.

Tea leaves are a particularly rich source of fluoride and fluoride is rapidly released into tea infusions, most of the release occurring in 5-10 min. Fluoride concentrations of brewed tea commonly range from 0.5 to 4 ppm.[11,15,36] As would be anticipated, concentrations have been found to be somewhat greater when fluoridated water is used in brewing than when water with low fluoride content is used.

Other dietary sources of fluoride intake

Among the non-beverage sources of dietary fluoride, in the USA the categories of meat, fish and poultry and of grain and cereal products account for about 6 or 7% of total fluoride intake from the diet, and all other foods account for about 12% of dietary intake (Table 3-1).

The fluoride concentration of a few items of meat, fish and poultry is extremely high. The fluoride content of canned sardines may be as high as 16 mg/kg,[60] and the fluoride content of mechanically deboned meat products is high because of the presence of bone particles (see **Infants**). However, the fluoride content of most meat, fish and poultry products is quite modest.

Use of fluoridated water in commercial food preparation increases somewhat the fluoride content of canned fruits, vegetables, soups and stews, but such foods in the aggregate do not contribute large amounts of fluoride to the diet.

Preschool children

For children from 1 to 6 years of age, as for older individuals, fluoride intake is predominantly from beverages rather than from food. Intake of fluoride is likely to be quite low when the predominant beverage is cow milk, but will be considerably greater when consumption of fruit juices, fruit-flavored drinks and carbonated beverages is high.

In a study of young children conducted in North Carolina,[46] consumption of milk and water accounted for less than 40% of total liquid consumption by children from 2 through 6 years of age. Much of the total liquid intake was from fruit juices, fruit-flavored drinks and carbonated beverages. Fluoride intake from liquids other than water and milk averaged 0.36 mg/day by 2- and 3-year-old children and 0.54 mg/day by 4-6-year-old children. However, because some children in each category consumed no liquids or very small amounts of liquids other than milk or water, the distribution of intake was skewed toward higher values. The mean +1SD value for fluoride intake from beverages other than water or milk was 1.06 mg/day and the maximum value was 2.39 mg/day. For an 18 kg 5-year-old child, a fluoride intake of 1.06 mg/day is 56 $\mu g \cdot kg^{-1} \cdot day^{-1}$ and an intake of 2.39 mg/day is 133 $\mu g \cdot kg^{-1} \cdot day^{-1}$. It is therefore evident that some children, even those living in communities with low fluoride concentrations in the drinking water, obtain generous amounts of fluoride from beverages.

In some cultures, tea is widely consumed and may be offered even to small children.[22,40] However, the number of small children who regularly consume tea is much smaller than the number who regularly consume fruit juices, fruit-flavored drinks and carbonated beverages.

Infants

Much of the infant's diet consists of human milk or milk of other mammals. Fluoride is poorly transported from plasma to milk. (see Chapter 4), and concentrations of fluoride in milk remain low even when the intake of fluoride by the woman (or other mammal) is high.[55] Infant formulas provide variable amounts of fluoride, the amount depending primarily on the fluoride content of the water used as a diluent. With few exceptions, beikost contributes little to total fluoride intake. Beikost is a collective term for foods other than milk or formula fed to infants.[27]

Breast-fed infants

As determined by modern analytic techniques, the fluoride concentration of human milk generally ranges from 5 to 10 μg/L (Table 3-2). An infant consuming 0.15 liter·kg^{-1}·day^{-1} of human milk with a fluoride concentration of 6 μg/L will obtain about 1 μg·kg^{-1}·day^{-1} from this source (Table 3-3).

The examples presented in Table 3-3 concern fluoride intake by infants consuming 0.17, 0.15 or 0.12 liter·kg^{-1}·day^{-1} of milk or formula. The examples of 0.17 and 0.15 liter·kg^{-1}·day^{-1} were chosen because mean energy intakes by formula-fed infants are approximately 114 kcal·kg^{-1}·day^{-1} from birth to 2 months of age and 98 kcal·kg^{-1}·day^{-1}, from 2 to 4 months of age,[23] and these energy intakes are provided by 0.17 and 0.15 liter·kg^{-1}·day^{-1}, respectively, of milk or formula providing 667 kcal/L. The example of 0.12 liter·kg^{-1}·day^{-1} (equivalent to 80 kcal·kg^{-1}·day^{-1}) is considered representative of the intake of milk or formula by many infants over 6 months of age who obtain only a portion of their energy intake from milk or formula.

Formula-fed infants

Commercially prepared formulas are available as ready-to-feed (667 kcal/L), concentrated liquid (1333 kcal/L) requiring the addition of an equal volume of water before feeding, and powder (generally requiring that 145 g of powder be mixed with 880 mL of water to provide a 667 kcal/L formula). In many countries, formulas marketed as liquids – either ready-to-feed (667 kcal/L) or concentrated (1333 kcal/L) – were at one time commercially prepared with the local water supply. In the USA, where the same formula was generally manufactured in a number of locations, the fluoride concentration of a ready-to-feed formula produced in a plant using fluoridated water was generally about 1 mg/L, whereas the fluoride content of the same

Table 3-2

Fluoride concentrations of infant foods
(Modified from Fomon and Ekstrand[24])

Food	Fluoride concentration* (μg/L)
Human milk	5-10
Formula	
Ready to Feed	100-300
Concentrated liquid	
Mild-based	100-300
Isolated soy protein-based	100-400
Powdered	
Milk-based	400-1000
Isolated soy protein-based	1000-1600
Cow milk	30-60
Beikost	
Most products other than dry cereals	100-300
Fruit juices	
Procuced with non-fluoridated water	10-200
Produced with fluoridated water	100-1700
Dry cereals	
Produced with non-fluoridated water	90-200
Produced with fluoridated water	4000-6000
Wet-pack cereal-fruit products	2000-3000
Poultry-containing products	100-5000

* Concentration ranges have been rounded off. Most reported values fall within the ranges listed in the table; Human milk from Esala et al.,[20] Spak et al.,[55] Ekstrand et al.[17] Cow milk from Ekstrand (unpublished); Formulas from Johnson and Bawden[35] and McKnight-Hanes et al.[39] Beikost from Singer and Ophaug[52] and Dabeka et al.[14]

Table 3-3
Estimated fluoride intakes from milks and formulas (Modified from Fomon and Ekstrand[25])

Milk or formula	Fluoride concentration (μg/L)			Fluoride intake[a] (μg·kg^{-1}· d^{-1})		
	Formula	Water	As fed	Formula intake 170 mL·kg^{-1}·d^{-1}	Formula intake 150 mL·kg^{-1}·d^{-1}	Formula intake 120 mL·kg^{-1}·d^{-1}
Human Milk			6	1	1	1
Formulas Ready to Feed Milk-based	200	–	200	34	30	24
Concentrated Liquid Milk-based	200	200	200	34	30	24
	200	1000	600	102	90	72
ISP-based[.b]	240	200	270	46	41	22
	240	1000	620	105	93	74
Powdered Milk-based	690[c]	200	276[d]	47	41	33
	690	600	628	107	94	75
	690	1000	980	167	147	118
Cow Milk			40	6	6	5

[a] Mean energy intakes are approximately 114 kcal·kg^{-1}·d^{-1} from birth to 2 months of age and 98 kcal·kg^{-1}·d^{-1} from 2 to 4 months of age.[23] An exclusively formula-fed infant consuming a 667 kcal/L formula will therefore consume approximately 0.17 L·kg^{-1}·d^{-1} from birth to 2 months of age and approximately 0.15 L·kg^{-1}·d^{-1} from 2 to 4 months of age. 0.12 L·kg^{-1}·d^{-1} is an estimate of formula intake by older infants.
[b] Isolated soy protein-based.
[c] μg/kg of formula powder
[d] Assumes that 145 g of formula is diluted with 880 mL of water make 1 liter.

formula made in a plant with low fluoride content of the water was generally 0.2-0.3 mg/L.[52] This situation was changed in 1978, and, at present, when infant formulas are produced in cities with fluoridated municipal water supplies, a major part of the fluoride is removed from the water before incorporating it into the infant formula.

The fluoride content of infant formulas as marketed at present is influenced only to a small extent by water used in commercial preparation but to a larger extent by the fluoride content of the mineral mix. Concentrations of fluoride are generally somewhat greater in isolated soy protein-based formulas and in protein hydrolysate-based formulas than in milk-based formulas, primarily because the sources of calcium that must be added to non-milk-based formulas contain appreciable amounts of fluoride. In the case of isolated soy protein-based formulas, additional fluoride is included as part of the isolated soy protein. As currently marketed in the USA and Canada, fluoride concentrations of *ready-to-feed formulas* generally range from 100 to 300 µg/L (Table 3-2) and provide modest intakes of fluoride. The fluoride intake of an infant consuming 0.17 liter·kg⁻¹·day⁻¹ of a ready-to-feed formula with fluoride concentration of 200 µg/L will be 34 µg·kg⁻¹·day⁻¹ (Table 3-3).

The fluoride concentrations of *concentrated liquid formulas* generally range from 100 to 300 µg/L in milk-based products and from 100 to 400 µg/L in isolated soy protein-based products (Table 3-2). Depending on the fluoride content of the water used for diluting the concentrated liquid formulas, fluoride concentrations of the formulas as fed commonly range from 200 to 620 µg/L (Table 3-3).

When a concentrated *liquid milk-based formula* providing 200 µg of fluoride per liter is mixed with an equal volume of water that provides 200 µg fluoride per liter, the concentration of fluoride in the formula as fed will be 200 µg/L. With formula intake of 0.17 liter·kg⁻¹·day⁻¹ fluoride intake will be 34 µg·kg⁻¹·day⁻¹ and with a formula intake of 0.15 liter·kg⁻¹·day⁻¹ fluoride intake will be 30 µg·kg⁻¹·day⁻¹ (Table 3-3). However, if the same formula is diluted with water providing 1000 µg of fluoride per liter, intake of fluoride from consumption of 0.17 liter·kg⁻¹·day⁻¹ will be 102 µg·kg⁻¹·day⁻¹ and intake of fluoride from consumption of 0.15 liter·kg⁻¹·day⁻¹ will be 90 µg·kg⁻¹·day⁻¹. If the intake of the formula is 0.12 liter·kg⁻¹·day⁻¹ (as might be the case for an older infant receiving 20% or more of energy intake from beikost) rather than 0.17 or 0.15 liter·kg⁻¹·day⁻¹, fluoride intake from the formula will be 0.72 µg·kg⁻¹·day⁻¹. As may be seen from Table 3-3, intake of fluoride from concentrated liquid isolated soy protein-based formulas is slightly greater than that from correspondingly prepared milk-based formulas.

Fluoride concentrations of milk-based *powdered formulas* as marketed commonly range from 400 to 1000 µg/kg and fluoride concentrations of isolated soy protein-based formulas as marketed range from 1000 to 1600 µg/kg (Table 3-2). As generally reconstituted with water to yield a liter of formula, the fluoride concentration of a milk-based formula will be about 276 µg/L if water providing 200 µg fluoride per liter is used as the diluent and about 980 µg/L if water providing 200 µg fluoride per liter is used as the diluent (Table 3-3).

The fluoride concentration of *cow milk* ranges from 30 to 60 µg/L (Table 3-2) and fluoride intake by infants fed cow milk is therefore quite low (Table 3-3).

With the exceptions of dry infant cereals and strained chicken and turkey, the fluoride concentration of *beikost* is relatively low (Table 3-2). Dry infant cereals are manufactured in a slurry and subsequently dried, with much of the fluoride content of the water adsorbed onto the dry cereal. The fluoride content of dry cereals may be as high as 5000 or 6000 µg/kg,[14,52] and the preparation of such cereal with powdered or concentrated liquid formula that has been diluted with fluoridated water may result in an appreciable contribution to total fluoride intake. For example, if an infant living in a community with fluoridated water is fed a 70 g serving of cereal (10 g of dry cereal diluted with 60 mL of formula), and the fluoride concentrations of cereal and formula are 5000 and 600 µg/L, respectively, the concentration of fluoride in the cereal as fed will be 1229 µg/kg and a feeding of 70 g will result in an intake of 86 µg fluoride – about 11 µg/kg for an 8 kg infant.

Among commercially prepared beikost items, chicken is also notable in its fluoride content. The source of this chicken is aged laying hens with high fluoride concentrations in the bones. The meat used in commercial preparation of strained chicken for infants is obtained by mechanically deboning the neck and spine. The fluoride content of the resultant product may be as high as 5000 µg/kg (Table 3-2). Turkey products may also be relatively high in fluoride. These products should be fed spar-

Table 3-4

Comparison of fluoride intakes from milks and formula during the 1960s and early 1970s
with those during the 1980s and early 1990s (From Fomon and Ekstrand,[24])

Age Interval	1960s and Early 1970s		1980s and Early 1990s	
	F intake* $\mu g \cdot kg^{-1} \cdot d^{-1}$	Estimated % of Infants	F Intake $\mu g \cdot kg^{-1} \cdot d^{-1}$	Estimated % of Infants
Birth - 1 months				
Feeding				
Human Milk	1-37	20	1-37	50-60
Infant Formula	34-167	80	34-167	40-50
Cow Milk	–	–	–	–
1-4 months				
Feeding				
Human Milk	1-29	< 10	1-29	35-40
Infant Formula	30-147	> 70	30-147	60-65
Cow Milk	6	20	–	–
4-10 months				
Feeding				
Human Milk	–	–	1-37	15
Infant Formula	24-118	< 20	24-118	55
Cow Milk	5	> 80	5	30

*Fluoride intakes by exclusively breast-fed infants do not exceed 1 $\mu g \cdot kg^{-1} \cdot d^{-1}$; however, many breast-fed infants also receive infant formula and the range of intakes in the table include those of partially breast-fed infants. Estimates of fluoride intake from infant formulas have been calculated from values in Table 3-3 and are therefore somewhat less than would be the case if calculations had been based on concentrations of fluoride in concentrated liquid and powdered infant formulas actually marketed in the 1960s and early 1970s.

ingly. Other strained foods containing chicken or turkey do not contain enough of the poultry to result in high concentrations of fluoride.

Comments on fluoride intake by infants

Ophaug et al.[43] determined the dietary intake of fluoride by 6-month-old formula-fed infants living in communities with fluoride concentrations in the drinking water in three categories: less than 0.3 ppm, 0.3-0.7 ppm, and more than 0.7 ppm. Fluoride intakes averaged 230, 320 and 490 μg/day respectively – approximately 29, 40, and 61 μg per kg of body weight for an 8 kg infant. The authors pointed out that concentrated liquid formula diluted with fluoridated water (1 ppm) may provide a fluoride intake greater than 100 $\mu g \cdot kg^{-1} \cdot day^{-1}$.

Fluoride intake by infants is best discussed in the context of estimates of intakes required to produce adverse effects. Various investigators[4,21,28,59] have estimated that the intake of fluoride associated with development of enamel fluorosis of the permanent teeth ranges from 40 to 100 $\mu g \cdot kg^{-1} \cdot day^{-1}$ (Chapter 9). Although these estimates are the best available, confidence in them must be limited because they

- are based on few data

- fail to distinguish between doses of fluoride resulting in high peak plasma fluoride concentrations (as occur with daily consumption of a supplement) and lower and more sustained plasma concentrations (as in infants fed infant formulas providing generous intakes of fluoride), and

- fail to indicate the duration of time over which the intakes must be sustained to produce adverse effects.

Because estimates of the threshold level for development of mild dental fluorosis are in the range of 40-100 $\mu g \cdot kg^{-1} \cdot day^{-1}$, it seems likely from the calculations presented in Table 3-3 that infants fed formulas made from concentrated liquids or powders diluted with water providing 1000 μg fluoride per liter are at risk of dental fluorosis. A major effort should be made to avoid use of fluoridated water for dilution of formula powders. In addition, when economically feasible, young infants fed formulas prepared from concentrated liquids should have these formulas made up with nonfluoridated water. For older infants who consume appreciable amounts of beikost, the daily intake of formula falls substantially below 0.15 liter/d, and the risk of using fluoridated water to dilute concentrated liquid formulas decreases.

Changing pattern of fluoride intake by infants
As reviewed elsewhere[24,25] the pattern of dietary intake of fluoride by infants in the USA has changed greatly since the 1970s. Because of the greater number of young infants breast fed now than in the 1950s, 1960s and early 1970s,[26] fluoride consumption by the infant population during the early months of life is less than in the past when nearly all infants were fed formulas for the first 2-4 months of life. However, fluoride exposure of older infants is now much greater.

Table 3-4 presents a comparison of fluoride intake from milks and formulas during the 1960s and early 1970s with that during the 1980s and early 1990s. In 1971, fresh cow milk was fed to 40% of 4-month-old infants, 75% of 6-month-old infants, and to nearly all infants 8 months of age or older.[26] As already mentioned, concentrations of fluoride in cow milk are low. Feeding practices of the 1950s, 1960s and early 1970s therefore resulted in a low intake of fluoride by most infants older than 4 months. In the late 1980s and early 1990s, about 80% of 6-month old infants, 60% of 8-month-old infants and 50% of 10-month-old infants were formula-fed.

Appreciation of these changes in fluoride exposure of infants is important because, as already mentioned, fluoride intake during infancy may be a factor in the development of fluorosis of the permanent teeth. Although several reports published during the past decade indicate that fluorosis has increased in the USA, most of the studies concern children whose patterns of fluoride intake during infancy differed considerably from the current pattern. Unfortunately, there is little information about the relative susceptibility of older and younger infants to the adverse effects of fluoride consumption.

Fluoride exposure from dental products and miscellaneous sources

Topical use of dental products such as fluoridated dentifrices, fluoridated mouthrinses, fluoridated lacquers and fluoridated gels is associated with ingestion of fluoride, and intake from

Table 3-5
Fluoride content of some common dental fluoride preparations

	Type of preparation		Fluoride concentration (ppm)	Amount used	Total fluoride dose (mg)
Topical by dental personal	2%	NaF sol.	9100	2-3 mL	18-27
	10%	SnF$_2$ sol.	24250	2-3 mL	49-73
	5%	NaF varnish	22600	0.5-1 g	11-23
	1.23%	APF gel	12300	3-4 g	37-49
	9%	SnF·ZnSiO$_4$	22500	2 g paste	45
Home treatment	0.05%	NaF sol.	226	10 mL/day	2.3
	0.2%	NaF sol.	910	10 mL/week	9.1
	0.5%	APF gel.	5000	3-4 g/tray	15-20
	0.4%	SnF$_2$	970	2 g/brush	2
Dentifrice	0.22%	NaF	1000	2 g[(1)]	2
	0.76%	MFP	1000	2 g[(1)]	2
	0.145%	F(NaF+MFP)	1450	2 g[(1)]	2.9

[(1)] 1 g twice daily

these sources should not be ignored in establishing recommendations for use of fluoride supplements. Table 3-5 identifies some common dental fluoride preparations.

Fluoridated dentifrices

In most of the industrialized countries of the western world, nearly all dentifrices sold (more then 90%) contain 1000 or 1500 ppm fluoride as sodium fluoride (NaF) or sodium monofluoro-phosphate (MFP). Various studies have indicated that in children less than 6 years of age, from 24 to 60% (mean 44%) of the dentifrice is swallowed,[5,19,31,41,48,50] and the swallowed quantity is almost completely absorbed[16] (see also Chapter 4).

Of the fluoride applied to the toothbrush, the quantity ingested appears to vary inversely with age and directly with the amount applied.[6,8,41,50,56] It is not surprising that rinsing of the mouth with water after the teeth are brushed will greatly decrease the amount of

dentifrice that is swallowed. When the mouth is rinsed three times with water, minimal amounts of fluoride are ingested.[54]

If an 18 kg 5-year-old child applies 0.5 g of dentifrice (0.5 mg fluoride) to the toothbrush and ingests 44%, fluoride ingestion will be 12 μg/kg. If the child brushes his teeth twice daily, ingestion will be 24 μg·kg^{-1}·day^{-1}. Some children will apply more than 0.5 g of dentifrice per brushing episode, resulting in considerably greater ingestion of fluoride from dentifrice.

Although a retrospective study failed to demonstrate an association between use of a fluoridated dentifrice early in life and subsequent fluorosis,[48] a controlled clinical trial demonstrated an association between use of fluoridated dentifrice before 2 years of age and subsequent mild fluorosis.[45] Additional controlled studies on the consequences of use of fluoridated dentifrices during early life are needed (see also Chapter 18).

Fluoride-containing mouthrinses

Exposure to fluoridated mouthrinses by young preschool children is less common than exposure to fluoridated dentifrices. Nevertheless, it has been estimated[63] that in preschool children from 3 to 5 years of age, use of a low potency mouth rinse (230 mg/L) may result in ingestion of 0.25-0.41 mg fluoride – 14-23 µg/kg per episode for a 18 kg 5-year-old child. Fluoride ingestion from use of a high potency rinse would be anticipated to be several times greater.

Gels

Fluoride-containing mouth gels may be applied, usually by the dental profession once yearly, to individuals living in communities with low concentrations of fluoride in the water supply. The quantity of fluoride ingested may be high,[18] but it seems unlikely that such infrequent exposure is an important contributor to dental fluorosis (see also Chapters 4 and 8).

Miscellaneous sources of exposure

The vessel used for cooking may also influence fluoride content of the food.[29] Teflon-coated vessels release fluoride whereas aluminum vessels absorb fluoride during cooking. When water containing 1 mg fluoride per kg of water was boiled for 15 minutes in a stainless steel or Pyrex vessel, there was little change in fluoride concentration. In a Teflon-coated vessel, fluoride concentration increased to about 3 mg/kg, whereas in an aluminum vessel fluoride concentration decreased to about 0.3 mg/kg.

Even for residents of heavily industrialized communities, airborne sources of fluoride contribute little to the daily fluoride intake. Similarly, fluoride exposure from the use of fluoride-containing tranquilizers (benzothiadiazines, fluorosteroids, phenothiazines and fluorobutyrophenones), fluoride-containing anesthetics (methoxyflurane, enflurane and halothane) or other fluoride-containing drugs rarely contributes substantially to fluoride intake.

Fluoride supplements

In the early 1960s, because the favorable effect of fluoride on decreasing the prevalence and severity of dental caries was believed to be predominantly systemic, and because it was known that dental caries prevalence was less among individuals living in communities in which the fluoride concentration of the drinking water was 1 mg/L or more, it seemed reasonable to provide fluoride supplements to children living in communities with low concentrations of fluoride in the drinking water.[3] Several fluoride supplementation programs were introduced in the 1960s and 1970s, each based on the assumption that the cariostatic effect of fluoride was solely or predominantly systemic rather than a local effect at the surface of the tooth. Suitable dose-response data were not available, and the recommended fluoride dosage was set to match the supposed fluoride intake of individuals of similar age living in communities with fluoridated water. In 1972, the Committee on Nutrition of the American Academy of Pediatrics recommended that fluoride supplements be given to infants and children living in communities in which the fluoride concentration of the drinking water was less than 0.5 mg/L.[12] It was recommended that the supplement be sufficient to provide an intake of 0.5 mg/day for infants and children less than 3 years of age and 1 mg/day for older children. However, in practice, the supplement alone commonly provided such intakes.

This level of fluoride supplementation was then shown to be associated with development of dental fluorosis,[1] and in 1979 a revised dosage schedule was proposed. In communities in which the fluoride concentration of the drinking water was less than 0.3 mg/L, a supplement of 0.25 mg/day was recommended for the first 2 years of life, a supplement of 0.5 mg/day for children 2-3 years of age, and a supplement of 1 mg/day for children 3-16 years of age.[13]

Even with doses of fluoride supplements in this range, several reports[30,32,61] have shown a significant association between fluoride supplementation and enamel fluorosis of the permanent teeth.

After review of the evidence, the participants of a workshop held in January 1994 under the auspices of the American Dental Association came to the conclusion that fluoride supplements should not be recommended for infants less than 6 months of age. For individuals more than 6 months of age living in communities in which the fluoride content of the drinking water was less than 0.3 mg/L, a daily supplement of 0.25 mg/day was recommended for individuals from 6 months to 3 years of age, a supplement of 0.5 mg/day for individuals 3-6 years of age, and a supplement of 1 mg/day for those 6-16 years of age. For children 6-16 years of age living in communities in which the fluoride content of the drinking water was 0.3-0.7 mg/L, a fluoride supplement of 0.5 mg/day was recommended. These recommendations were subsequently accepted by the American Academy of Pediatrics (AAP News 11: 4, 1995) and presumably by the American Dental Association (J Am Dent Assoc 125; 336, 1994).

In the opinion of the authors, even this modified dosage schedule may provide excessive amounts of fluoride. For infants 6-12 months of age living in a community with fluoride content of the water less than 0.3 mg/L, fluoride intake may be 24-41 $\mu g \cdot kg^{-1} \cdot day^{-1}$ from formula alone (Table 3-3) and beikost will provide small additional amounts of fluoride. Thus, total dietary intake of fluoride is likely to be 30-50 $\mu g \cdot kg^{-1} \cdot day^{-1}$. There is therefore some question about the desirability of providing a fluoride supplement of 0.25 mg/day (31 $\mu g \cdot kg^{-1} \cdot day^{-1}$ for an 8 kg infant) (see also Chapter 9).

The justification for use of fluoride supplements for preschool children is also questionable. As has been discussed, intake of fluoride by 5-year-old children is not infrequently more than 50 $\mu g \cdot kg^{-1} \cdot day^{-1}$ from beverages other than water and dairy products, and small additional amounts of fluoride are obtained from other dietary sources. Twice daily use of a fluoridated dentifrice is likely to result in fluoride ingestion of about 24 $\mu g \cdot kg^{-1} \cdot day^{-1}$. Fluoride intake of many children living in communities with low fluoride content of the drinking water will therefore be generous without the use of a supplement. A fluoride supplement of 0.5 mg given to an 18 kg 5-year-old results in an additional 28 $\mu g \cdot kg^{-1} \cdot day^{-1}$. Thus, for many preschool children given supplements, total fluoride intake will be more than 100 $\mu g \cdot kg^{-1} \cdot day^{-1}$.

Literature cited

1. Aasenden R, Peebles TC. Effects of fluoride supplementation from birth on human deciduous and permanent teeth. Arch Oral Biol 1974; 19: 321-6.

2. Allen HE, Halley-Henderson MA, Hass CN. Chemical composition of bottled mineral water. Arch Environ Health 1989;44: 102-16.

3. Arnold FA Jr, McClure FJ, White CL. Sodium fluoride tablets for children. Dent Prog 1960; 1: 8-12.

4. Baelum V, Fejerskov O, Manji F, Larsen MJ. Daily dose of fluoride and dental fluorosis. Dan Dent J 1987; 91: 452-6.

5. Barnhart WE, Hiller KL, Leonard GJ, Michaels SE. Dentifrice usage and ingestion among four age groups. J Dent Res 1974; 53: 1317-22.

6. Baxter PM. Toothpaste ingestion during toothbrushing by school children. Br Dent J 1980; 148: 125-8.

7. Beals TL, Anderson GH, Peterson RD, Thompson GW, Hargreaves JA. Between-meal eating by Ontario children and teenagers. J Canad Diet Assoc 1981; 42: 242-7.

8. Bruun C, Thylstrup A. Dentifrice usage among Danish children. J Dent Res. 1988; 67: 1114-7.

9. Chan JT, Stark C, Jeske AH. Fluoride content of bottled waters: implications for dietary fluoride supplementation. Texas Dent J 1990; 107: 17-21.

10. Chao ESM, Anderson, GH, Thompson, GW, Hargreaves JA, Peterson RD. A longitudinal study of the dietary changes of a sample of Ontario children II: Food intake. J Can Diet Assoc 1984; 45: 112-8.

11. Clovis J, Hargreaves JA. Fluoride intake from beverage consumption. Community Dent Oral Epidemiol 1988; 16: 11-5.

12. Committee on Nutrition: Fluoride as a nutrient. Pediatrics 1972; 49: 456-9.

13. Committee on Nutrition: Fluoride supplementation: revised dosage schedule. Pediatrics 1979; 63: 150-2.

14. Dabeka RW, McKenzie AD, Conacher HBS, Kirkpatrick BS. Determination of fluoride in Canadian infant foods and calculation of fluoride intake by infants. Can J Public Health 1982; 73: 188-91.

15. Duckworth SC, Duckworth R. The ingestion of fluoride in tea. Br Dent J 1978; 145: 368-70.

16. Ekstrand J, Ehrnebo M. Absorption of fluoride from fluoride dentifrices. Caries Res 1980; 14: 96-102.

17. Ekstrand J, Hardell LI, Spak C-J. Fluoride balance studies on infants in a 1-ppm-water-fluoride area. Caries Res 1984; 18: 87-92.

18. Ekstrand J, Koch G, Lindgren LE, Pettersson LG. Pharmacokinetics of fluoride gels of children and adults. Caries Res 1981; 15: 213-20.

19. Ericsson Y, Forsman B. Fluoride retained from mouthrinses and dentifrices in preschool children. Caries Res 1969; 3: 290-9.

20. Esala S, Vuori E, Helle A. Effect of maternal fluorine intake on breast milk fluorine content. Br J Nutr 1982; 48: 201-4.

21. Farkas CS, Farkas EJ. Potential effect of food processing on the fluoride content of infant foods. Sci Total Environ 1974; 2: 399-405.

22. Farkas CS. Body iron status associated with tea consumption. Can Med Assoc J 1979; 121: 706 (letter).

23. Fomon SJ, Bell EF. Chapter 7. Energy. In: Fomon SJ. Nutrition of normal infants. St. Louis: Mosby 1993; 103-20.

24. Fomon SJ, Ekstrand J. Fluoride intake by infants. J Public Health Dent 1996; (in press).

25. Fomon SJ, Ekstrand J. Chapter 18. Fluoride. In: Fomon SJ. Nutrition of normal infants. St. Louis: Mosby 1993; 299-310.

26. Fomon SJ. Chapter 3. Trends in infant feeding since 1950. In: Fomon SJ. Nutrition of normal infants. St. Louis: Mosby 1993; 15-35.

27. Fomon SJ. Infant nutrition, 2nd. edn. Philadelphia: Saunders 1974; 408.

28. Forsman B. Early supply of fluoride and enamel fluorosis. Scand J Dent Res 1977; 85: 22-30.

29. Full CA, Parkins FM. Effect of cooking vessel composition on fluoride. J Dent Res 1975; 54: 192.

30. Granath L, Widenheim J, Birkhed D. Diagnosis of mild enamel fluorosis in permanent maxillary incisors using two scoring systems. Community Dent Oral Epidemiol 1985; 10: 273-6.

31. Hargreaves JA, Ingram GS, Wagg BJ. A gravimetric study of the ingestion of toothpaste by children. Caries Res 1972; 6: 237-43.

32. Holm A-K, Anderson R. Enamel mineralization disturbances in 12-year-old children with known early exposure to fluorides. Community Dent Oral Epidemiol 1982; 10: 335-9.

33. Ismail AI, Burt BA, Eklund SA. The cariogenicity of soft drinks in the United States. JADA 1984; 109: 241-5.

34. Jenkins GN. Fluoride intake and its safety among heavy tea drinkers in a British fluoridated city. Proc Finn Dent Soc 1991; 87: 571-9.

35. Johnson J, Bawden JW. The fluoride content of infant formulas available in 1985. Pediatr Dent 1987; 9: 33-7.

36. Kumpulainen J, Koivistoinen P. Fluorine in foods. Residue Rev 1977; 68: 37-57.

37. MacFadyen EE, McNee SG, Weetman DA. Fluoride content of some bottled spring water. Br Dent J 1982; 153: 423-4.

38. McGuire S. Fluoride content of bottled water. N Engl J Med 1989; 321: 836-7 (letter).

39. McKnight-Hanes MC, Leverett DH, Adair SM, Shields CP. Fluoride content of infant formulas: soy-based formulas as a potential factor in dental fluorosis. Pediatr Dent 1988; 10: 189-94.

49. Merhav H, Amitai Y, Palti H, Godfrey S. Tea drinking and microcytic anemia in infants. Am J Clin Nutr 1985; 41: 1210-3.

41. Naccache H, Simard PL, Trahan L, Demers M, Lapointes C, Brodeur J-M. Variability in the ingestion of toothpaste by preschool children. Caries Res 1990; 24: 359-63.

42. Nowak A, Nowak, MV. Fluoride concentration of bottled and processed water. Iowa Dent J 1989 75: 28.

43. Ophaug RH, Singer L, Harland BF. Dietary fluoride intake of 6-month and 2-year-old children in four dietary regions of the United States. Am J Clin Nutr 1985; 42: 701-7.

44. Osis D, Wiatrowski E, Samachson J, Spencer H. Fluoride analysis of the human diet and of biological samples. Clin Chim Acta 1974; 51: 211-6.

45. Osuji OO, Leake JL, Chipman ML, Nikiforuk G, Locker D, Levine N. Risk factors for dental fluorosis in a fluoridated community. J Dent Res 1988; 67: 1488-92.

46. Pang DTY, Phillips CL, Bawden JW. Fluoride intake from beverage consumption in a sample of North Carolina children. J Dent Res 1992; 71: 1382-8.

47. Rao GS. Dietary intake and bioavailability of fluoride. Ann Rev Nutr 1984; 4: 115-36.

48. Ripa LW. A critique of topical fluoride methods (dentifrices, mouthrinses, operator-, and self-applied gels) in an era of decreased carious and increased fluorosis prevalence. J Public Health Dentistry 1991; 51: 23-41.

49. Schulz EM, Jr, Epstein, JS, Forrester DJ. Fluoride content of popular carbonated beverages. J Prev Dent 1976; 3: 27-9.

50. Simard PL, Lachapelle D, Trahan L, Naccache H, Demers M, Brodeur J-M. The ingestion of fluoride dentifrices by young children. J Dent Child 1989; 56: 177-81.

51. Singer L, Ophaug RH, Harland BF. Dietary fluoride intake of 15-19-year-old male adults residing in the United States. J Dent Res 1985; 64: 1302-5.

52. Singer L, Ophaug R. Total fluoride intake of infants. Pediatrics 1979; 63: 460-6.

53. Singer L, Ophaug RH, Harland BF. Fluoride intake of young male adults in the United States. Am J Clin Nutr 1980; 33: 328-32.

54. Sjögren K, Ekstrand J, Birkhed D. Effect of water-rinsing after toothbrushing on fluoride ingestion and absorption. Caries Res 1994; 29: 455-9.

55. Spak CJ, Hardell LI, De Chateau P. Fluoride in human milk. Acta Paedatr Scand 1983; 72: 699-701.

56. Szpunar SM, Burt BA. Dental caries, fluorosis, and fluoride exposure in Michigan schoolchildren. J Dent Res 1988; 67: 802-6.

57. Tamacas JC, Ramsey AC, Hardwick JL. Fluoride contents of beverages commonly used in England. J Dent Res 1974; 53: 1088 (abstract).

58. Tate WH, Snyder R, Montgomery EH, Chan JT. Impact of source of drinking water on fluoride supplementation. J Pediatr 1990; 117: 419-21.

59. Toth K. Fluoride ingestion related to body weight. Caries Res 1975; 9: 290-1 (abstract).

60. Trautner K, Siebert G. An experimental study of bio-availability of fluoride from dietary sources in man. Archs Oral Biol 1986; 31: 223-8.

61. von der Fehr FR, Larsen MJ, Bragelien J. Dental fluorosis in children using fluoride tablets. Caries Res 1990; 24: 102-3 (abstract).

62. Walton JL, Messer LB. Dental caries and fluorosis in breast-fed and bottle-fed children. Caries Res 1981; 15: 124-37.

63. Wei SH, Kanellis MJ. Fluoride retention after sodium fluoride mouthrinsing of preschool children. J Am Dent Assoc 1983; 106: 626-9.

Section II

PHYSIOLOGY AND TOXICOLOGY OF FLUORIDES

CHAPTER 4

FLUORIDE METABOLISM

J. Ekstrand

Introduction – Absorption – Fluoride in blood plasma
Pharmacokinetics of fluoride – Distribution – Excretion

Introduction

The human organism is exposed to fluoride in a number of ways. In many countries fluoride is added to the drinking water supplies for the prevention of dental caries. Fluoride is also an important component of most dentifrices and a large number of other commercially available dental preparations. These products can be divided into two main categories, namely, those intended to be swallowed and absorbed into the systemic circulation, such as tablets and drops, and those intended for topical application to the tooth surfaces only - fluoride dentifrices, mouthrinses, gels and varnishes. Various quantities of topically applied fluoride are, however, swallowed and subsequently absorbed.

Apart from its positive cariostatic properties, fluoride is a hazardous substance. An acute intake of a large dose or chronic ingestion of lower doses of fluoride can result in a variety of side effects such as acute gastric and kidney disturbances, dental and skeletal fluorosis or even death. This is discussed in Chapter 8.

In order to understand the biological effects of fluoride on the human organism, a thorough knowledge of fluoride metabolism is necessary. Generally, the subject can be divided into ab-

sorption, distribution and elimination. The main features of fluoride metabolism are illustrated in Fig. 4-1.

In an overall description of fluoride metabolism, blood plasma is considered the central compartment into which fluoride must pass for its subsequent distribution and elimination. Roughly 50% of an ingested fluoride dose in an adult will be excreted in the urine and most of the remainder will be taken up by mineralized tissues. Fluoride is not irreversibly bound and is released from these tissues during normal remodeling of bone or following substantial changes in daily fluoride exposure. In soft tissues, fluoride establishes a steady state distribution between the intracellular and extracellular fluids. As a consequence, when the plasma level of fluoride rises or falls there is a proportional and parallel change in the intracellular fluids. The major route for the elimination of fluoride from the body is the kidney. In the following text the major features of fluoride metabolism will be discussed in greater detail.

Absorption

The major route of fluoride absorption is ingestion via the gastrointestinal tract. Fluoride may

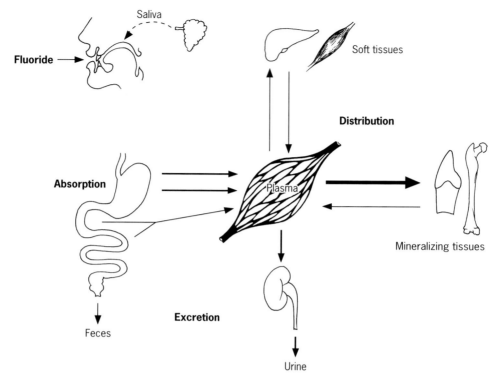

Fig. 4-1. Schematic representation of fluoride metabolism.

also be inhaled from airborne fluoride (see Chapter 1) or as a result of the biotransformation of fluoride-containing general anesthetics such as methoxyflurane, halothane, enflurane and isoflurane.

The fluoride source may be inorganic or organic. There are soluble compounds such as NaF, HF, H_2SiF_6, Na_2PO_3F and less soluble compounds like CaF_2, MgF_2 and AlF_3. Depending on their solubilities, fluoride ions are released, except for Na_2PO_3F, which is first hydrolyzed by enzymatic activity and subsequently absorbed. Regarding the biological effect of fluoride, only the fluoride ion is important in dentistry, medicine and public health.

Fluoride is generally ingested in a beverage, in food or as a pharmaceutical preparation such as NaF tablets. Depending on the physical and chemical properties of the compound and its solubility, varying amounts of the ingested fluoride dose will be absorbed and enter the systemic circulation.

Rate and degree

After intake of a NaF tablet or solution, fluoride is rapidly absorbed (Fig. 4-2). Only a few minutes after the dose is swallowed, there is a detectable rise in the plasma fluoride concentration.[2] The height of the plasma peak is proportional to the fluoride dose ingested and the rate of absorption, but is also determined by the body weight (volume of distribution) of the subject, i.e. the larger the body weight, the lower plasma peak and *vice versa*. The plasma peak usually occurs within 30 minutes; the time

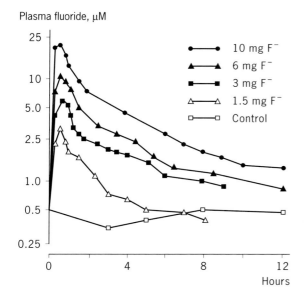

Fig. 4-2. Plasma fluoride concentrations after oral intake of four different doses of fluoride to a young adult. The plasma fluoride concentration during a control day on standardized low-fluoride diet is also shown.[4]

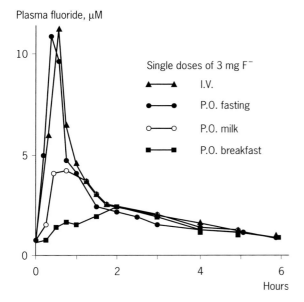

Fig. 4-3. Plasma fluoride concentration after intake of 3 mg fluoride on four separate occasions: intravenously, orally, orally + a glass of milk, and orally + a calcium-rich breakfast.[6]

for its occurrence is independent of the amount of fluoride ingested.

Readily soluble fluoride compounds, such as NaF tablets or aqueous solutions of NaF, are almost completely absorbed, whereas compounds with lower solubility, such as CaF_2, MgF_2, and AlF_3, are less completely absorbed.[4,26,31]

The ingestion of fluoride with food also retards its absorption,[6,37] as demonstrated in Fig. 4-3. When fluoride ingested as NaF tablets is taken on a fasting stomach the degree of ab-

57

Plasma fluoride, µM

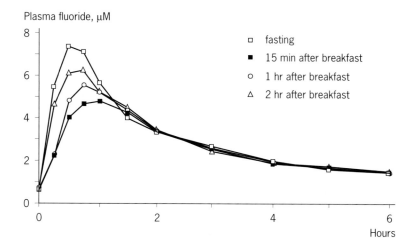

Fig. 4-4. Mean plasma fluoride concentration (n = 6) after swallowing 3 mg F in the form of a $Na_2 PO_3F$ (MFP) toothpaste.[14]

sorption of fluoride is almost 100%, but when the same dose is taken together with a glass of milk it decreases to 70%. The same dose taken together with a calcium-rich breakfast will further reduce the degree of absorption to 60%. The decrease in absorption associated with the ingestion of milk or food is probably due to binding of fluoride with certain food constituents, including calcium and other di- and trivalent cations. When this occurs, the fecal excretion of fluoride will increase.

The timing of fluoride ingestion in relation to a meal is critical with respect to fluoride bioavailability, as shown in Fig. 4-4. When a fluoride dentifrice is ingested on a fasting stomach the plasma peak is recorded within 30 minutes, but when the dentifrice is swallowed 15 minutes after a meal, the peak does not occur until after 1 hour. Not only the peak time but also the peak height will be reduced.[14] The clinical implication is that if toothbrushing occurs soon after a meal, fluoride absorption will be inhibited to some extent, and high plasma fluoride peaks will not occur. This might be important for small children, who tend to retain and ingest more of the toothpaste applied to the brush (see also Chapters 3 and 8).

Mechanism and site of absorption

The absorptive process occurs by passive diffusion; there is no convincing evidence that active transport processes are involved. Fluoride is absorbed from both the stomach and the intestine. The mechanism and the rate of gastric absorption of fluoride are related to gastric acidity.[40] There are data showing that fluoride is absorbed in the form of the undissociated weak acid hydrogen fluoride, HF, which has a pK_a of 3.45. That is, when ionic fluoride enters the acidic environment of the stomach lumen, it is largely converted into HF ($H^+ + F^- \Leftrightarrow HF$), an uncharged molecule which readily passes through biologic membranes, including the gastric mucosa (see also Chapter 8). Most of the fluoride that is not absorbed from the stomach will be rapidly absorbed from the small intestine, which has an enormous reserve capacity for absorption.

Absorption from food and dental fluoride preparations

Soluble fluorides in aqueous solutions are nearly completely absorbed. The fluoride compounds which occur naturally or are added to the drinking water, yield fluoride ions which are almost completely absorbed from the gastrointestinal tract. Dietary fluoride is also well absorbed with high bioavailability. In a balance study in infants it was found that the bioavailability of the fluoride in the infant's diet was about 90%.[15]

The fluoride from NaF tablets and fluoride from most dental products intended for topical application is almost completely absorbed when swallowed.[4,5,11,12] The bioavailability of fluoride from NaF dentifrices has been reported to be close to 100% but somewhat less for Na_2PO_3F (MFP).[5] However, this may vary among the various brands of dentifrice, as different abrasive systems might bind some of the fluoride. It would be expected, for example, that calcium-containing abrasive systems would reduce the rate and the degree of absorption. As pointed out in Chapter 3, small children may swallow various amounts of toothpaste during brushing; the ingested fluoride dose has been reported to range from .10 mg up to 2 mg and even more.[23] Since most of the ingested fluoride in the dentifrice is absorbed and distributed to the blood, the ingestion of fluoride dentifrice among small children should be kept to a minimum to prevent the occurrence of fluorosis (see also Chapter 8). A thorough rinsing after toothbrushing will minimize the ingestion of fluoride following toothbrushing with fluoridated toothpaste.[30]

The fluoride from acidulated phosphate fluoride gels (APF gels) which contain NaF dissolved in phosphoric acid (pH 3.5) is also well absorbed.[11] The fluoride concentration of most of these products is 1.23% (12,300 ppm or 647 mM). During a normal clinical procedure using trays, 2 g to as much as 5 g of the gel may be inserted into the oral cavity, corresponding to a fluoride dose of 24-60 mg fluoride (se also Table 3-5). From a toxicologic point of view, the ingestion of these gels thus has important clinical implications because of the possibility of acute side effects. Gastric disturbances, nausea, vomiting and subtoxic plasma fluoride levels fol-

lowing ingestion of these gel has been reported[34] (see also Chapter 8).

Other fluoride products that contain high fluoride concentrations include the fluoride varnishes. One such product, Duraphat®, contains 5% NaF. After the varnish is painted on the tooth surfaces, it remains there for up to 12 hours, during which time fluoride is deposited in the enamel. Some of the fluoride also diffuses into the saliva and is swallowed. A very modest increase in plasma fluoride concentration, comparable to that which occurs after the ingestion of about 1.0 mg fluoride, is associated with the application of fluoride varnishes.[12] The ingestion of the varnish following a routine clinical procedure should not result in any toxic side effects.

Fluoride in blood plasma

Plasma is the biological fluid into which and from which fluoride must pass for its distribution elsewhere in the body and for its elimination from the body. For these reasons, plasma is often referred to as the central compartment. In plasma, fluoride exists in two general forms: ionic fluoride (also called inorganic fluoride or free fluoride) and non-ionic or bound fluoride. Ionic fluoride, which is sensed by the fluoride ion-specific electrode, is the one of significance in dentistry, medicine and public health. The biologic significance of the non-ionic forms has not been determined. Together, the ionic and the non-ionic fractions are called "total" plasma fluoride.[19] The non-ionic forms of fluoride, ionic fluoride, is not bound to any plasma proteins.[8,36] In the blood, the ion is asymmetrically distributed between plasma and the blood cells so that the plasma concentration is approximately twice as high as that associated with the cells.[41] The scientific literature contains a rather wide range (0.7-2.4 µM for "normal" plasma fluoride levels.[19] Some of the disparate results may have been due to the use of fasting sub-

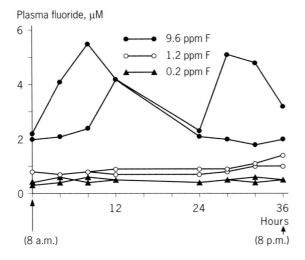

Fig. 4-5. The diurnal variation in plasma fluoride levels in subjects resident in areas with different fluoride concentrations in the drinking water.[16]

jects in some studies and non-fasting subjects in others. Undetected but substantial differences in the amounts of fluoride ingested chronically, or differences in fluoride metabolism, may also contribute to the explanation. It is virtually certain that problems with the analysis of fluoride have been contributory. This is especially likely when only the fluoride electrode is used for the analysis of samples with low concentrations. The use of preparative methods that concentrate the fluoride in small volumes, such as the acid-HMDS microdiffusion method, is recommended when such low levels of fluoride are to be measured (see also Chapter 2).

Chronic fluoride exposure and plasma levels

Plasma fluoride concentrations are not homeostatically regulated but instead they rise and fall according to the pattern of fluoride intake, among other factors.[2,19] The earlier concept of fluoride homeostasis was based on findings showing that plasma fluoride concentrations were similar among persons living in places with widely different water fluoride levels.[29] It was later established that these findings were due to the use of inappropriate analytic methods.[35] Since plasma fluoride levels

are not homeostatically regulated, there is no "normal" physiologic concentration. The plasma fluoride level expected in a healthy, fasting, long-term resident of a community with water fluoridation (1 ppm) is approximately 1 μM (0.019 ppm). As illustrated in Fig. 4-5 there is a considerable fluctuation during the day in plasma fluoride levels in subjects living in an area with a high fluoride concentration in the drinking water, particularly in adults. Variations in plasma levels were also observed in the 1.2 ppm area, although they were not as evident.[16]

In addition to the level of chronic fluoride intake, as well as recent intake, plasma fluoride levels are influenced by the relative rates of bone accretion and dissolution and by the renal clearance rate of the ion. In the long term, there is a direct relationship between the concentrations of fluoride in bone and in plasma and with age.[20,25]

Pharmacokinetics of fluoride

The absorption, soft tissue distribution, mineralized tissue uptake and renal excretion of fluoride are, in principle, simultaneous: the dif-

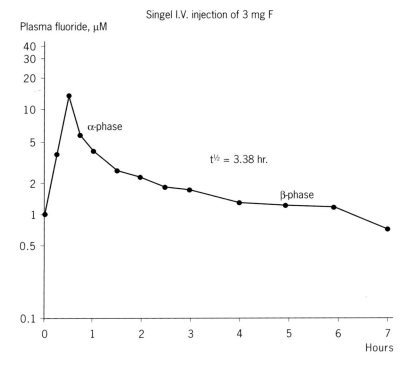

Fig. 4-6. The plasma fluoride concentration plotted on a logarithmic scale versus time after i.v. injection as a 30 min infusion of 3 mg. The plasma half-life is calculated from the β-phase (elimination phase) and was found to be 3.38 hr.[2]

ferent rates for each of these processes will influence the plasma fluoride concentration at any given time after fluoride intake. A pharmacokinetic analysis of the plasma fluoride concentration curve after intake of a single dose of fluoride will quantitatively describe the cumulative influence of the various metabolic processes and provide important information about the kinetics of fluoride in the human body.

By plotting the plasma concentration of fluoride as a function of time on a semilogarithmic scale (Fig. 4-6), three exponential phases can be distinguished: an initial increase, followed by a rapid fall for about 1 hour and thereafter a slower decline. These phases represent absorption, distribution and elimination and can be described quantitatively by using pharmacokinetic models. Theoretically, the body can be regarded as being composed of one or more compartments: the two-compartment open model has been utilized to describe the pharmacokinetics of fluoride (Fig. 4-7).

It should be pointed out that these models represent only theoretic spaces postulated to account for the experimental finding that drugs are distributed into various body fluids and tissues at various rates. In the two-compartment open model, fluoride enters the system via the central compartment; it is then distributed to the peripheral compartment: elimination of the ion occurs from the central compartment.

The initial increase in the plasma fluoride concentration in Fig. 4-2 reflects the absorption of fluoride from the gastrointestinal tract into the blood. The straight line indicates a first-order process, i.e. fluoride is absorbed from the gastrointestinal tract by first-order kinetics; the amount absorbed per unit time is proportional

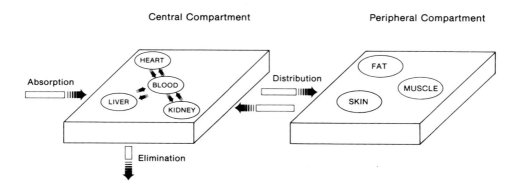

Fig. 4-7. The two-compartment open model.

to the amount present. When the plasma peak is reached, the absorption gradually decreases and the distribution of fluoride from the blood to the tissues increases. Both distribution and elimination of the ion start during the initial absorption phase but are of less quantitative importance at this stage.

The declining portion of the curve can be separated into two exponential phases. The early phase is commonly known as the distribution phase (α-phase) and the latter, the elimination phase (β-phase). During the α-phase, distribution to the soft tissues primarily determines the rapid decline in plasma fluoride concentration. Fluoride is rapidly distributed to well-perfused tissues, such as the heart, kidneys, liver and, because fluoride is a mineralized tissue seeker, to the bone. These tissues belong to the central compartment. Fluoride is more slowly distributed to poorly perfused tissues such as resting skeletal muscle and adipose tissue, which belong to the peripheral compartment. The concentration of fluoride then increases in the peripheral compartment until a steady-state is reached. This is followed by a net flux from the peripheral compartment to the central compartment, as fluoride is con-

tinuously eliminated from the central compartment. The curve then enters the β-phase (the elimination phase) in which the curve is monotonic but with a less pronounced slope compared to the α-phase. This decline in plasma concentration reflects the elimination of fluoride from the body and can be characterized by the elimination half-life ($t\frac{1}{2}$) which is the time required for the plasma fluoride concentration to fall by one-half. The plasma half-life for fluoride in human adults, which typically ranges from 4 to 10 hours, is calculated from this final exponential slope.[2] Since the α-phase and the β-phase can be described by exponential equations, it can be assumed that the overall pharmacokinetics of fluoride occurs by first-order kinetics. That is, the rate of elimination is proportional to the plasma concentration; the higher the plasma concentration of fluoride the faster elimination and *vice versa*.

The fact that the pharmacokinetics of fluoride can be described by first-order processes has several important implications. One of these concerns the question of fluoride homeostasis. According to this concept, which was advanced about 35 years ago, plasma fluoride levels are maintained over time, within a

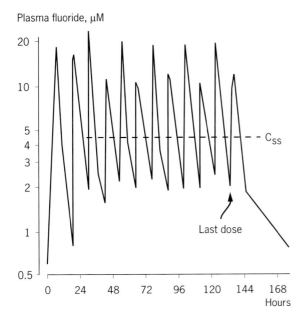

Plasma fluoride, µM

Fig. 4-8. Semilogarithmic plot of the plasma fluoride concentration after repeated intake (at 8 a.m. and 8 p.m.) of 4.5 mg fluoride as NaF tablet for 4 days. C_{SS} indicates the mean steady-state level.[2] Note that the plasma peak at C_{SS} is less at 8 p.m. compared to at 8 a.m. due to non-fasting condition at 8 p.m.

relatively narrow range, regardless of the amount of fluoride intake.[29] This would not be predicted from, nor is it supported by, the observation of first-order kinetics, which in general points to passive diffusion as the underlying transport mechanism. The data contained in Fig. 4-8 show the plasma fluoride level after multiple doses of 4.5 mg fluoride every 12 hours over 4 days.[2] The plasma level rises and falls during each dosage interval. That is, the fluctuation of the plasma fluoride concentration depends on the fluoride dose ingested, dose frequency and the plasma half-life of fluoride.

Distribution

Distribution in soft tissues
Fluoride is distributed from the plasma to all tissues and organs. The rates of delivery are generally determined by the blood flow to the tissues in question. Consequently steady-state fluoride concentrations are achieved more rapidly between plasma and well-perfused tissues, such as the heart, lungs and liver, than for less well perfused tissues such as resting skeletal muscle, skin and adipose tissue.

In general, steady-state tissue-to-plasma fluoride concentration ratios fall between 0.4 and 0.9 regardless of the rates at which the steady-state levels are achieved (Table 4-1).[39] Some notable exceptions to this range include the kidney, brain and adipose tissue. Fluoride is concentrated to high levels within the kidney tubules so that taken as a whole, this organ has a higher concentration than that of plasma. The blood-brain barrier is effective in restricting the passage of fluoride into the central nervous system where the fluoride concentration, like that of fat, is only about 20% that of plasma.[32] It is noteworthy that, in the absence of ectopic mineralization such as may occur in the large arteries or in the placenta near term, the soft tissues do not accumulate fluoride.

63

Table 4-1

Tissue-to-plasma (T/P) fluoride (^{18}F)
concentration ratios of some soft tissues of the rat.[39]

Tissue	T/P ratio
Liver	0.98
Lung	0.83
Kindney	4.16
Tongue	0.69
Diaphragm	0.61
Heart	0.46
Brain	0.08
Fat	0.11
Skin	0.43
Salivary gland	0.63

The fact that the fluoride concentrations of plasma and the extracellular fluid are higher than those of the intracellular fluids is consistent with the hypothesis that it is HF, and not ionic fluoride, which is in diffusion equilibrium across cell membranes. This hypothesis and the physiologic and toxicologic consequences is discussed in detail in Chapter 8. This concept largely accounts for the different T/P ratios shown in Table 4-1, for the pH-dependence of the absorption of fluoride from the stomach and for the pH-dependence of its reabsorption from the kidney tubules.

Distribution to mineralized tissues

Fluoride is an avid mineralized tissue seeker, its clearance rate from plasma by bone is even higher than that of calcium. Approximately 99% of all fluoride in the human body is found in mineralized tissues. Following an injection of radioactive fluoride in laboratory animals, the skeleton is clearly labeled within a few minutes.[18]

The selective affinity of fluoride for mineralized tissues is, in the short-term, due to uptake on the surface of bone crystallites by the processes of isoionic and heteroionic exchange. In the long run, it is actually incorporated into the crystal lattice structure in the form of fluorapatite or fluorhydroxyapatite (see Chapters 5 and 6).

During the growth phase of the skeleton, a relatively high portion of an ingested fluoride dose will be deposited in the skeleton. Further, a larger fraction of a single dose given to a very young individual will be deposited in skeleton compared with the same dose given to an adult.

The "balance" of fluoride in the body, i.e. the difference between the amount of fluoride ingested and the amount of fluoride excreted in the urine and the feces, can be positive or negative. When the fluoride is derived from human milk or cow's milk, biologic fluids with a low fluoride content (see Chapter 3), urinary excretion generally exceeds intake i.e. there is a negative fluoride balance. In infants when fluoride intakes are extremely low sufficient fluoride is released from bone to extracellular fluid to result in urinary excretion higher than intake.[10] This is in great contrast to when a fluoride dose, i.e. a fluoride supplement or an infant formula diluted with fluoridated water, is given to infants. Studies on metabolism in infants show that the retention will be strongly correlated with fluoride intake (Fig. 4-9).[9] Retention of fluoride following intake of a fluoride supplement of 0.25 mg given to infants has been shown to be as high as 80%.[9]

This is in strong contrast to the situation in an adult. In a study in which young adults (aged 23-27 years) were given fluoride as a single intravenous injection, about 40% of the injected fluoride dose was found in the urine.[14] Thus, under normal conditions approximately one-half of the daily fluoride intake by adults will be deposited in the skeleton and the rest excreted in the urine.

Fluoride is not irreversibly bound to bone. This has been demonstrated in individuals who moved from an area with a high fluoride con-

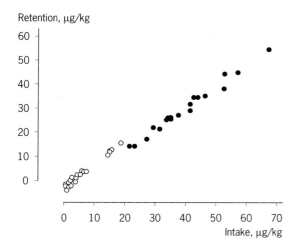

Fig. 4-9 Relationship of retention of fluoride to intake of fluoride in infants aged 37-410 days old. Each open circle indicates the results when only food with a low fluoride content was given. The filled circles indicate the results when a fluoride dose of 0.25 mg was given as drops .[9]

centration in the drinking water to an area with a lower water fluoride level. The urinary fluoride concentration in these individuals was shown to remain unusually high for long periods.[24,42] Thus, fluoride was mobilized slowly but continuously from the skeleton. Similar findings have been noted among workers with chronic occupational exposure to fluoride who were subsequently employed elsewhere.[1] Their plasma fluoride levels reflected their bone fluoride concentrations for long periods after the industrial fluoride exposure. This relationship is largely due to the fact that bone is not static but, instead, continuously undergoes a remodeling, whereby old bone is resorbed and new bone is formed.

Hence, the plasma concentrations and the urinary excretions mirror a physiologic balance that is determined by earlier fluoride exposure, the degree of accumulation of the ion in bone, the mobilization rate from bone and the efficiency of the kidneys in excreting fluoride.[2]

Distribution to the fetus

There are several published views about the passage of fluoride across the placenta. Some authors have postulated that the placenta acts as a total barrier to fluoride; others have suggested that it is only partial. Some have claimed that the placenta acts as a barrier only when there are sudden increases in the maternal plasma fluoride level. It has been claimed that the fact that primary dentition exhibits less severe degrees of dental fluorosis than the permanent dentition indicates the presence of a placental barrier, but, as will be shown in Chapter 8, this is erroneous.

Recent data from human studies have shown, however, that the placenta is not in any sense a barrier to the passage of fluoride to the fetus.[28] There is a direct relationship between the serum fluoride concentrations of the mother and the fetus, and the cord serum concentration is 75% that of the maternal fluoride concentration. From the fetal blood, fluoride is readily taken up by the mineralizing fetal bones and teeth.

Excretion

Renal handling of fluoride

The major route for the removal of fluoride from the body is by the kidneys. Because ionic fluoride is not bound to plasma proteins,[8,36] its concentration in the glomerular filtrate is undoubtedly the same as in plasma water. After entering the renal tubules, a variable amount of the ion will be reabsorbed and returned to the systemic circulation. The remainder will be excreted in the urine.

On this basis, it is apparent that the first determinant of the amount of fluoride excreted in the urine is the glomerular filtration rate. If this rate is reduced for any reason, such as chronic renal failure, this will be reflected in increased plasma and bone fluoride levels. Several studies have shown that if the glomerular filtration rate is severely reduced (to about 30% of normal or less) on a chronic basis, the plasma fluoride levels are markedly elevated.[27,38]

The renal clearance of fluoride in the adult typically ranges from 30 to 50 mL/minute,[13,27,38] whereas clearance rates of the other halogens, chloride, iodide and bromide, are usually less than 1.0 mL/minute.

The percentage of the filtered fluoride reabsorbed from the renal tubules can range from about 10% to 90%. The degree of reabsorption depends largely on the pH of the tubular fluid and urinary flow. Thus the clearance rate can be increased or decreased by changes in urine flow rate[22] as well as changes in urinary pH.[7,13]

The pH-dependence of the renal clearance of fluoride is best explained by the hypothesis that it is the undissociated acid, HF, which diffuses across the tubular epithelium. Thus, as the tubular fluid becomes more acidic, more of the ionic fluoride is converted into HF. This increases the chemical potential (concentration gradient) for HF and promotes its diffusion out of the tubules. Conversely, as the tubular fluid becomes more alkaline, more of the fluoride exists in the ionic form. The ion is considered relatively impermanent, remaining within the tubules to be excreted (see also Chapter 8).

A wide variety of factors can influence urinary pH, including the composition of the diet, high altitudes, certain drugs and many respiratory or metabolic diseases. Any of these factors could have a significant impact on the overall metabolism of fluoride through modifications of urinary pH. For example, a vegetarian diet promotes a more alkaline urine than does a diet mainly composed of meats.[13] Compared with a meat diet, therefore, a vegetarian diet would cause a less positive fluoride balance. That is, proportionately less of the fluoride ingested daily would remain within the body to be deposited in the teeth and bones.

Excretion via breast milk

As discussed in Chapter 3, the fluoride content of human breast milk represents a reference point for the natural daily fluoride intake during the first 6 months of life.[10,33] This is especially important when comparing the daily fluoride intake by formula-fed and breast-fed infants. The fluoride concentration of colostrum and mature breast milk is reported to be the same; about 0.4 µM.[33] There is very little difference in fluoride concentration of milk from mothers living in a 1 ppm F area or a 0.2 ppm F area, even though the plasma concentration would be substantially different. Further, there seems to be no diurnal variation in the fluoride concentration. Studies of lactating mothers have shown that there is a limited transfer of fluoride from plasma to breast milk.[3,17]

Excretion via feces and sweat

Other routes of fluoride excretion are via sweat and feces, but are of less quantitative importance. It is generally accepted that most of the fluoride in the feces was never absorbed. Fecal fluoride usually accounts for less than 10% of the amount ingested each day; that is, more than 90% is typically absorbed.[10,15] If the diet contains high concentrations of certain divalent or trivalent cations, however, the absorption of fluoride may be diminished.

In temperate climates, excretion by sweating is usually negligible. In a study of volunteers who spent a few hours in a sauna, the fluoride concentrations were measured both in plasma and sweat after an intake of 10 mg fluoride. After 2 hours the fluoride concentration in sweat was only 1/5 (1.6-2.6 μM) compared to plasma (7.9-13 μM).[21] In tropical climates, during periods of prolonged and heavy exercise or in occupational exposure to elevated temperatures, where the fluid loss from the body via sweat may approach as much as 4-6 L/day, the excretion of fluoride via sweat will be about a tenth of a milligram of fluoride.

Literature cited

1. Boillat MA, Baud CA, Lagier R, et al. Fluorose industrielle. Etude multidisciplinare de 43 ouvriers de l'industrie de l'aluminium. Schweiz Med Wochenschr 1979; 109, Fasc. 19, Suppl. 8: 4-28.

2. Ekstrand J, Alván G, Boréus LO, Norlin A. Pharmacokinetics of fluoride in man after single and multiple oral doses. Eur J Clin Pharmacol 1977; 12: 311-7.

3. Ekstrand J, Boréus LO, de Chateau P. No evidence of transfer of fluoride from plasma to breast milk. Br Med J 1981; 283: 761-2.

4. Ekstrand J, Ehrnebo M, Boréus LO. Fluoride bioavailability after intravenous and oral administration: importance of renal clearance and urine flow. Clin Pharmacol Ther 1978; 23: 329-37.

5. Ekstrand J, Ehrnebo M. Absorption of fluoride from fluoride dentifrices. Caries Res 1980; 14: 96-102.

6. Ekstrand J, Ehrnebo M. Influence of milk products on fluoride bioavailability in man. Eur J Clin Pharmacol 1979; 16: 211-5.

7. Ekstrand J, Ehrnebo M. Whitford GM, Järnberg PO. Fluoride pharmacokinetics during acid – base changes in man. Eur J Clin Pharmacol 1980; 18: 189-94.

8. Ekstrand J, Ericsson Y, Rosell S. Absence of protein-bound fluoride from human blood plasma. Arch Oral Biol 1977; 22: 229-32.

9. Ekstrand J, Fomon S, Ziegler EE, Nelson S. Fluoride pharmacokinetics in infancy. Pediatr Res 1994; 35: 157-63.

10. Ekstrand J, Hardell LI, Spak CJ. Fluoride balance studies on infants in a 1 ppm fluoride area. Caries Res 1984; 18: 87-92.

11. Ekstrand J, Koch G, Lindgren LE, Petersson LG. Pharmacokinetics of fluoride gels in children and adults. Caries Res 1981; 15: 213-20.

12. Ekstrand J, Koch G, Petersson LG. Plasma fluoride concentration and urinary fluoride excretion in children following application of the fluoride-containing varnish Duraphat. Caries Res 1980; 14: 185-9.

13. Ekstrand J, Spak CJ, Ehrnebo M. Renal clearance of fluoride in a steady state condition in man: influence of urinary flow and pH changes by diet. Acta Pharmacol Toxicol 1982; 50: 321-5.

14. Ekstrand J, Spak CJ, Vogel G. Pharmacokinetics of fluoride in man and its clinical relvance. J Dent Res 1990; 69 (Spec Iss): 550-5.

15. Ekstrand J, Ziegler EE, Nelson SE, Fomon SJ. Absorption and retention of dietary and supplemental fluoride by infants. Adv Dent Res 1994; 8: 175-80.

16. Ekstrand J. Relationship between fluoride in the drinking water and the plasma fluoride concentration in man. Caries Res 1978; 12: 123-7.

17. Ekstrand J, Spak C-J, Falch J, Afseth J, Ulvestad H. Distribution of fluoride to human breast milk following intake of high doses of fluoride. Caries Res 1984; 18: 93-5.

18. Ericsson Y, Hammarström L. Mouse placenta transfer of F18 in comparison with Ca45. Acta Obstet Gynecol Scand 1962; 41: 144-58.

19. Guy WS. Inorganic and organic fluorine in human blood. In: Johansen E, Taves D, Olsen TO, eds. Continuing evaluation of the use of fluorides. AAAS Selected Symp 11. Boulder, CO: Westview Press 1976; 125-47.

20. Hanhijärvi H. Comparison of free unionized fluoride concentration in plasma and renal clearance in patients in artificially fluoridated and non-fluoridated drinking water areas. Proc Finn Dent Soc 1974; 70: 1-67.

21. Henschler D, Büttner W, Patz J. Absorption, distribution in body fluid and bioavailability of fluoride. In: Kuhlencordt F, Kruse HP, eds. Calcium

metabolism, bone and metabolic diseases. Berlin: Springer Verlag 1975: 111-21.

22. Järnberg PO, Ekstrand J, Ehrnebo M. Renal excretion of fluoride during water diuresis and induced urinary pH changes in man. Toxicol Lett 1983; 18: 141-6.

23. Levy SM. A review of fluoride intakes from fluoride dentifrice. J Dent Child 1993; 2: 115-24.

24. Linkins R, McClure FJ, Steere AC. Urinary excretion of fluoride following defluoridation of a water supply. Public Health Rep 1956; 71: 217-20.

25. Parkins FM, Tinanoff N, Moutinko M, Ansley MB, Wazin MH. Relationships of human plasma fluoride and bone fluoride to age. Calcif Tissue Res 1974; 16: 335-8.

26. Patz J, Henschler D, Fickenscher H. Bioverfügbarkeit von Fluorid aus verschiedenen Salzen und unter dem Einfluz verschiedener Nahrungsbestandteile. Dtsch Zahnaertzl Z 1977; 32: 482-6.

27. Schiffel HH, Binswanger U. Human urinary fluoride excretion as influenced by renal functional impairment. Nephron 1980; 26: 69-72.

28. Shen YW, Taves DR. Fluoride concentrations in the human placenta and maternal and cord blood. Am J Obstet Gynecol 1974; 119: 205-7.

29. Singer L, Armstrong WD. Regulation of human plasma fluoride concentration. J Appl Physiol 1960; 15: 508-12.

30. Sjögren K, Ekstrand J, Birkhed D. Effect of water rinsing after tooth brushing on fluoride ingestion and absorption. Caries Res 1994; 29: 455-59.

31. Spak CJ, Ekstrand J, Zylberstein D. Bioavailability of fluoride added to baby formula and milk. Caries Res 1982; 16: 249-56.

32. Spak CJ Ekstrand J, Ericsson S, Leksell LG. Distribution of fluoride to the central nervous system. Caries Res 1986; 20: 157 (Abstr).

33. Spak CJ, Hardell LI, de Chateau P. Fluoride in milk. Acta Paediatr Scand 1983; 72: 699-701.

34. Spak CJ, Sjöstedt S, Eleborg L, Veress P, Perbeck L, Ekstrand J. Studies on human gastric mucosa after application of 0.42% fluoride gel. J Dent Res 1990; 69: 426-9.

35. Taves DR, Guy WS. Distribution of fluoride among body compartments. In: Johansen E, Taves D, Olsen TO, eds. Continuing evaluation of the use of fluorides. AAAS Selected Symp 11. Boulder, CO: Westview Press 1976; 159-85.

36. Taves DR. Electrophoretic mobility of serum fluoride. Nature 1968; 220: 582-3.

37. Trautner K, Einwag J. Influence of milk and food on fluoride bioavailability from NaF and Na_2FPO_3 in man. J Dent Res 1989; 68: 72-7.

38. Waterhouse C, Taves DR, Munzer A. Serum inorganic fluoride: Changes related to previous fluoride intake, renal function and bone resorption. Clin Sci 1980; 58: 145-52.

39. Whitford GM, Pashley DH, Reynold KE. Fluoride tissue distribution: short term kinetics. Am J Physiol 1979; 236: F141-F148.

40. Whitford GM, Pashley DH. Fluoride absorption: the influence of gastric acidity. Calcif Tissue Int 1984; 36: 302-7.

41. Whitford GM. Fluoride distribution between plasma and blood cells. Zahn Mund Kieferheilkd 1981; 69: 732.

42. Zipkin I, Linkins R, McClure FJ, Steere AC. Urinary fluoride levels associated with use of fluoridated waters. Public Health Rep 1956; 71: 767-72.

CHAPTER 5

FLUORIDE IN TEETH AND BONE

C. Robinson • J. Kirkham • J.A. Weatherell

General principles – Concentrations of fluoride in dental enamel
Concentrations of fluoride in dentin – Concentrations of fluoride in cementum
Concentrations of fluoride in bone – Concentrations of fluoride in calculus

General principles

Factors governing fluoride concentration and distribution

The retention of fluoride in the body is due almost entirely to the capacity of apatite (the mineral form that comprises over 99% of the skeleton) to bind and integrate fluoride ion into its crystal lattice. Fluoride concentrations in the unmineralized soft tissues and in the body fluids are relatively low and fairly consistent. Where high levels do occur, they are invariably transient.[2,31,63,65,76,82,83]

Concentrations in the mineralized tissues are variable due to i) the level of fluoride intake, ii) the duration of exposure and iii) interrelated factors, e.g. the stage of tissue development, its rate of growth, vascularity, surface area and reactivity of mineral crystallites, porosity and degree of mineralization.[32,84,95] In all mineralized tissues, fluoride levels tend to be greatest at the surface since this region is the closest to tissue fluid supplying fluoride (Fig. 5-1). The distribution and concentration in surfaces, however, will change differentially with age (Fig. 5-2).[35,63,82]

Mechanisms of fluoride uptake

Although F^- binding to organic components[13] is possible, body fluoride seems to be invariably present as inorganic fluoride. As the pKa of HF is 3.4, fluoride in blood, saliva and tissue fluid will be present in the fully ionized form as F^-. However, any fluoride present at low pH, e.g. in the stomach (pH of approximately 2.0) will exist almost totally in the undissociated form, i.e. HF.

In the mineralized tissues, some fluoride is incorporated within the interior of the mineral crystallites[94] as an integral part of the crystal lattice (see Chapter 6). However, fluoride may also be more superficially located, perhaps absorbed on crystal surfaces,[96] or loosely entrapped in the hydration shells of the mineral crystallites and some will be temporarily present in blood and tissue fluids.[55] The formation of CaF_2 and other fluoride-rich species is also possible. For example, when fluoride is applied to a tooth surface in a highly concentrated form (often at low pH), part of the apatite mineral may be destroyed. Phosphate and hydroxyl ions from the tooth mineral will enter the solution and fluoride will be deposited as CaF_2 or other fluoride-rich phases on or in the outer

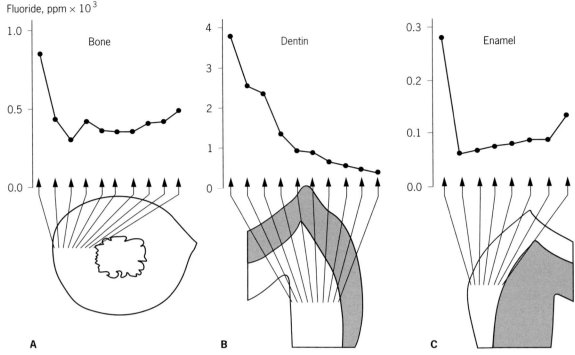

Fig. 5-1. **A** Fluoride distribution across human femur, showing relatively high concentrations of fluoride in periosteal and endosteal regions, with a typically high concentration in the periosteal region. **B** Fluoride distribution across section of molar dentin. The fluoride concentration falls steeply from the pulpal surface to the enamel-dentin junction. **C** Fluoride distribution across section of human molar enamel. The fluoride concentration is high in the surface region and falls to a plateau in the enamel interior.

enamel[5,23,28,41,55] (see Chapter 12). This same phenomenon has been claimed for developing bones at high levels of fluoride intake. The true status of fluoride at the outer extremities of apatite crystals is still unclear. While the precise ultrastructural location of fluoride in relation to the mineral lattice, especially the surface, is uncertain, most of the F^- which enters the apatite lattice probably replaces an OH^- ion or at least occupies an equivalent space.[17,40] This does not preclude the possibility that a small fraction of the fluoride might occupy other regions in the lattice. It has been suggested that F^- (perhaps together with CO_3^{2-}) may replace the larger PO_4^{3-} ion and it seems that fluoride is also able

to substitute for CO_3^{2-} or HCO_3^- present in the mineral (for details see Chapter 6).[15,56,58] The progress of fluoride in the first and second stages is very rapid. The third stage, however, involves migration through the crystal lattice itself and is presumably extremely slow, requiring the disposition of appropriate sites throughout the crystal lattice. The extent to which this occurs at body temperature is likely to be extremely small. Most of the fluoride buried within the mineral crystallites will, therefore, have been acquired during the period of crystal growth, a process sometimes known as "accretion". Being built into the crystal as it forms, such fluoride is quickly buried and will remain

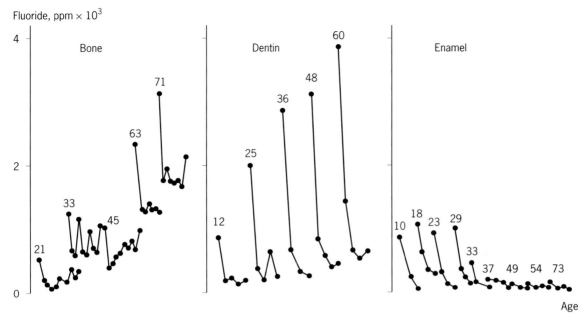

Fig. 5-2. Differential changes between bone, dentin and enamel in individuals from the same low-fluoride district (fluoride content of the drinking water < 0.1 ppm). The gradients shown represent fluoride distributions from the surface to the interior of each tissue; the numbers above the curves refer to the age of the subject from which the tissue was obtained.

locked in the lattice interior for as long as the crystal exists. However, even during periods of active crystal growth, acquisition of fluoride by exchange or adsorption will also be important.

Fluoride loss from bones and teeth

Not all of the fluoride acquired by a mineralized tissue will be present in the apatite crystal lattice or permanently bound by the mineral.[3,12,30,72] Some superficially located fluoride may be lost again, by back exchange, back-diffusion and migration from the mineral to the surrounding tissue fluid, blood, saliva or plaque fluid.[5,10,48,51] Even some of the firmly bound fluoride within the apatite crystallites might also be lost as crystals are destroyed e.g. by osteoclastic resorption of mesenchymal tissues (bone, cementum and dentin),[9,30,45] by

wear[26,85,90] or, in the case of the dental tissues, by severe acid erosion.

Effect of fluoride on the crystallinity and reactivity of the mineral

The incorporation of fluoride can significantly alter the properties of mineralized tissues since the inclusion of any extraneous element in a crystalline lattice will alter its reactivity.[25] When situated in the position normally occupied by a hydroxyl group, fluoride can greatly increase lattice stability, presumably by attracting the protons of adjacent apatite hydroxyl ions.[40] This changes the sense of one of the hydroxyls so that both now face towards the fluoride ion, thereby increasing the degree of hydrogen bonding in the so-called "hydroxyl column".[17,94] In addition, compared with hydroxyl, the fluoride ion is better aligned within the plane formed by the three adjacent calcium II ions. The electrostatic attractions between these calcium ions and the highly electronegative fluoride ion will, therefore, be greater than that which could exist between calcium and hydroxyl.[64] The result is that the fluoridated apatite lattices are more crystalline,[20,57,97] more stable and therefore less soluble in acid.[7,36,44,81,94] Fluoridated apatite will also form more easily because of a lower ionic product. Both effects are probably highly significant with regard to dental caries.[8,14,19,37,81] (see also Chapters 6 and 12).

In contrast, fluoride which is more superficially located may have relatively little effect on the behavior of the crystallite lattice. It can, however, dramatically affect fluid-crystal equilibria which involve the interaction between ions at crystal surfaces and those in solutions.[7,62] Such equilibria will affect fluoride concentrations in tissue fluids which could have an important effect on nearby cells involved in tissue development and mineralization,[52,79,92] and presumably upon enamel remineralization.[1,42,74,80]

Effect of fluoride on tissue composition

Whatever site it occupies, the presence of fluoride in the tissue will introduce changes in composition. A decrease in carbonate content is generally found in highly fluoridated bone and tooth mineral.[58,97] This is probably due to direct substitution of carbonate by fluoride, although more highly crystalline fluoridated apatites may be less able to incorporate carbonate. Citrate concentrations are also reduced,[95,97] perhaps for similar reasons. However, an increase in the tissue's magnesium content is also frequently observed.[49,91] It has been suggested that some magnesium-fluorophosphate complex might form, but there is still no direct evidence in support of this idea. Fluoride is, however, known to prolong or delay enamel maturation. Magnesium is known to accumulate se-

lectively at this stage, so it is possible that high magnesium content is associated with a prolonged period of uptake.

Concentrations of fluoride in dental enamel

Developing enamel

At the beginning of enamel formation the enamel forming cells (ameloblasts) lay down a partially mineralized (30% by weight) protein matrix, the thickness of which delineates the external form of the tooth. At this stage, fluoride has already been taken up by the tissue (Fig. 5-3) and, if fluoride is administered in the diet or drinking water, the small crystallites in this region take up fluoride readily.

Extracellular matrix processing occurs throughout the stage of matrix secretion. This is followed by matrix withdrawal, which is completed during the maturation stage. The resulting pores are occupied by fluid which, when removed by drying in air, produces an area of chalky white appearance.[29,66] The extent, shape and location of this porous area vary with tooth type and species of animal. This porous enamel readily accumulates ions and other molecules and it has been demonstrated that fluoride is also preferentially absorbed at this stage. A fluoride peak is usually found at or just before the enamel begins to mineralize rapidly, i.e. at the maturation stage (Fig. 5-3).

The discovery of relatively high concentrations of fluoride in this region is not surprising in view of the tissue's porosity[18,86] due to matrix degradation and loss (see Fig. 5-4) since it has long been known that, posteruptively, fluoride concentrations are high wherever enamel is porous. In view of the changes which fluoride can bring about in the development and mineralization of dental enamel, the presence of a relatively high concentration of fluoride

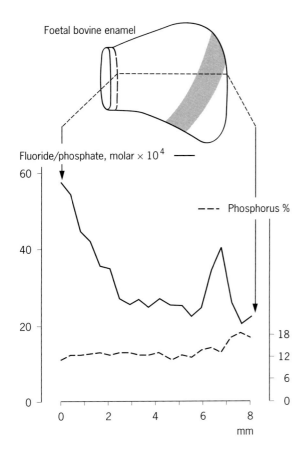

Foetal bovine enamel

Fluoride/phosphate, molar × 10^4 ——

– – – Phosphorus %

Fig. 5-3. Fluoride and phosphorus concentrations at each stage of development in the enamel of a developing bovine primary mandibular incisor. Fluoride is expressed as F:P molar ratio and phosphorus is expressed as P% by weight (see also Fig. 5-4).

during this sensitive stage of enamel formation may be of special significance. It is generally considered that fluoride associated with mineralized tissues (being bound to the mineral) would not be hazardous to the nearby cells, but the fluoride present in the porous enamel might be an exception. At least some of this fluoride is not tightly bound by the mineral, as fluoride concentrations fall again to approach background levels as the tissue matures.[21]

The crystals in enamel are highly ordered and regular and their growth is probably controlled by a protein fraction of the enamel matrix, since experiments have shown that removal of controlling protein is a prerequisite to crystal growth.[67,68] These proteins can be released from the crystallites when the enamel is incubated in a cell-free medium and this release is inhibited by fluoride.[69] If, *in vivo*, the (loosely bound) fluoride in the porous region of developing enamel were similarly to inhibit the release of modulating proteins from crystallites, it could prevent crystal growth and delay enamel maturation. Removal of modulating proteins can also be effected by proteolytic enzymes which are specifically expressed at the transition/maturation stage.[70,71] Fluoride at this stage might well impair crystal growth by increased adsorption of modulating proteins to a fluoridated apatite, or via a direct effect on the enzyme activity.

Erupted enamel
Fluoride is not homogeneously distributed

Chapter 5

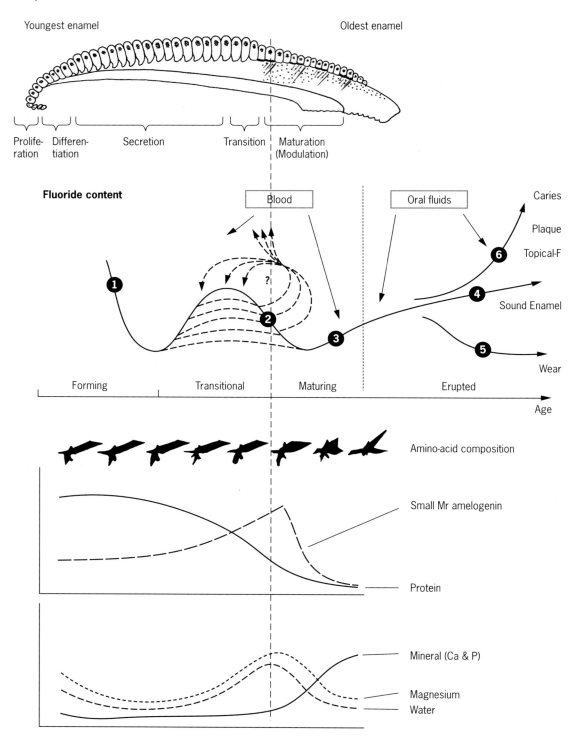

Youngest enamel

Oldest enamel

Proliferation · Differentiation · Secretion · Transition · Maturation (Modulation)

Fluoride content

Blood

Oral fluids

Caries

Plaque

Topical-F

Sound Enamel

Wear

Forming · Transitional · Maturing · Erupted

Age

Amino-acid composition

Small Mr amelogenin

Protein

Mineral (Ca & P)

Magnesium

Water

⇐ Fig. 5-4. Summary of current information regarding fluoride content of enamel throughout the life of the tooth. Fluoride concentrations are relatively high in the earliest formed enamel (1). Preferential accumulation then seems to occur at the transition/maturation interface. In this region the organic matrix (mainly amelogenin) is breaking down rapidly and is removed with a concomitant increase in the tissue water content (2). Fluoride concentrations rise in the surface region during late maturation when ameloblasts modulate between ruffled and smooth- ended morphologies (3). This continues until after eruption, little fluoride being taking up by fully mineralized sound enamel (4). Some fluoride is lost by wear (5). Fluoride can be acquired by sound fully mineralized enamel only at high concentrations of topical application or if the enamel becomes porous due to carious attack (6).

across the thickness of enamel even at the earliest stages of development. In the incompletely mineralized state, fluoride concentrations are highest at the tooth surface and low at the interior. In all erupted teeth, fluoride concentrations increase exponentially from a plateau level in the enamel interior to high concentrations at the tooth surface[34,38,87] (Fig. 5-5). Concentrations also vary topographically in a consistent way in the tooth surface and the pattern changes with age and dental experience. In a study of young anterior teeth, surface fluoride concentrations were found to be highest in the first-formed enamel near the incisal edge and decreased steeply towards the more recently formed cervical region (Fig. 5-6a). In older teeth, the pattern is inverted. Fluoride concentrations in the cervical region of the enamel surface increase, while the high surface concentration near the incisal edge is gradually reduced by wear (Fig. 5-6b). In individuals over the age of 30, fluoride concentrations in the enamel surface were highest near the cervical margin and lowest near the incisal edge.[85]

Acquisition of fluoride by the enamel surface appears to continue while the tissue remains porous. The time taken to occlude the spaces in this developmental porosity on the surface of the newly erupted tooth varies considerably with tooth type. Any factors which can interfere with this process of posteruptive maturation will prolong the length of time during which the enamel is porous and will extend the period of fluoride uptake. Fluoride itself may

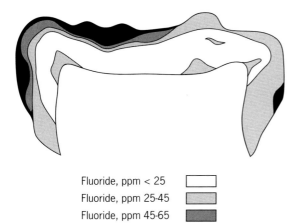

Fluoride, ppm < 25

Fluoride, ppm 25-45

Fluoride, ppm 45-65

Fluoride, ppm > 65

Fig. 5-5. Distribution of fluoride in a single section of human molar enamel. Fluoride concentrations can be seen to be highest at the enamel surface falling to a plateau in the interior and rising slightly again at the junction with the dentin.

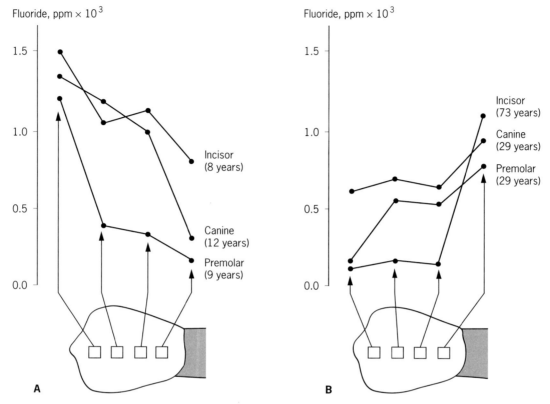

Fig. 5-6. Fluoride distribution in surface enamel of teeth from individuals living in the West Riding of Yorkshire (fluoride concentration of the drinking water < 0.1 ppm). **A** Fluoride distribution in the labial or buccal surfaces of three young anterior teeth. The fluoride concentration falls from the biting edge to the cervical margin. **B** Fluoride distribution in the labial or buccal surfaces of older anterior teeth. The fluoride concentration rises from the biting edge to the cervical margin.

prolong the process of maturation and since high concentrations of fluoride can accumulate in porous tissue, this may explain the fluoride levels found in the outermost region of fluorotic enamel.[50]

Penetration of fluoride into fully mineralized enamel is very slow. Fully mineralized enamel has a density of about 2.98 g/mL with a porosity as low as about 0.1% space by volume. Under normal circumstances fluoride does not appreciably penetrate such sound, mature enamel. The creation of porosity or the chemical destruction of the apatite lattice is necessary before the concentration of fluoride in highly mineralized enamel can be significantly increased. This happens when solutions, gels or pastes containing high concentrations of fluoride are applied to the tooth surface especially at low pH, as described previously, resulting in the formation of CaF_2 via double decomposition. The formation of fluoridated apatite or calcium fluoride cannot, however, be the sole mechanism by which fluoride may be taken up at the surfaces of dental tissues. Anomalous

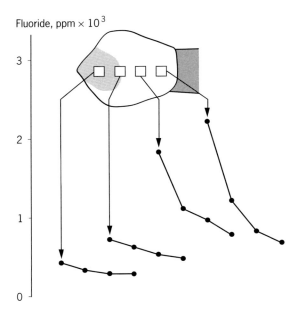

Fig. 5-7. Fluoride distribution curves in four regions of the labial surfaces of a mandibular premolar from a person resident in an area with a fluoride content of the drinking water of 1.9 ppm. The tooth showed signs of severe wear, possessing a marked facet on the enamel near the biting edge; this facet is represented by a stippled area.

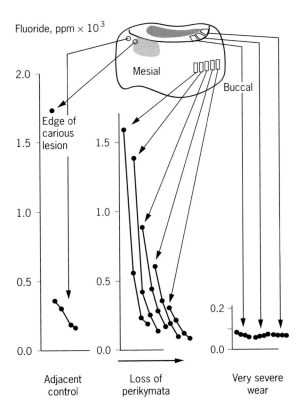

Fig. 5-8. Variations in the fluoride concentration in the surface region of a premolar from a 44-year-old individual. Each curve represents the gradient in fluoride concentration from surface to interior of enamel. Each point corresponds to the concentration in a layer of enamel about 20 μm thick. At the occlusal surface, where the enamel was severely worn, the high fluoride concentration originally present in the enamel surface has been lost. Even the slight wear occurring towards the buccal surface (this was indicated by a gradual disappearance of perikymata) was associated with a clear reduction in the fluoride concentration of the enamel surface. Near the occlusal surface the presence of an approximal carious lesion was associated with a relatively high surface fluoride concentration, due perhaps both to uptake by the more porous enamel of the lesion as well as to an absence of wear.

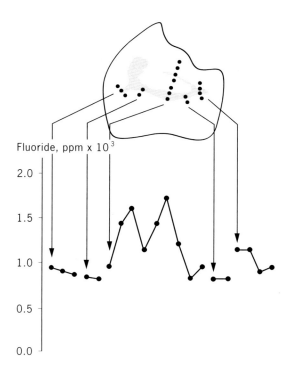

Fluoride, ppm x 10^3

Fig. 5-9. Concentration of fluoride in layers of enamel about 20 µm thick removed from small areas on the approximal aspect of a premolar tooth, as indicated by the black circles on the diagram. The hatched area on the tooth surface represents the area which was covered by plaque on the tooth (Weatherell & Newman, unpublished work).

solubility behavior of surface deposits leads to studies of mineral deposits on enamel after various treatments.[43,54] Such compounds often dissolved faster than calcium fluoride.[59] Chemical and physical studies of these materials revealed a calcium fluoride/phosphate complex approximating to $CaF_{1.8}(HPO_4)_{0.1}$ or $CaF_{1.7}(HPO_4)_{0.1}$. Infrared and x-ray analysis[11, 46,47] confirmed the presence of phosphate in these materials. Changes in pH during precipitation and dissolution of such phases may be of considerable significance in the case of dental caries.

Difficulties in quantitating CaF_2 at the tooth surface stimulated studies which revealed a further possible mechanism of fluoride uptake. Fast Magic Angle Spinning investigations using ^{19}F originally carried out by Jesinowski,[93] exploited ^{19}F homonuclear bipolar interactions. Using rapid spinning techniques, a res-

onance peak was observed which did not correspond to FAP or CaF_2. This would correspond to nonspecifically adsorbed fluoride, attached via hydrogen bonds to acid phosphates which dominate the apatite surfaces at physiologic pH. Interestingly, this occurred on apatite surfaces treated with only small amounts of NaF and was followed by the appearance of a resonance peak corresponding to fluorapatite.

It is likely that incorporation of fluoride into enamel and indeed mineralized tissues in general occurs initially by nonspecific adsorption to acid phosphates in the stern layer, followed by slower migration into the apatite lattice proper. It also raises the question that much of the surface fluoride in skeletal tissues may be in this form and is perhaps more available to solution than was previously thought.

The exposure of sound, fully mineralized enamel to low levels of fluoride normally present in the diet and drinking water has very little effect on overall enamel fluoride concentrations. This is demonstrated by the fact that worn facets of enamel show relatively little fluoride increase (Fig. 5-7), indicating that sound enamel does not normally reaccumulate appreciable amounts of fluoride. Even archaeologic specimens of teeth contain the concentrations of fluoride characteristic of worn enamel[71] and also exhibit the shallow surface-to-interior concentration gradients typical of abraded sites in recently extracted teeth. Such shallow concentration gradients are found wherever sound enamel has been lost by abrasion, e.g. at normal occlusal surfaces (Fig. 5-8).

Porosity in previously sound enamel, however, seems to be invariably associated with an increase in the fluoride content of enamel (e.g. Fig. 5-9). As a result of the absorption of fluoride by porous enamel, carious lesions exhibit high fluoride concentrations, even when very little seems to be available from dietary sources (Fig. 5-9); for further details see Chapter 11.

Concentrations of fluoride in dentin

Dentin, like cementum and bone, is a mesenchymal tissue. Unlike enamel, which is ectodermal, mesenchymal tissues have collagenous matrices and these are retained during the process of mineralization. The apatite crystallites are considerably smaller than those of enamel and much less crystallized. The capacity for fluoride uptake in dentin is therefore much greater because of the increased surface area of the crystallites, the tubular structure and higher degree of tissue hydration.[16,75,88] Dentin is also metabolically active and continues to grow throughout the life of the tooth.

In permanent teeth, the average concentrations of fluoride in dentin increase up to the age of about 40 and then plateau at a level related to the concentration of fluoride in the environment. This average data conceals more complex, though consistent, distribution patterns in the tissue itself. Fluoride concentrations are highest at or near the surface limits (i.e. the pulpal surfaces) of the tissue[77] (Fig. 5-10). Here, fluoride continues to be absorbed and probably increases in concentration throughout life, partly because dentin continues to form and will constantly accumulate fluoride by accretion during mineralization, where exchange also tends to be maximal. While newly formed dentin, primary or secondary, will avidly incorporate fluoride, it may be present for a relatively short time and might therefore have a relatively low fluoride concentration. This is presumably why fluoride concentrations tend to be low in secondary dentin, which has had relatively little time to accumulate the element. Conversely, a totally quiescent dentin surface may passively absorb and accumulate very large amounts of fluoride, provided that sufficient time is available to incorporate fluoride by exchange.

The distribution pattern of fluoride in the primary tooth dentin, while reflecting overall exposure to fluoride (for example in the drinking water) is complicated by the process of physiologic resorption which occurs at the pulpal surface prior to exfoliation.[27,89] The fluoride concentration in the pulpal surface of primary dentin therefore rises during the period of root formation but falls during the period of resorption. This is seen in all primary teeth but the greatest rise and fall in fluoride concentrations is found in the pulpal surfaces of multi-rooted teeth, presumably because such teeth take a long time both to form and to resorb the roots before the teeth are shed.

Concentrations of fluoride in cementum

Cementum forms a thin layer (50-100 µm) on the surfaces of tooth roots. Like bone and den-

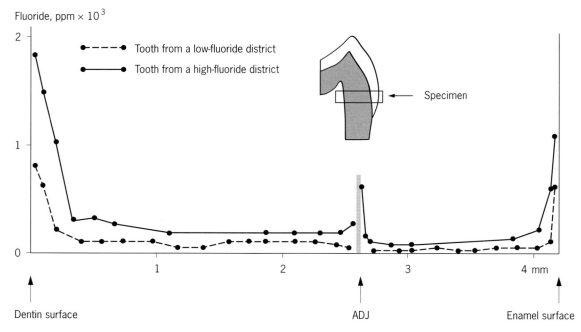

Fig. 5-10. Distribution of fluoride across the enamel and dentin of a tooth from a low and a tooth from a high-fluoride district. The concentration of fluoride is highest at the outer surface of the enamel and at the pulpal surface of the dentin. Throughout the tooth, the concentration of fluoride in the dentin is higher than that of enamel and the level reflects the different concentrations in the drinking water (Nakagaki & Weatherell, unpublished work).

tin, it is a collagenous mesenchymal tissue. It is much closer to bone than dentin, however, in terms of its histologic structure. The small crystal size and poor crystallinity characteristic of mesenchymal tissues facilitates fluoride uptake in cementum compared with dental enamel. This is further increased by the lower mineral content and greater tissue porosity compared with enamel.

As with all of the other mineralized tissues, the highest fluoride concentrations of cementum tend to be found near the outer surfaces, falling towards the interior of the tissue (Fig. 5-11).[39,53] This would appear to be a function of accessibility of tissue fluid to the outer cemental surface and would also probably explain the tendency for higher fluoride concentrations at the interface with the dentin. A relationship be-

tween cementum thickness and fluoride content also suggests that the rate of cementum deposition could affect fluoride concentrations such that rapidly forming tissue would not have sufficient time to accumulate fluoride. Fluoride content could also reflect the structure of the tissue in that a highly mineralized layer is often found near to the junction with the dentin which is associated with a high fluoride content.[53]

Concentrations of fluoride in bone

Nowhere does the complexity of fluoride uptake and concentration become more apparent than in bone (see Chapters 6 and 7). While it is developing, the tissue is highly vascularized

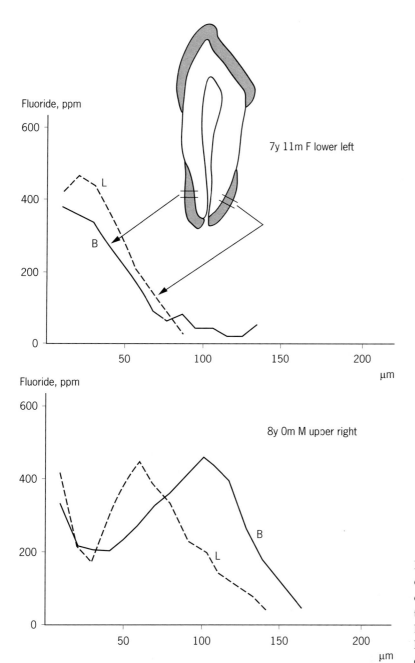

Fluoride, ppm

7y 11m F lower left

Fluoride, ppm

8y 0m M upper right

Fig. 5-11. Distribution of fluoride in buccal and lingual cementum of the same canine teeth. F = Female; M = Male; B = Buccal; L = Lingual. From Kato et al.[39] with the permission of the publishers.

Fluoride, ppm × 10³

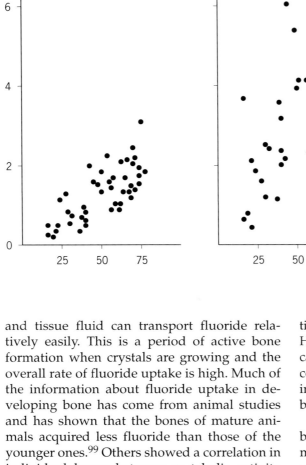

Fig. 5-12. Fluoride concentrations in cortical compacta and cancellum from ribs, postmortem, from individuals resident in a low fluoride district (fluoride concentration in the drinking water < 0.1 ppm). Cancellous bone invariably contains much higher concentrations of fluoride than the associated compact bone.

and tissue fluid can transport fluoride relatively easily. This is a period of active bone formation when crystals are growing and the overall rate of fluoride uptake is high. Much of the information about fluoride uptake in developing bone has come from animal studies and has shown that the bones of mature animals acquired less fluoride than those of the younger ones.[99] Others showed a correlation in individual bones between metabolic activity and fluoride uptake; i.e. metabolically active metaphyseal cortex and periosteal bone took up more than midcortical compact bone and cancellous bone incorporated more than the cortical compacta (Fig. 5-12).[91] Recent microanalytic studies have shown that this may be due to the relatively high proportion of available surface in cancellous bone. The distribu-

tion of fluoride is, in fact, similar. In compact Haversian bone, the picture is more complicated because of the variable numbers of incompletely mineralized osteons and the growing crystallites will take up fluoride rapidly both by accretion and exchange.

After the period of growth has ended, the bone fluoride concentration continues to rise more slowly towards a plateau.[78] Two phases of uptake have been identified,[30] an initial rapid phase followed by a slower uptake as new exchangeable sites become available.

The situation in man, however, is less clear. Fluoride accumulation by developing bones and teeth begins during fetal development (see Chapter 4).[6,18,22,33] Significant fluoride concentrations are seen in human fetal bones and the concentration reflects levels of fluoride intake.[22] At concentrations of fluoride in the drinking water between 0.5 and 1 ppm, fluoride concentrations appear to rise with foetal age. This effect was not observed in fetuses from areas where drinking water fluoride concentrations were low (< 0.2 ppm).[73]

In the adult skeleton the precise relationship between the fluoride concentration in bone and the age of the individual is still not clear. Early studies[24] clearly showed that fluoride levels in postmortem specimens of human rib rose with age in both cancellous and compact bone (Fig. 5-12). However, other investigators[35] reported that the fluoride levels in rib cancellum reached a plateau at the age of 55.

The explanation of age-related changes in bone fluoride content is complex. Metabolic activity of human bone decreases with age and a gradual reduction in the rate of fluoride incorporation might, therefore, be expected. It is also known that bone resorption accelerates after the fifth decade.[4] How this affects the concentration of bone fluoride will depend upon whether removal is site-specific. For example, where resorption involves bone surfaces, (where fluoride tends to accumulate) average fluoride concentrations might be expected to be reduced. However, removal of bone in senile osteoporosis proceeds from the endosteal to the periosteal surface, leaving an increased amount of fluoride-rich periosteal bone in older individuals (Fig. 5-2).

Removal of fluoride

As in the other tissues, not all the fluoride absorbed by bone is firmly held and early animal studies showed that some is subsequently lost again. Such loss might be partly due to back-exchange between fluoride ions, perhaps nonspecifically bound in the stern/hydration layer or the outer layer of the crystallites and hydroxyls in adjacent tissue fluids. Loss will also occur due to physiologic resorption of bone during development, remodeling and senile osteoporosis. It has been suggested[30] that removal by exchange is relatively rapid and would take place over weeks, whereas osteoclastic resorption is much slower and may extend over years.

In skeletal fluorosis (see Chapter 7) there are abnormally high fluoride concentrations of fluoride in the bone. Analysis of postmortem fluorotic bone indicated a threshold level of 5000-6000 ppm dry fat-free compact bone above which fluorosis might be expected.[35] A "critical threshold", in relation to bone fluoride, however, is misleading since most of this fluoride is inertly bound in the apatite lattice and will not affect cellular control or mineralization of the hard tissues. The concentration of fluoride in bone therefore provides an indication of past history of fluoride exposure but there is no evidence that fluoride deeply incorporated in bone causes fluorosis.

Concentration of fluoride in calculus

The mineralized deposits on the teeth, while not a tissue as such, do contain fluoride and may be useful in monitoring fluoride availability to the dentition. Only one study has reported detailed fluoride distribution in calculus.[60] In both supra- and subgingival calculus, the outer surfaces tended to contain more fluoride than the inner portion, although this was less well defined in the subgingival material. This can be related to availability of fluoride from the external environment, i.e. from saliva on the outer surface and from enamel on the inner. In addition, the rate of formation may be slower towards the surfaces, permitting more time for fluoride accumulation. Concentrations varied from approximately 100 ppm in the interior to 1000 ppm towards the surfaces.

Literature cited

1. Arends J, Christoffersen J, Christoffersen MR, Schutof J. Influence of fluoride concentration on the progress of demineralization in bovine enamel at pH 4.5. Caries Res 1983; 17: 455-7.

2. Armstrong WD, Singer L, Ensinck J, Rich C. Plasma fluoride concentrations of patients treated with sodium fluoride. J Clin Invest 1964; 43: 555.

3. Armstrong WD. The significance of the skeletal deposition of fluoride. Trans Fourth Macy Conf Metab Interrelations 1952; 4: 257.

4. Atkinson PJ, Weatherell JA. Variations in the density of the femoral diaphysis with age. J Bone Joint Surg 1967; 49: 781-8.

5. Baud CA, Bang S. Electron probe and x-ray diffraction microanalysis of human enamel treated in vitro by fluoride solution. Caries Res 1970; 4: 1-13.

6. Bawden JM, Wolkoff AS, Flowers CE. F18 recovery from fetal lambs following intravenous injections into the ewe. J Dent Res 1965; 44: 1013-4.

7. Brown WE, Gregory TM, Chow LC. Effects of fluoride on enamel solubility and cariostasis. Caries Res 1977; 11: 118-41.

8. Brudevold F, Gardner DE, Smith FA. The distribution of fluoride in human enamel. J Dent Res 1956; 35: 420-9.

9. Casarett LJ, Doull J. In: Doull J, Klaassen CD, eds. Toxicology. New York; Macmillan 1980.

10. Caslavska V, Moreno EC, Brudevold F. Determination of the calcium fluoride formed from in vitro exposure of human enamel to fluoride solutions. Archs Oral Biol 1975; 20: 333-9.

11. Christoffersen J, Christoffersen MR, Kibalczyc W, Perdok WA. Kinetics of dissolution and growth of calcium fluoride and effects of phosphate. Acta Odontol Scand 1988; 46: 325-36.

12. Costeas A, Woodard HG, Laughlin JS. Depletion of ^{18}F from blood flowing through bone. J Nucl Med 1970; 11: 43-5.

13. Crenshaw MA, Bawden JW. Fluoride binding by organic matrix from early and late developing bovine fetal enamel determined by flow rate dialysis. Arch Oral Biol 1981; 26: 473-6.

14. Dowse CM, Jenkins GN. Fluoride uptake in vivo in enamel defects and its significance. J Dent Res 1957; 36: 816.

15. Eanes ED. Enamel apatite: chemistry, structure and properties. J Dent Res 1979; 58: 829-34.

16. Elliott CG, Smith MD. Dietary fluoride related to the fluoride content of teeth. J Dent Res 1960; 39: 93-8.

17. Elliott JC. Recent progress in the chemistry, crystal chemistry and structure of the apatites. Calcif Tissue Res 1969; 3: 293-307.

18. Ericsson Y, Ullberg S. Autoradiographic investigations of the distribution of ^{18}F in mice and rats. Acta Odontol Scand 1958; 16: 363-74.

19. Feagin F, Patel PR, Koulourides T, Pigman W. Study of the effect of calcium, phosphate, fluoride and hydrogen ion concentrations on the remineralization of partially demineralized human and bovine enamel surfaces. Arch Oral Biol 1971; 16: 535-48.

20. Frazier PD. X-ray diffraction analysis of human enamel containing different amounts of fluoride. Arch Oral Biol 1967; 12: 35-42.

21. Fukae M. Alkaline phosphatase extracted from porcine immature enamel. In: Fearnhead RW, Suga S, eds. Tooth enamel, IV. Amsterdam: Elsevier 1984: 120-4.

22. Gedalia I, Brzezinski A, Portuguese N, Berkovici B. The fluoride content of teeth and bones of human foetuses. Arch Oral Biol 1964; 9: 331-40.

23. Gerould CH. Electron microscope study of mechanism of fluorine deposition on teeth. J Dent Res 1945; 24: 223-33.

24. Glock GE, Lowater F, Murray MM. The retention and elimination of fluorine in bones. Biochem J 1941; 35: 1235-9.

25. Gruner JW, McConnell D, Armstrong WD. The relationship between crystal structure and chemical composition of enamel and dentin. J Biol Chem 1937; 121: 771-81.

26. Hallsworth AS, Weatherell JA. The micro-distribution uptake and loss of fluoride in human enamel. Caries Res 1969; 3: 109-18.

27. Hargreaves JA, Weatherell JA. Variation of fluoride concentration in human deciduous teeth. In: Advances in fluoride research and dental

caries prevention. Oxford: Pergamon Press 1965; 247-54.

28. Hercules DM, Craig NL. Composition of fluoridated dental enamel studied by x-ray photoelectron spectroscopy (ESCA). J Dent Res 1976; 55: 829-35.

29. Hiller CR, Robinson C, Weatherell JA. Variations in the composition of developing rat incisor enamel. Calcif Tissue Res 1975; 18: 1-12.

30. Hodge HC. The significance of the skeletal deposition of fluoride. In: Transactions of the Fourth Conference on Metabolic Interrelations. Josiah Macy Foundation, 1952.

31. Hodge HC. Fluoride metabolism: its significance in water fluoridation. J Am Dent Assoc 1956; 52: 307-14.

32. Hodge HC. Metabolism of fluorides. J Am Dent Ass 1961; 177: 313-6.

33. Hudson JT, Stookey GK, Muhler JC. The placental transfer of fluoride in the guinea pig. Arch Oral Biol 1967; 12: 237-46.

34. Iijima Y, Katayama T. Fluoride concentration in deciduous enamel in high- and low-fluoride areas. Caries Res 1985; 19: 262-5.

35. Jackson D, Weidmann SM. Fluorine in human bone related to age and the water supply of different regions. J Path Bact 1958; 76: 451-9.

36. Jenkins GN, Venkateswarlu P, Zipkin I. Fluoride and Human Health. Geneva: WHO Monograph 1970.

37. Jenkins GN. Theories on the mode of action of fluoride in reducing dental decay. Proc Natl Acad Sci 1963; 22: 97-104.

38. Jenkins GN, Spiers RC. Distribution of fluoride in human enamel. Proceedings of the Physiological Society of London 1953; 121: 21.

39. Kato K, Nakagaki H, Weatherell JA, Robinson C. Distribution of fluoride in the cementum of human deciduous canines. Caries Res 1991; 25: 406-9.

40. Kay MI, Young RA, Posner AS. Crystal structure of hydroxyapatite. Nature 1964; 204: 1050-2.

41. Kerebel B, Daculsi G. Recherches recentes sur l'action du fluor en odontologie. Med Hyg 1978; 36: 3202-5.

42. Koulourides T, Cueto H, Pigman W. Rehardening of softened enamel surfaces of human teeth by solutions of calcium phosphate. Nature 1961; 189: 226-7.

43. Kreinbrink AT, Sazavsky CD, Pyrz JW, Nelson DGA, Honkonen RS. Fast-magic-angle-spinning ^{19}F NMR of inorganic fluorides and fluoridated apatitic surfaces. J Magn Reson 1990; 88: 267-76.

44. Kutnerian K, Kuyper AC. The influence of fluoride on the solubility of bone salt. J Biol Chem 1957; 233: 760-3.

45. Largent EJ, Heyroth FF. Absorption and excretion of fluoride: 3. Further observations on the metabolism of fluorides at high levels of intake. J Indust Hyg Toxicol 1949; 31: 134-8.

46. LeGeros RZ, Zhang R, Retino M, Slott P, LeGeros JP. Synthetic CaF_2-like materials: preparation and characterisation. Part 2. J Dent Res 1992; 24: 522.

47. LeGeros RZ, Zhang R, Torres W, LeGeros JP. Effect of phosphate on crystal growth of CaF_2. Caries Res 1990; 24: 407.

48. Lott HV. Fluorine release from enamel. Helv Odontol Acta 1962; 6: 10-4.

49. McCann HG, Bullock FA. The effect of F-ingestion on the composition and solubility of mineralized tissues of rat. J Dent Res 1957; 236: 391-8.

50. McClure FJ, Likins RC. Fluorine in human teeth studied in relation to fluorine in the drinking water. J Dent Res 1951; 30: 172-6.

51. Mellberg JR, Laakso PV, Nicholson CR. The acquisition and loss of fluoride by topically fluoridated human tooth enamel. Arch Oral Biol 1966; 11: 1213-20.

52. Moreno EC, Kresak M, Zahradnik RT. Physicochemical aspects of fluoride apatite systems relevant to the study of dental caries. Caries Res 1977; 11: 142-71.

53. Nakagaki H, Weatherell JA, Strong M, Robinson C. Distribution of fluoride in human cementum. Arch Oral Biol 1985; 30: 101-4.

54. Nelson DGA, Jongbloed WL, Arends J. Morphology of enamel surfaces treated with topical fluoride agents: SEM considerations. J Dent Res 1983; 62: 1201-8.

55. Neuman WF, Neuman MW, Main ER, O'Leary J, Smith FA. The surface chemistry of bone. II. Fluoride deposition. J Biol Chem 1950; 187: 655-61.

56. Neuman WF, Neuman MW. The chemical dynamics of bone mineral. Chicago:University of Chicago Press 1958.

57. Newesley JW, McConnell D, Armstrong WD. The nature of carbonate contents in tooth mineral. Experientia 1963; 19: 620.

58. Nikiforuk G, Grainger RM. Fluoride – carbonate – citrate interrelation in enamel. In: Stack MV, Fearnhead RW, eds. Tooth enamel, IV. Bristol: John Wright & Sons 1964: 26-31.

59. Ögaard B. Applicability of acid-etching techniques for fluoride determination on enamel after topical fluoride treatment. Acta Odontol Scand 1988; 46: 337-40.

60. Okumura H, Nakagaki H, Kato K, Ito F, Weatherell JA, Robinson C. Distribution of fluoride in human dental calculus. Caries Res 1993; 27: 271-6.

61. Overall CM, Limeback H. Identification and characterisation of enamel proteinases isolated from developing enamel. Biochem J 1988; 256: 965-72.

62. Pak CY, Diller EC. Effect of MG, Citrate, F^- and SO_4 on the solubility, dissolution and growth of bone mineral. Calcif Tissue Res 1969; 4: 69-77.

63. Perkinson JD, Whitney IB, Monroe RA, Lotz WE, Comar CL. Metabolism of fluorine-18 in domestic animals. Am J Anat 1955; 182: 383-9.

64. Posner AS, Eanes ED, Harper RA, Zipkin I. X-ray diffraction analysis of the effect of fluoride on human bone apatite. Arch Oral Biol 1963; 8: 549-70.

65. Robinson C, Kirkham J. Effect of fluoride in developing enamel. J Dent Res 1990; 69: 685-91.

66. Robinson C, Kirkham J. The dynamics of amelogenesis as revealed by protein compositional studies. In: Butler WT, ed. The chemistry and biology of mineralized tissues. Birmingham, AL: Ebsco Media 1985; 248-63.

67. Robinson C, Kirkham J, Stonehouse NJ, Shore RC. Control of crystal growth during enamel maturation. Conn Tissue Res 1989; 22: 139-45.

68. Robinson C, Shore RC, Kirkham J, Stonehouse NJ. Extracellular processing of enamel matrix proteins and the control of crystal growth. J Biol Buccale 1990; 18: 355-61.

69. Robinson C, Kirkham J. Enamel matrix components, alterations during development and possible interactions with the mineral phase. In: Fearnhead RW, Suga S, eds. Tooth enamel, IV. Amsterdam: Elsevier 1984; 261-5.

70. Robinson C, Kirkham J, Stonehouse NJ, Shore RC. Extracellular processing of enamel matrix and origin and function of tuft protein. In: Fearnhead RW, ed. Tooth enamel, V. Japan: Florence Publishers 1989; 59-63.

71. Robinson C, Kirkham J, Weatherell JA, Strong M. Dental enamel – a living fossil. In: Cruwys E, Foley RA, eds. Teeth and anthropology. Oxford: BAR Publishers 1986; 31-54.

72. Savchuck WB, Armstrong WD. Metabolic turnover of fluoride by the skeleton of the rat. J Biol Chem 1951; 193: 575-85.

73. Schraad JF, Bergmann KE, Gawlik D, Gatschke W, Vogel M. Die Accretion von Fluorid im Skelett wahrend der Foetalperiode. Dtsch Zahnaerztl Z 1984; 39: 965-7.

74. Silverstone LM. Remineralization of human enamel in vitro. Proc Roy Soc Med 1972; 65: 906-8.

75. Singer L, Armstrong WD. Relation between the fluoride contents of rat calcified tissues. J Dent Res 1969; 48: 947-50.

76. Smith FA, Gardner DE, Hodge HC. Investigations on the metabolism of fluoride. II. Fluoride content of blood and urine as a function of the fluorine in drinking water. J Dent Res 1950; 29: 596-600.

77. Sugimoto M. Distributions of fluoride and magnesium in the human dentin as revealed by electron microprobe. Jap J Oral Biol 1981; 23: 790-808

78. Suttie JW, Phillips PH. The effect of age on the rate of fluoride deposition in the femur. Arch Biochem Biophys 1959; 83: 355-9.

79. Taves DR, Newman WF. Factors controlling calcification. AEC Research and Development Report 1963; UR 628.

80. Ten Cate JM, Duijsters PPE. Influence of fluoride in solution on tooth demineralization. I. Chemical data. Caries Res 1983; 17: 193-9.

81. Volker JF. Effect of fluorine on solubility of enamel and dentin. Proc Soc Exp Biol Med 1939; 42: 725-7.

82. Wallace-Durbin P. The metabolism of fluorine in the rat using F-18 as a tracer. J Dent Res 1954; 33: 789-800.

83. Weatherell JA, Deutsch D, Robinson C. Fluoride

and its relation to bones and teeth. In: Kuhlencordt F, Kruse HP, eds. Calcium metabolism, bone and metabolic bone Diseases. Berlin: Springer-Verlag 1975.

84. Weatherell JA, Weidmann SM. The distribution of organically bound sulphate in bone and cartilage during calcification. Biochem J 1963; 89: 265-7.

85. Weatherell JA, Hallsworth AS, Robinson C. Effect of tooth wear in the distribution of fluoride in the enamel surface of human teeth. Arch Oral Biol 1973; 18: 1175-89.

86. Weatherell JA, Deutsch D, Robinson C, Hallsworth AS. Assimilation of fluoride by enamel throughout the life of the tooth. Caries Res 1977; 11: 85-115.

87. Weatherell JA, Hargreaves JA. The microsampling of enamel in thin layers by means of strong acids. Arch Oral Biol 1965; 10: 139-42.

88. Weatherell JA, Robinson C, Best JS. Influence of anatomical site on fluoride levels in rat molars. Caries Res 1981; 15: 386-98.

89. Weatherell JA, Hargreaves JA. Effect of resorption on the fluoride content of deciduous dentin. Arch Oral Biol 1966; 11: 749-56.

90. Weidmann SM. Uptake and retention of fluoride by teeth of animals under experimental fluorosis. Arch Oral Biol 1962; 7: 63-72.

91. Weidmann SM, Weatherell JA. The uptake and distribution of fluorine in bones. J Path Bact 1959; 78: 243-55.

92. Yardeni J, Hermel J. The anticariogenic effect of sodium fluoride. J Dent Res 1969; 48: 965.

93. Yesinowski JP, Wolfgang RA. Mobley MJ. Adsorption on and surface chemistry of hydroxyapatite. New York: Plenum 1983.

94. Young RA. Biological apatite vs. hydroxyapatite at the atomic level. Clin Orthop 1975; 113: 249-62.

95. Zipkin I, McClure FJ, Lee WA. Relation of the fluoride content of human bone to its chemical composition. Arch Oral Biol 1960; 2: 190-5.

96. Zipkin I. Mobilization of fluoride from the bones and teeth of growing and mature rats. Arch Oral Biol 1972; 17: 479-94.

97. Zipkin I, Posner AS, Eanes ED. The effect of fluoride on the X-ray diffraction pattern of the apatite on human bone. Biochim Biophys Acta 1962; 59: 255-8.

98. Zipkin I, Schraer H, Lee WA. The effect of fluoride on the citrate content of the bones of the growing rat. Arch Oral Biol 1963; 8: 119-26.

99. Zipkin I, McClure FJ. Deposition of fluorine in bones and teeth of growing rats. J Dent Res 1952; 31: 494-5.

THE EFFECT OF FLUORIDE ON BONE MINERALIZATION

A.S. Posner

Introduction – Isomorphous substitution in $Ca_{10}(PO_4)_6(OH)_2$– Precipitated hydroxyapatites
Bone mineral – Mineralization mechanisms – Observations on bone
Fluoride treatment of osteoporosis

Introduction

The hardness and mechanical strength of bone, unlike other connective tissues, is a result of the deposition of calcium phosphate within its organic matrix. This highly specialized connective tissue serves as a support framework for and enters into metabolic interrelationship with the body. About 35% of the dry, fat-free weight of mature bone is the organic matrix while the remainder is the mineral phase. Collagen comprises about 90% of the organic phase of bone with the remaining organic substances consisting of non-collagenous proteins, lipids and carbohydrates. The composition of bone changes with growth and the mineralization process, but, mature bone in a given species is fairly constant in composition.

It was shown as early as 1926[4] by x-ray diffraction that bone mineral is an analog of the basic calcium phosphate mineral, hydroxyapatite. Crystallographers delineate the structure of a crystalline material by calculating from single crystal x-ray (or neutron) diffraction data the three-dimensional space and vibrational parameters of the atoms in the structural unit. For hydroxyapatite the structural unit is written $Ca_{10}(PO_4)_6(OH)_2$. However, hydroxyapatite is often given the simplest formula, $Ca_5(PO_4)_3(OH)$. We will employ the structurally related formula, not the latter, in this Chapter.

Isomorphous substitution in $Ca_{10}(PO_4)_6(OH)_2$

Hydroxyapatite is distinguished by the abundance of isomorphous substitution in its structure. For example, fluoride often appears as a substitute for hydroxyl and strontium can substitute for calcium. Thus, we have a whole family of apatites of similar structure but different formulas, such as fluorapatite and strontium apatite. The calcium positions in apatite can be filled by the divalent cations of Pb, Sr, Fe, Mg, Ba, Sn, Mn, Cd, Y, La, Ce and others, and, even by the monovalent cations of Na and K, with appropriate adjustment for electrical neutrality.

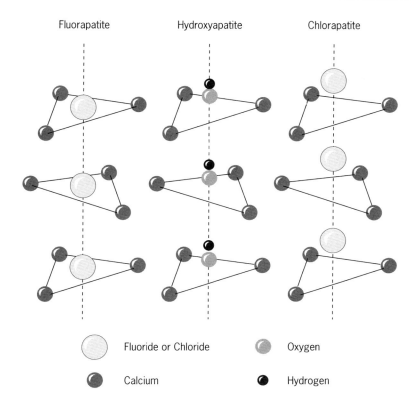

Fluorapatite   Hydroxyapatite   Chlorapatite

○ Fluoride or Chloride   ◐ Oxygen

● Calcium   ◑ Hydrogen

Fig. 6-1. Partial structures of fluorapatite, $Ca_{10}(PO_4)_6F_2$, hydroxyapatite, $Ca_{10}(PO_4)_6(OH)_2$ and chlorapatite, $Ca_{10}(PO_4)_6Cl_2$, respectively, which show the differences in F, OH and Cl positions in these isomorphous structures. Redrawn from Posner.[16]

The tetrahedral PO_4 groups can be substituted for by SO_4, VO_4, SiO_4 and even the planar CO_3 group. The OH position can be filled by F, Cl and, under certain conditions, the CO_3 group. Carbonate ion substitution is of particular interest to bone apatite and will be treated in more detail below.

In some cases, isomorphous substitution of even minor amounts in hydroxyapatite can change its properties measurably. Our knowledge of the three-dimensional atomic structure helps explain this phenomenon. Fig. 6-1 illustrates the substitution for OH by F and Cl ions. It can be seen that when F replaces OH it is more tightly bonded to the three adjacent calcium ions because it is closer to them than the OH. In turn, the Cl is situated further away from the plane of the calcium ions and so is more weakly bonded by the Coulombic forces which hold all of these ions to the calcium ions. The effect of F substitution for OH in bone will be discussed later.

Carbonate ion is the third most abundant chemical group found in the apatites after phosphorus and calcium. The carbonate-fluorapatite mineral francolite contains 4.5% CO_3 by weight,[15] about the same amount of carbonate found in bone mineral. Well crystallized hydroxyapatites have been synthesized with as much as 9.5% CO_3.[12] The structural position of the CO_3 group in well crystallized apatites helps define its role in bone mineral. Well crystallized apatites have low surface areas and thus very little carbonate appears as a surface constituent. In poorly crystallized apatites, such as bone apatite, much of the carbonate is

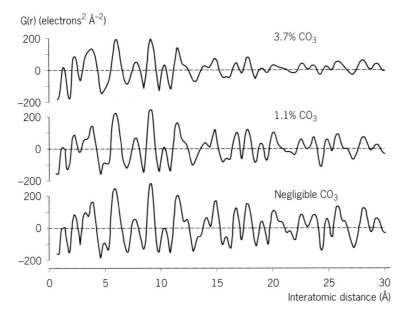

G(r) (electrons^2 Å^{-2})

3.7% CO$_3$

1.1% CO$_3$

Negligible CO$_3$

Interatomic distance (Å)

Fig. 6-2. Reduced radial distribution functions, G(r), calculated from the x-ray diffraction patterns of hydroxyapatites of increasing CO$_3$ content. The decrease in G(r) amplitude and resolution at high interatomic distances result from the atomic distortion due to inclusion of CO$_3$ ions in the structures. Redrawn from Posner & Betts.[17]

situated on their large specific surfaces (see below).

It has been shown by infrared data[12,15] that in well crystallized hydroxyapatites the divalent, planar CO$_3^2$ group substitutes for the trivalent, tetrahedral PO$_4^3$ group. It is believed that electrical neutrality is achieved by some combination of (a) calcium deficiency and (b) Na^{+1} substitution for Ca^{+2}. Under certain high temperature conditions CO$_3$ substitutes for the OH ion.[6] The mechanism by which neutrality is obtained in the rare case when CO$_3$ substitutes for OH is not known.

Infrared spectroscopy[2,12] and radial distribution function analysis of x-ray diffraction data[2] have shown that carbonate substitution for phosphate results in internal induced strain (i.e. structural distortion due to atomic misalignment) even in well crystallized apatites. Compounds with structural distortion are more reactive chemically than their structurally correct counterparts. Fig. 6-2 shows the effect of increasing the carbonate content of well crystallized synthetic hydroxyapatites on the x-ray

radial distribution function.[16] No structural studies have been made of the effect of carbonate substitution for OH. The studies of the atomic structure of well crystallized hydroxyapatites will provide a basis for the investigation of chemically precipitated, poorly crystallized hydroxyapatites.

Precipitated hydroxyapatite

When hydroxyapatite is precipitated from a highly supersaturated solution of calcium phosphate an unstable amorphous calcium phosphate precursor is observed.[5] This noncrystalline material, which normally has a Ca/P ratio of 3/2 rather than the 10/6 value of apatite, converts autocatalytically to a finely divided, non-stoichiometric hydroxyapatite. In aqueous suspension the latter slowly improves in crystal size and stoichiometry. When hydroxyapatite is precipitated from solutions of low supersaturation the precursor is not seen and fine dot-like crystals of non-stoichiometric hydroxyapatite are precipitated initially.[5] Precipitated hydroxyapatites differ from high temperature preparations because of their submicroscopic crystal size, which results in large and reactive surfaces, and by their non-stoichiometry, which also accounts for their high reactivity. They are usually calcium- and hydroxyl-deficient and contain internal hydrogen bonds between orthophosphate oxygens for chemical neutrality.[23] A general formula suggested for these apatites is: $Ca_{10x}H_x(PO_4^- CO_3)_6(OH)_{2x}$ with x varying from zero to almost 2. This formula is based on the amount of pyrophosphate produced when a series of non-stoichiometric hydroxyapatites were heated to 600°C.[1] Further, calcium-deficient hydroxyapatites when heated above 900°C decompose into beta-tricalcium phosphate (whitlockite). Ca-deficient apatites improve in stoichiometry when in contact with calcium solutions and thus decrease in solubility.[13] The large and reactive specific surfaces of precipitated hydroxyapatites make them suitable for use as catalysts and in column chromatography as adsorbents.

Bone mineral

Bone mineral is a single phase consisting of submicroscopic, non-stoichiometric crystals of hydroxyapatite similar to chemically precipitated hydroxyapatites. This makes for a reactive material which satisfies the need for the normal resorption and redeposition accompanying bone growth, repair and turnover.

Human adult bone crystals are generally reported to be plate-like, 25-35 nm at their longest with a thickness of 2.5-5.0 nm.[16] In each species the average crystal increases in size with maturity, after which the average size remains the same.[14,22] In the resorption and redeposition procedure, which continues throughout life, the newly deposited crystals are smaller than the more mature crystals.[16] In adult bone the mature crystals far outnumber the newly deposited ones and so the average adult crystal size does not change with time, even though certain actively mineralizing areas of bone contain smaller crystals than the average.

Definitive proof of the occurrence of a non-apatitic calcium phosphate precursor in bone mineral deposition remains to be shown. The nature of a possible precursor will reveal something about the chemical milieu of the earliest mineral deposition. If an amorphous precursor appears, it is likely that bone mineral precipitates from highly supersaturated solution. If an acid calcium phosphate is the precursor, as suggested for octocalcium phosphate,[3] then the mineralizing solution is probably slightly acidic. There is some evidence that an amorphous phase appears in the earliest mineralization of certain species.[9-11] More work is needed to clear up this problem.

Bone mineral improves not only in crystal size with maturity but in chemical stoichiometry, never achieving the hydroxyapatite stoichiometry.[14] Heating to 300°C produces pyrophosphate and heating to 900°C produces beta-tricalcium phosphate, showing that bone apatite is a non-stoichiometric hydroxyapatite similar in properties to the chemically precipitated apatites.

Bone apatite contains about 4% carbonate present as CO_3 ion with about half on the crystal surfaces, easily exchangeable with body fluids. The remainder of the carbonate is thought to occupy phosphate positions, thereby inducing structural distortion as in the case of carbonate substitution in synthetic and mineral apatites cited above. This is corroborated by the fact that the x-ray diffraction radial distribution function of bone apatite resembles the function of carbonate-containing synthetic apatite and not that of carbonate-free apatite function.[17] It is assumed that the reactivity of bone apatite is related, in part, to the structural distortion induced by carbonate.

Like the synthetic apatites, bone apatite has

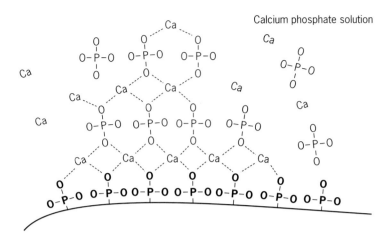

Fig. 6-3. Diagram illustrating a possible mechanism of nucleation of bone apatite by a phosphoprotein substrate. The substrate is in bold face, while the solution ions are in lighter type. Redrawn from Posner.[16]

been shown to have a high and reactive surface. The *in vitro* chemisorption of a variety of molecules on inorganic bone apatite surfaces strongly suggests that the organic matrix of bone is bound to the inorganic mass. This bonding could account, in great part, for the biomechanical strength of bone. The high surface reactivity of bone mineral is needed for the metabolic role of this tissue.

Mineralization mechanisms

In the mineralization process the organic matrix is first formed by the cell and then is infused extracellularly with mineral. There is no unified theory of the mechanism of bone mineralization. Many diverse experiments have shown that a number of individual chemical processes accompany the deposition of mineral in the matrix. The mechanisms proposed fall into three general categories:

- Raising of local supersaturation causing spontaneous precipitation;

- Provision of heterogeneous nucleators in the matrix and

- Removal or neutralization of mineral inhibitors.

These processes can occur separately or simultaneously, intracellularly and/or extracellularly.

An example of the first category can be seen in the early suggestion[21] that alkaline phosphatase, present at all mineralization sites, produces an excess of free phosphate, and thus apatite supersaturation, by the hydrolysis of phosphate esters. While alkaline phosphatase is always present at mineralization sites, it is also found in non-mineralizing tissue, making the role of this enzyme in bone mineralization unclear.

The following have been proposed as nucleating substrates for the mineralization of bone: collagen, gamma carboxyglutamate containing proteins, phosphoproteins, glycoproteins, calcium acidic phospholipid-phosphate complexes and proteolipids. The diagram in Fig. 6-3 illustrates how phosphoproteins may

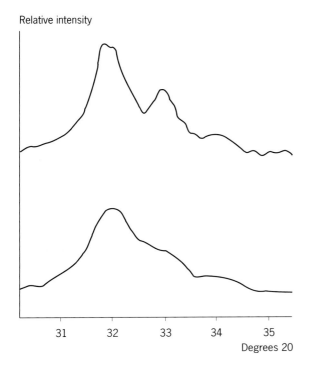

Relative intensity

31   32   33   34   35

Degrees 2θ

Fig. 6-4. Comparison of x-ray diffraction power patterns (Copper K-alpha radiation) of low fluoride (below) and high fluoride (above) human iliac crest bone; the fluoride values were 0.224% and 0.870%, respectively. The better resolved x-ray diffraction pattern of the high fluoride bone is indicative of crystal growth. Drawn from Posner et al.[18]

act as heterogeneous nucleators of bone apatite. Finally, the molecular species which are the major inhibitor of tissue mineralization are the high molecular weight proteoglycans. All of these observations have been discussed more fully in earlier reviews.[8, 24]

Observations on bone

A number of bone disorders result from improper formation of the organic matrix, particularly collagen. Abnormal cellular or extracellular formation of the collagen matrix can result in diseases characterized by improper mineralization. On the other hand, some disorders (e.g. rickets) are the result of insufficient mineralization of a normal organic matrix, often due to a calcium-deficient diet or lack of vitamin D.

The ingestion of high amounts of fluoride can result in the malformation of bone known as fluorosis. This disease is often seen in areas where the drinking water contains over 10 ppm fluoride. Fluoride levels as high as 4 ppm do not result in fluorosis but do affect the nature of the bone crystals. Ingestion of fluoride affects the solubility, and therefore the reactivity, of bone apatite crystals by substitution of F for OH, by improving the apatite stoichiometry and by increasing the crystal size. A post-mortem study of the bones of a number of individuals of advanced age who lived in areas where fluoride in the drinking water ranged from 0 to 4 ppm showed an increase in crystal size with increasing fluoride content of bone (Fig. 6-4).[18]

Fluoride lowers the solubility of bone apatite when it substitutes for hydroxyl ion. Thus, the supersaturation of the fluid involved in bone mineralization is increased with regard to the F-substituted bone apatite as opposed to F-free bone apatite. This increase in supersaturation

93

gives an increase in crystal size with fluoride substitution. In fact, bone crystals are of the order of size where a slight increase in crystal size will decrease the solubility measurably. The classical Gibbs-Kelvin equation deals with the relationship between crystal size and solubility. Above a certain size, the solubility of a solid does not change. Below that critical size the solubility rises markedly, due to the increased input of surface effects as the crystal diminishes in size. Finally, another reason for stabilization is the concomitant improvement in apatite stoichiometry with fluoride-induced crystal growth.

Fluoride treatment of osteoporosis

Osteoporosis is the abnormal decrease in bone mass and increased bone fragility seen most commonly in the elderly, particularly in post-menopausal women (see Chapter 7). The decrease in bone mass leading to fractures in this disease is the result of an imbalance between resorption and formation in the lifelong process of bone remodeling. A treatment of osteoporosis should increase bone mass by the inhibition of resorption or the stimulation of bone formation. The United States Food and Drug Administration approved treatments of this disease by estrogen, calcitonin and calcium result mainly in inhibition of bone resorption.[19] Fluoride treatment, on the other hand, results

in an increase in bone mass as a result of the stimulation of bone formation.[7]

Oral sodium fluoride therapy for osteoporosis has been widely evaluated. In addition to stimulating osteoblast activity, fluoride stabilizes bone mineral by substitution of F for OH in bone apatite and by increasing the average bone crystal size, as noted above. It seems uncertain whether the mineral stabilization alone results in the increase in bone mass accompanying the ingestion of therapeutic doses of fluoride.[7]

A recent 4-year study of the daily treatment of osteoporosis failed to show a decrease in fracture rate for either the experimental and placebo group, in spite of the increase in bone mass.[20] Apparently, the bone formed by fluoride treatment is more brittle than normal bone. In the subsequent Chapter, other aspects of this will be discussed.

Note added in proof: A recent study by Pak and co-workers of a 12-month treatment of osteoporosis, which combined an oral slow-release fluoride dose with calcium citrate, showed increased bone deposition which was mechanically sound. Apparently the 2-month fluoride free period with only calcium citrate treatment, which followed the year-long, low-dose fluoride ingestion, cleared the body of fluoride toxicity allowing time for normal bone formation (Trends in Endocrinology, September 1995).

Literature cited

1. Berry EE. The structure and composition of some calcium-deficient apatites. J Nucl Chem 1967; 29: 317-27.

2. Blumenthal NC, Betts F, Posner AS. Effect of carbonate and biological macromolecules on formation and properties of hydroxyapatite. Calcified Tissue Res 1975; 18: 81-90.

3. Brown WE, Chow LC. Chemical properties of bone mineral. Ann Rev Mat Sci 1976; 6: 213-326.

4. DeJong WF. La substance minerale dans les os. Rec Trav Chim 1926; 45: 445-6.

5. Eanes ED, Gillessen IH, Posner AS. Intermediate stages in the precipitation of hydroxyapatite. Nature 1965; 208: 365-7.

6. Elliott JC. The problems of the composition and structure of the mineral components of hard tissues. Clin Orthopaed 1973; 93: 313-45.

7. Eriksen EF, Hodgson SF, Riggs BL. Treatment of osteoporosis with sodium fluoride. In: Riggs BL, Melton LJ, eds. Osteoporosis, etiology, diagnosis and management. New York: Raven Press 1988: 415-32.

8. Glimcher MJ. Composition, structure and organization of bone and other mineralized tissues and the mechanism of calcification. In: Greep R, ed. Handbook of physiology-endocrinology. Baltimore: Williams and Wilkins 1976: 25.

9. Landis WJ, Boyan-Salyers BE. Characterization of mineral deposits in bacterionema matruchotii using anhydrous methods of specimen preparation. Trans Orthopaed Res 1981; 63: 325.

10. Landis WJ, Geraudie J, Paine MC, Neuringer JR, Glimcher MJ. An electron optical and analytical study of mineral deposition in the developing fin trout, salmo gaidneri. Trans Orthopaed Res 1981: 63: 271.

11. Landis WJ, Glimcher MJ. Electron diffraction and electron probe microanalysis of the mineral phase of bone tissue prepared by anhydrous techniques. J Ultrastruc Res 1978; 63: 188-97.

12. LeGeros RZ, Trautz O, LeGeros JP, Klein E. Carbonate substitution in apatite structure. Bull Soc Chim, Spec No. 1968: 1712-8.

13. Likins RC, Posner AS, Steere AC. Effect of calcium treatment on solubility of synthetic hydroxyapatite and rat molar enamel. J Am Dent Assoc 1958; 57: 335-9.

14. Menczel J, Posner AS, Harper RA. Age changes in the crystallinity of rat bone apatite. Isr J Med Sci 1965; 1: 251-2.

15. Montel G. Conceptions nouvelles sur la physico-chimie des phosphate de structure apatitique. Bull Soc Chim, Spec No. 1968: 1693-700.

16. Posner AS. The mineral of bone. Clin Orthopaed 1985; 200: 87-99.

17. Posner AS, Betts F. Synthetic amorphous calcium phosphate and its relation to bone mineral. Acc Chem Res 1975; 8: 273-81.

18. Posner AS, Eanes ED, Harper RA, Zipkin I. X-ray diffraction analysis of the effect of fluoride on human bone apatite. Arch Oral Biol 1963; 8: 549-70.

19. Raisz LG, Kream BE. Regulation of bone formation, Part 2. New Engl J Med 1983; 309: 83-9.

20. Riggs BL, Melton LJ. The prevention and treatment of osteoporosis. New Engl J Med 1992; 327: 620-7.

21. Robison R. The possible significance of hexophosphoric esters in ossification. Biochem J 1923; 17: 286-93.

22. Sillen A, Smith P. Weaning patterns are reflected in strontium/calcium ratios of juvenile skeletons. J Archaeol Sci 1984; 11: 237-45.

23. Stutman JM. Posner AS, Lippincott ER. Hydrogen bonding in calcium phosphates. Nature 1962; 193: 368-70.

24. Veis A. The role of acidic proteins in biological mineralization. In: Everett DH, Dickson I, eds. Ions in macromolecular and biological systems. Bristol: Scientechnica 1978: 259.

CHAPTER 7

CLINICAL ASPECTS OF FLUORIDE IN BONE

F. Melsen • E.F. Eriksen • L. Mosekilde

Introduction – Mechanisms of action of fluoride on bone – Osteofluorosis
Fluoride treatment in osteoporosis

Introduction

The effect of fluoride on human bone was first described in 1932 by Møller & Gudjonsson[48] and 5 years later characterized in detail in Danish cryolite workers. This industrial type of fluorosis revealed radiologic signs of systemic osteosclerosis with a thickened skeleton due to appositionally formed bony tissue, spur formations at tendon insertions and ossification of ligaments. These changes were most pronounced in the central skeleton and to a lesser degree in the peripheral parts and the skull. Postmortem findings in two of the cryolite workers comprised heavy white and fragile bones with thickened and irregular cortical and cancellous structures with signs of hypomineralization and mineralization defects. Similar findings in industrial fluorosis have later been reported from Switzerland among workers in the aluminum industry[3] and in areas of endemic fluorosis caused by high fluoride content in the drinking water.[73] On the basis of these milestone reports and several additional papers describing the effects of fluoride treatment in osteoporotic patients, it is possible to charac-terize osteofluorosis radiographically and morphologically. These descriptions may lead to a better understanding of how fluoride affects the human skeleton.

Mechanisms of action of fluoride on bone

Effects on bone resorption

There is some evidence that fluoride may affect bone resorption. *In vitro*, fluoride decreases the solubility of bone mineral,[14] and fluoride pretreatment decreases the bone resorption induced by parathyroid hormone.[20] On the other hand, Baylink *et al.*[4,5] reported increased resorptive activity in endosteal areas of bone formed prior to initiation of fluoride therapy. Whether the increased resorption is caused directly by fluoride or by secondary hyperparathyroidism is still unknown. The long-term effects of fluoride on bone resorption seem to differ. In osteoporotic patients treated with fluoride for 2 and 5 years in combination with calcium and vitamin D, a decrease in bone resorptive activity has been demonstrated by both calcium kinetic and histomorphometric methods.[11,15]

Changes in apatite crystallinity could explain the inhibition of bone resorption seen after fluoride treatment.[14] Increased resistance to dissolution by osteoclastic enzymes as well as high levels of fluoride liberated from fluoride-containing bone during the resorptive process, however, might inhibit osteoclastic activity and explain the discrepancy between the acute and chronic therapeutic effects.

Effects on bone formation

Sodium fluoride stimulates bone formation at the cellular,[36,37] tissue[15] and organ level[11] in most species, leading to a positive balance per remodeling cycle,[15] an increase in trabecular bone volume[9,15,18,19,22] and a positive overall calcium balance.[11] The effect of sodium fluoride on bone formation is also reflected in a rise in serum alkaline phosphatase levels[16,27,59] and bone Gla-protein (BGP).[59] Apparently, the *in vitro* effects of sodium fluoride on cultured osteoblasts are species-specific and related to dose and the developmental stage of the osteoblasts.[6,7] Sodium fluoride stimulates proliferation and differentiation of osteoblasts derived from embryonic chicken calvaria[16] and induces osteogenesis of embryonic mesenchyme in chicken.[23] However, the effects on mature human osteoblast-like cells cultured from trabecular explants have been variable.[38,40,78]

We have recently tested the influence of sodium fluoride on marrow stromal cell cultures that contain a population of osteogenic stem cells from human marrow stroma.[37] In this study, sodium fluoride 10^5 M stimulated proliferation to 180% of that of the controls (Fig. 7-1). Fluoride also affected cellular differentiation. This effect was particularly evident in the presence of $1,25(OH)_2D_3$, where sodium fluoride stimulated production of alkaline phosphatase, bone Gla-protein and, most importantly, collagen synthesis as reflected in carbox-

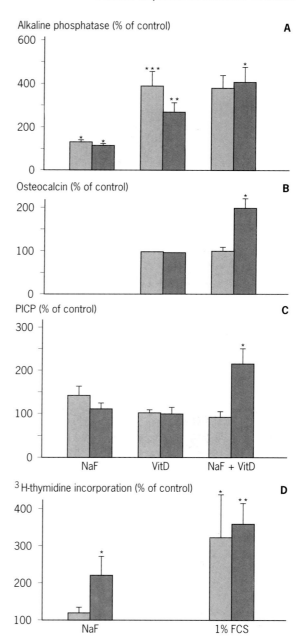

Fig. 7-1. Effects of sodium fluoride *in vitro* on cell proliferation as reflected in thymidine incorporation and synthesis of osteocalcin, alkaline phosphatase and type I procollagen extension peptide (P1CP).

yterminal propeptide of type I collagen concentrations in the conditioned medium[36,37] (Fig. 7-1). The effects of fluoride also seemed to be more pronounced for less differentiated stromal cells than for osteoblasts.[37]

Both direct and indirect cellular mechanisms have been implicated in the observed increase in bone formation during chronic fluoride administration. Bone cells are responsive to changes in electrical currents in their environment.[17] Bone crystals may act as transducers for mechanical stress, generating piezoelectric currents in bone that may affect osteoblast activity. The increased rigidity of crystalline fluorohydroxyapatite may enhance these piezoelectric currents. It has been hypothesized that such mechanisms could explain the more pronounced effect of fluoride on the weight-bearing axial skeleton (vertebral column and os ilium) than on non-weight-bearing bones such as the radius[59].

Effects on bone structure

The effects of fluoride treatment on bone structure have only been partially characterized. Vesterby et al.[75] reported a decrease in the marrow star volume of cancellous bone after fluoride treatment. The marrow star volume is a structural parameter which increases with increasing trabecular perforations and disintegration of the trabecular network. Thus, this finding suggests that fluoride treatment improves trabecular structure. One should bear in mind, however, that a mere thickening of trabeculae would also tend to decrease the marrow star volume, without actually bridging the gap between trabeculae. So far, no analyses of cortical bone structure have been published.

Effects on bone mineralization

The cause of the fluoride-induced mineralization defect is unknown. Studies performed in the late 1960s and early 1970s strongly suggested that the excessive osteoid formation and incomplete mineralization of new bone seen after fluoride therapy could be diminished by giving vitamin D and calcium supplements.[33,55,63,64] The severity of the mineralization defect seems to increase with increasing dose of fluoride. At 60 mg of sodium fluoride per day to adults, tetracycline labels in bone are sharp and uniform, but at 90 mg/day the newly formed bone fails to incorporate tetracycline labels.[33] However, the mechanism by which fluoride inhibits bone mineralization and how calcium (and vitamin D) ameliorates this abnormality has not been established. The $Ca \times PO_4$ product in serum shows no major changes during fluoride treatment and changes in vitamin D-metabolites mainly reflect concomitant vitamin D therapy. Fluoride does not seem to be a crystal poison either; on the contrary, it enhances crystal growth.[14] After incorporation of fluoride, apatite crystals are larger (see previous chapter). This structural change in bone crystals might affect their binding to organic matrix constituents. Johnson[31] hypothesized that the osteoid tissue formed during fluoride therapy does not calcify normally. Furthermore, fluoride increases the bone matrix content of termatan sulfate, a mineralization inhibitor.[70] Using a subcutaneous endochondral bone formation model in rats, Eanes & Reddi[14] found delayed uptake of ^{45}Ca in fluoride-treated animals. On the basis of histologic and biochemical data, they suggested that the mineralization defect was caused by retarded matrix development, leading to a decreased number of matrix sites for crystal nucleation.

The fluoride-induced mineralization defect and the beneficial effects of calcium and vitamin D supplementation are related to the duration of therapy. In the early studies reporting beneficial effects of calcium and vitamin D supplementation, treatment periods were less than 2 years.[2,33] Briancon & Meunier[9] found that only 8 of 74 patients had mineralization defects when studied histologically after 2-3 years of treatment. By contrast, in histologic studies

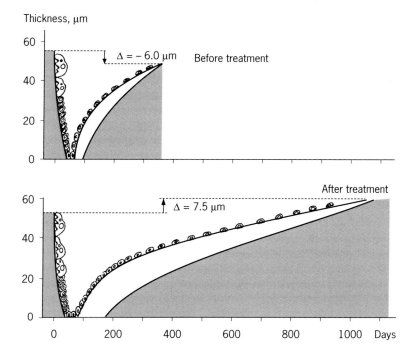

Thickness, μm

Fig. 7-2. Bone remodeling in osteoporotics before and after treatment with sodium fluoride (60 mg/day), calciferol (18,000 IU/day) and calcium phosphate (2 g/day) over a period of 5 years. Note the change in bone balance from negative to positive after treatment and the prolongation of the remodeling period after fluoride treatment.

after 4-5 years of treatment, most patients had mineralization defects despite calcium and vitamin D supplementation.[15,50] In the study by Eriksen *et al.*[15] the bone formation period was prolonged from 302 days to 1020 days in the posttreatment biopsies. The mineralization lag time (an index describing the time from initiation of bone matrix synthesis to mineralization of the matrix), normally 25-50 days, was prolonged to 108 days in the posttreatment biopsies, indicating the presence of a mineralization defect (Fig. 7-2). Moreover, a decrease in the rate of osteoblastic matrix synthesis could be demonstrated. Despite the inhibition of bone formation, however, a positive balance between resorption and formation per remodeling cycle and an increase in trabecular bone volume were demonstrated.

Osteofluorosis

The most common feature of osteofluorosis is the osteosclerosis in the central skeleton with irregular thickening of the bones due to periosteal sleeves of abnormally structured osseous tissue, osteophytosis, mineralization of tendons and muscle attachments, and bridging between the edges of the vertebral bodies. These changes may be radiographically diagnosed in the peripheral skeleton. A similar thickening and new bone formation may be observed in the tubular bones, and mineralization of interosseous membranes seems to be an important diagnostic feature radiologically. The cortical bone may further show radiologic signs of cancellization and cortical erosions. These radiologic changes correspond rather precisely to the gross anatomic findings.

Although the micromorphology of osteoflu-

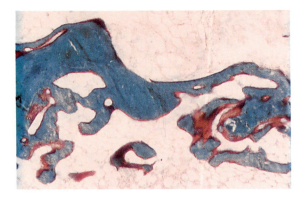

Fig. 7-3. Thickening of cancellous bone due to newly formed bone with woven pattern.

orosis by some authors is considered non-pathognomonic,[3] the combination of changes in the bone is so characteristic that other diseases can be excluded.

Microscopically the amount of bone tissue is increased due to a thickening of both cortical and cancellous structures (Fig. 7-3). The mineralized bone is a mixture of preexisting lamellar bone and newly formed bone with a woven pattern surrounding more or less randomly oriented osteocytes. The "fluorotic bone" may, in contrast to normal bone, occur on smooth surfaces which do not exhibit signs of previous resorption. Within the fluorotic bone, which on microradiograms is usually hypomineralized (Fig. 7-4), areas of non-mineralized matrix may be found. Apart from this apposition of fluorotic bone on surfaces of cancellous bone and on the periosteal and endosteal surfaces of the cortex, *de novo* bone formation without relation to preexisting bone can be found in the marrow cavity. The formation of fluorotic bone often occurs as very wide seams of irregular bone, indicating a long-lasting continuous formation. Concomitant with bone formation, remodeling takes place in both preexisting lamellar bone and in the newly formed fluorotic bone. The remodeling or internal reorganization of bone comprises sequences of resorption and subsequent formation, leading to new structural lamellar units (osteons). In contrast to the nor-

mal adult remodeling in which the balance between resorption and formation is negative, the balance in fluorotic bone remodeling is positive.[15] Both the positive remodeling balance and the formation of fluorotic bone leads to an increase in bone mass and trabecular continuity.[15,75] From a theoretical point of view this should benefit the biomechanical competence of bone. It is therefore surprising that biomechanical investigations of fluorotic bone from animal studies[47] and from osteoporotic humans after 5 years of sodium fluoride therapy[71] show a reduction in mechanical strength, indicating a different quality of bone induced by fluoride.

The increase in bone mass after fluoride exposure has been the rationale for introducing fluoride in the treatment of osteopenic conditions, especially osteoporosis. Since the introduction of fluoride as a drug about 30 years ago, the results of many studies have been reported, leading to a more profound understanding of how fluoride affects bone and calcium metabolism.

Fluoride treatment in osteoporosis

Several drugs or combinations of drugs are at present used or under investigation for the prevention and treatment of osteoporosis. According to their predominant pharmacologic

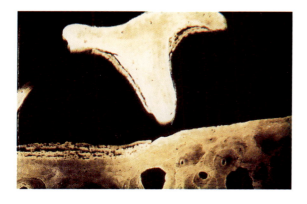

Fig. 7-4. Microradiogram shows hypomineraliza-tion of the fluorotic bone on cortical and cancellous surfaces.

action they can be divided into *antiresorptive* and *anabolic* drugs.[60]

The antiresorptive drugs inhibit recruitment, activation or activity of new or existing osteo-clasts. The activation of new remodeling cycles is reduced and the work performed by the os-teoclasts may be diminished. Unfortunately, because of the coupling between resorption and formation, osteoblast number, activity and work are also reduced after a couple of month-s.[51] The resulting increase in bone mass or bone mineral content is therefore limited to a few per cent. However, the risk of trabecular perfor-ations may be reduced because of a decreased number of resorptive cavities or a reduced re-sorption depth.[52] This will improve conserva-tion of an intact trabecular structure over time and support the maintenance of trabecular bone biomechanical competence. Estrogen, cal-citonin and bisphosphonates are typical antire-sorptive drugs.[60]

Anabolic drugs characteristically initiate *de novo* bone formation without previous resorp-tion or create a positive balance per remodeling cycle without reducing the activation of new remodeling cycles. These effects will result in a continuous growth in bone mass over time. At present, fluoride is the only drug available with this potency.[33,59,60,69]

Fluoride preparations for therapeutic use
Sodium fluoride is available in Europe in 10-25 mg coated or uncoated tablets whereas in the USA, only low-potency (2-5 mg) tablets are available. Slow-release formulations have been introduced in order to minimize gastrointesti-nal discomfort. *Sodium monofluorophosphate* is a more complex compound from which fluoride is released during intestinal absorption.[7] Meta-bolism and effects of fluoride after absorption from this compound are similar to sodium flu-oride, but the number of gastrointestinal side effects are reduced.

Pharmacokinetics of fluoride
After an oral sodium fluoride load, more than 90% is absorbed by simple diffusion mainly from the duodenum and the upper jeju-num.[13,44,66] Intestinal absorption is enhanced by gastric acidity[79] and is proportional to the solubility of the fluoride compound (see Chap-ter 4). Concomitant calcium ingestion decreases intestinal absorption, necessitating an increase in the fluoride dosage of approximately 25% to achieve the same net absorption.[32] Magnesium and aluminum also compromise fluoride ab-sorption. Fluoride is detectable in the blood within 10 min after an oral load and reaches peak levels after 30-60 minutes[10]. Around 50% of the absorbed dose is rapidly deposited in the skeleton. Most of the remainder is excreted in

the urine. Plasma half-life ranges from 2 to 9 hours.[10] The ability to excrete fluoride decreases with impaired renal function.[8,76]

In bone, fluoride substitutes for hydroxyl in the apatite crystal lattice, forming fluorohydroxyapatite[14] (see previous chapter). Skeletal fluoride content is proportional to dietary intake over a wide range.[43] Fluoride concentrations in bone and serum are in equilibrium, which means that fasting serum and urine fluoride levels reflect previous fluoride intake.[77]

Fluoride dosages

Fluoride appears to have a narrow therapeutic window. Early studies on iliac crest biopsies using microradiography showed that sodium fluoride dosages below 50 mg/day to adults stimulated bone formation inconsistently, whereas dosages above 80 mg/day induced mineralization defects, formation of abnormal bone and increased occurrence of side effects.[33] This is in accordance with recent investigations demonstrating that a daily oral dose of 75 mg/day lacks antifracture efficacy in spite of exceptional increases in spinal bone mineral content,[59] whereas 50 mg/day seems to reduce fracture rate compared to other treatment modalities for spinal osteoporosis.[46]

The individual therapeutic dosage of sodium fluoride depends on renal function and body size. For osteoporotic patients with normal kidney function we usually recommend an initial dosage of 40-60 mg/day. After 3-6 months the dosage is then adjusted on the basis of regular fasting serum fluoride measurements. The optimal therapeutic range in plasma is considered to be 5-10 M measured 24 hours after the last sodium fluoride dose.[27,72]

Treatment modalities

Studies performed 20-30 years ago strongly suggested that the incomplete mineralization induced by high dose fluoride mono-therapy could be reduced by giving oral vitamin D and calcium supplements.[2,33,34,45,53] By microradio-graphic examination of serial bone biopsies, Jowsey et al.[33] demonstrated that poorly mineralized bone formed during fluoride mono-therapy was followed by formation of normal lamellar bone during combined fluoride, calcium and vitamin D therapy. Oral calcium supplementation also decreased the enhanced bone resorption.[28,33] Most clinical studies therefore combine fluoride treatment with oral calcium supplementation but there is no consensus regarding the concomitant use of vitamin D. Some studies have demonstrated that addition of vitamin D or its 25-hydroxylated metabolites does not decrease the extent of the fluoride-induced mineralization defect[41] or further decrease fracture rate.[58] On the other hand, recent observations of a direct advantageous effect of $1,25\text{-}OH_2D_3$ on human osteoblast-like cells exposed to fluoride[36] suggest that addition of 1,25-dihydroxylated vitamin D metabolites to the treatment regimen may be indicated.

The effects of concomitant calcium and vitamin D supplementation on osteoid mineralization appear to be related to the duration of therapy. Beneficial effects have been reported following treatment periods of less than 2-3 years.[2,9,34] By contrast, in studies of treatment lasting more than 4-5 years, most patients had mineralization defects despite calcium and vitamin D administration.[15,50]

Another approach to reduce mineralization defects and the frequency of side effects is to give fluoride intermittently. Theoretically, such regimens may decrease the risk of side effects because fluoride levels in serum are increased for shorter periods. Moreover, a potential maximal effect on mitogenesis when fluoride is given combined with an increased mineralization of bone matrix in the fluoride-free periods may reverse the negative bone balance in osteoporotics even more than observed with continuous treatment regimens.

number of nonvertebral fractures was higher in the treatment group. Comparable results have been found in a smaller controlled study.[39] These two studies have been criticized on the grounds that the dosage used (75 mg sodium fluoride/day) was too large and may have resulted in qualitative changes in bone that would not have occurred with lower dosages. Indeed, recalculation in patients taking less than 50 mg/day of sodium fluoride have shown a significant reduction in fracture risk compared to placebo. However, the criticism cannot be resolved by debate or recalculation of available data but only by well-designed studies employing lower dosages of sodium fluoride.

The question of the effect of fluoride treatment on peripheral fractures is also unsolved. In a randomized series of elderly patients treated with either placebo or sodium fluoride (50 mg/day) for only 6 months, the fluoride-treated group had a significantly higher incidence of hip fractures.[29] Another unrandomized study[21] compared 16 patients treated with sodium fluoride, calcium, and vitamin D for 4 years with a control group followed for 3 years. A total of 11 femoral fractures occurred in 5 patients in the treated group compared to no fractures in the control group, However, other studies oppose these findings.[54,57] In a recent multicenter study on the occurrence of hip fractures 418 fluoride-treated osteoporotic patients were observed for more than patient-years.[57] They were compared with 120 osteoporotics who had been followed prospectively for 3 years prior to initiation of fluoride therapy. No significant difference could be demonstrated between the occurrence of hip fractures in the two groups (1.6 and 1.8%, respectively). The expected incidence of hip fracture in non-osteoporotic women of the same age in the general community was found to be 0.5%. Thus, according to this study untreated osteoporotics were at greater risk for hip fractures but fluoride treatment did not appear to add to this risk. Power & Gay[54] also found no relationship between hip fracture and fluoride treatment.

Because of the seriousness of hip fractures, the question of increased risk for hip fracture in fluoride-treated patients is a key issue in assessing the risks and benefits of sodium fluoride treatment. Prospective studies evaluating changes in bone mineral density of the hip and fracture risk are currently underway.

Differences in individual responsiveness to fluoride

About 25% of patients undergoing treatment with fluoride fail to respond adequately.[9,15, 30,61] The cause of this variability in response is not well understood. Neither dosage or bioavailability of fluoride appear to be significant determinants of responsiveness.[61]

In 28 patients receiving fluoride treatment iliac crest trabecular bone volume doubled in the group as a whole, but 7 patients showed no response at all.[9] The same trend was observed among 24 patients treated with fluoride, calcium and vitamin D for 5 years.[15] Apparently, patients with low bone mass respond better than patients with high bone mass.[42] In another study based on spinal x-rays from patients with postmenopausal osteoporosis treated with fluoride, it was shown that trabecular thickening increased in 15 of 27 patients[61]. New vertebral fractures occurred less frequently in these patients than in the other patients. However, no differences between responders and nonresponders could be demonstrated in terms of number of initial vertebral fractures.

Serial measurements of serum alkaline phosphatase activity from osteoporotic patients receiving fluoride demonstrated that 42% had a fine response, with a brisk and continuous increase in alkaline phosphatase activity, 32% had a medium response, with a slow, steady increase within normal range, and 21% did not respond or responded only insignificantly.[30] It has been claimed that a sparse response in serum alkaline phosphatase activity may predict a poor clinical response.[7] However, this concept has not been supported by other studies[27] and, at present, no standard has been established on which prediction of "responders" and "nonresponders" can be based.

Side effects
Symptomatic skeletal fluorosis has not occurred after fluoride treatment for up to 6 years. However, side effects have occurred in 30-50% of treated patients in several large series. The two main types, periarticular and gastrointestinal side effects, affected a mean of 34.6% and 20.5% of treated patients, respectively (Table 7-1).[27]

A *lower extremity pain syndrome*, with periarticular or foot pain and occasionally tenderness around the large joints, has been described. The underlying mechanism is unknown. Scintigraphic findings suggest the possibility of a chemical periostitis,[76] but this concept has not been supported by more detailed investigations.[49,58] Radiographs taken within 2 weeks after onset of symptoms are always negative.[65] However, repeated investigations 4 weeks after onset often show radiographic changes suggestive of healing stress microfractures at the sites of increased bone scan activity.[49,65,67] Other radiographic studies have shown evidence of new periosteal and endosteal bone growth in 67% of fluoride-treated osteoporotics with periarticular pain but have failed to detect stress fractures.[68]

The incidence of the pain syndrome increases with increased serum fluoride levels.[72] It has also been claimed by some investigators,[7,35] but not all,[27] that very large increases in serum alkaline phosphatase activity predict the occurrence of the pain syndromes. The symptoms always disappear within several weeks after discontinuation of treatment. In nearly half of the patients, they may recur after therapy is reinstituted even at a lower fluoride dosage.

Table 7-1

Frequency of side effects during treatment of osteoporosis with fluoride, calcium and vitamin D over 460 patient-years (*Modified from Hasling* et al.[20])

Articular or periarticular pains	37%
Ankle regions	34%
Knees	7%
Toes	3%
Plantar regions	2%
Wrists	2%
Fingers	1%
Heels	1%
Gastrointestinal distress	25%
Gastric pyrosis	17%
Nausea	9%
Hemorrhage	1%
Chronic anemia	0%
Alopecia	1%
Renal stone symptoms	0%
Hypercalcemic symptoms	0%

Gastrointestinal symptoms comprise upper intestinal discomfort, epigastric pain, nausea, vomiting and, occasionally, iron-deficiency anemia due to subclinical gastrointestinal bleeding.[27] A few cases of ulceration and hematemesis have been reported. The symptoms are probably induced by a direct irritating effect of the fluoride ion on the gastric mucosa or by the local formation of hydrofluoric acid. The frequency of gastric symptoms can be reduced by concomitant administration of calcium carbonate, by administration of the fluoride with meals or by the use of enteric-soluble tablets or sodium-monofluorophosphate.

Other clinical side effects are observed more rarely. Loss of hair and growth of small bone spurs have been reported occasionally. More unusual findings are optic neuritis, peripheral neuritis[18,58] and degenerative diseases of the central nervous system.[58] These isolated events are most likely to be coincidences.

Small but significant decreases in serum levels of coagulation factors has been reported in patients receiving fluoride, calcium and vitamin D.[27] Other liver function tests remained normal. Furthermore, no adverse effects on thyroid or renal function could be demonstrated. In this study it was found that 40% of the side-effects occurred during the first year, 14% during the second year, and 12% during the third and final year of the study. Thus the accumulation of fluoride in the skeleton does not appear to increase the incidence of side effects. Over a 5-year period, only 5-10% of patients had to discontinue treatment because of side effects.

The results of studies on side effects related to vitamin D and calcium supplementation are conflicting. No case of persistent or symptomatic hypercalcemia was found[27] in a group of 163 patients with a mean observation time of 2.8 years. In fact, the mean serum calcium level for the entire group decreased during treatment. Urinary excretion of calcium remained unchanged, and no case of kidney stones developed. However, other studies have observed more frequent hypercalcemia and hypercalciuria in patients treated with vitamin D and calcium, compared with patients treated with calcium alone.[58]

Contraindications to fluoride treatment
Chronic renal failure and osteomalacia are contraindications to fluoride therapy. Because the kidney is the main route of fluoride excretion, renal failure may lead to toxic accumulation of fluoride. In azotemic patients treated with fluoride, severe fluorosis with bilateral hip fractures has been reported.[19] Osteomalacia may be aggravated by fluoride-induced inhibition of mineralization. Previous hip fracture may constitute a relative contraindication.

Literature cited

1. Bang S, Baud CA, Boivin G, Demeurisse C, Gössi M, Tochon-Danguy HJ, Very JM. Morphometric and biophysical study of bone tissue in industrial fluorosis. In: Courvoisier B, Donath A, Baud CA, eds. Fluoride and bone. Bern: Hans Huber 1978: 168-75.

2. Baud CA, Lagier R, Bang S, Boivin G, Gössi M, Tochon-Danguy HJ. Treatment of osteoporosis with NaF, calcium or/and phosphorus, and vitamin D: histological, morphometric and biophysical study of the bone tissue. In: Courvoisier B, Donath A, Baud CA, eds. Fluoride and bone. Bern: Hans Huber 1978: 290-2.

3. Baud CA, Lagier R, Boivin G, Boillat MA. Value of the bone biopsy in the diagnosis of industrial fluorosis. Virchows Arch (A) 1978; 380: 283-97.

4. Baylink, DJ, Bernstein DS. The effects of fluoride therapy on metabolic bone disease: a histologic study. Clin Orthop 1967; 55: 51-85.

5. Baylink D, Wergedal J, Stauffer M, Rich C. Effects of fluoride on bone formation, mineralization, and resorption in the rat. In: Vischer TL, ed. Fluoride and medicine. Bern: Hans Huber 1970: 37-69.

6. Baylink DJ, Farley SM, Smith L. Characterisation of skeletal response to fluoride (abstract). Clin Res 1983; 31: 543A.

7. Baylink DJ, Duane PB, Farley SM, Farley JR. Monofluorophosphate physiology: the effects of fluoride on bone. Caries Res 1983; 17S: 56-76.

8. Berman LB, Taves DR. Fluoride excretion in normal and uremic humans (abstract). Clin Res 1973; 21: 100.

9. Briancon D, Meunier PJ. Treatment of osteoporosis with fluoride, calcium, and vitamin D. Orthop Clin North Am 1981; 12: 629-48.

10. Carlson CH, Armstrong WD, Singer L. Distribution and excretion of radiofluoride in the human. Proc Soc Exp Biol Med 1960; 104: 235-9.

11. Charles P, Mosekilde L, Taagehøj Jensen F. The effects of sodium fluoride, calcium phosphate, and vitamin D_2 for one to two years on calcium and phosphorus metabolism in postmenopausal women with spinal crush fracture osteoporosis. Bone 1985; 6: 201-6.

12. Dambacher MA, Lauffenburger T, Lämmle B, Haas HG. Long term effects of sodium fluoride in osteoporosis. In: Courvoisier B, Donath A, Baud CA, eds. Fluoride and bone. Bern: Hans Huber 1978: 238-41.

13. Dustin JP. Monitoring of fluoride dosage during treatment of bone disease. In: Vischer TL, ed. Fluoride and medicine. Bern: Hans Huber 1970: 178-89.

14. Eanes ED, Reddi AH. The effect of fluoride on bone mineral apatite. Metab Bone Dis Rel Res 1979; 2: 3-10.

15. Eriksen EF, Mosekilde L, Melsen F. Effect of sodium fluoride, calcium, phosphate, and vitamin D_2 on trabecular bone balance and remodeling in osteoporotics. Bone 1985; 6: 381-9.

16. Farley SM, Wergedal J, Smith L et al. Fluoride therapy for osteoporosis. Characterisation of the skeletal response by serial measurements of serum alkaline phosphatase. Metabolism 1987; 36: 211-8.

17. Fitzsimmons R, Farley JR, Adey RA, Baylink DJ. Evidence that action of electric field (EF) exposure to increased bone cell proliferation in vitro is selective for alkaline phosphatase (ALP) rich cells and dependent on mitogenic activity release (abstract). J Bone Miner Res 1986; S1: 157.

18. Franke J. Our experience in the treatment of osteoporosis with relatively low sodium-fluoride doses. In: Courvoisier B, Donath A, Baud CA, eds. Fluoride and bone. Bern: Hans Huber 1978: 256-62.

19. Gerster JC, Charhon SA, Jaeger P, Boivin G, Briancon D, Rostan A, Baud CA, Meunier PJ. Bilateral fractures of femoral neck in patients with moderate renal failure receiving fluoride for spinal osteoporosis. Brit Med J 1983; 287: 723-5.

20. Goldhaber P. The inhibition of bone resorption in tissue culture by nontoxic concentrations of sodium fluoride. Isr. J Med Sci 1967; 3: 617-26.

21. Gutteridge DH, Price RI, Nicholson GC, Kent GN, Retallack RW, Devlin RD, Worth GK, Glancy JJ, Michell P, Gruber H. Fluoride in osteoporotic vertebral fractures - trabecular increase, vertebral protection, femoral fractures. In: Christiansen C, Arnaud CD, Nordin BEC, Parfitt AM, Peck WA, Riggs BL, eds. Osteoporosis. Aalborg: Aalborg Stiftsbogtrykkeri 1984: 705-7.

22. Haas HG, Lauffenburger T, Guncaga J, Lentner C, Olah AJ, Dambacher MA. Bone turnover in osteoporosis, studied with sodium fluoride (abstract). Eur J Clin Invest 1973; 3: 235.

23. Hall BK. Sodium fluoride as an initiator of osteogenesis from embryonic mesenchyme in vitro. Bone 1987; 8: 111-6.

24. Hansson T, Roos B. Osteoporosis: effect of combined therapy with sodium fluoride, calcium, and vitamin D on the lumbar spine in osteoporosis. Am J Roentenol 1976; 126: 1294-6.

25. Harrison JE, Bayley TA, Josse RG. The relationship between fluoride effects on histology and on bone mass in patients with postmenopausal osteoporosis. Bone Miner 1986; 1: 321-5.

26. Harrison JE, McNeill KG, Sturtridge WC, Bayley TA, Murray TM, Williams C, Tam C, Fornasier V. Three-year changes in bone mineral mass of postmenopausal osteoporotic patients based on neutron activation analysis of the central third of the skeleton. J Clin Endocrinol Metab 1981; 52: 751-8.

27. Hasling C, Nielsen HE, Melsen F, Mosekilde L. The safety of osteoporosis treatment with sodium fluoride, calcium phosphate and vitamin D. Miner Electrolyte Metab 1987; 13: 96-103.

28. Hauck HM, Steenbock H, Parsons HT. The effect of the level of calcium intake on the calcification of bones and teeth during fluorine toxicosis. Am J Physiol 1933; 103: 489-93.

29. Inkovaara J, Keikinheimo R, Jarvinen K, Kasurinen U, Hanhijarvi H, Iisalo E. Prophylactic fluoride treatment and aged bones. Brit Med J 1975; 3: 73-4.

30. Ivey JL, Farley JR, Baylink DJ. Alkaline phosphatase response in sodium fluoride-treated osteoporotics (abstract). Clin Res 1981; 29: 95.

31. Johnson LC. Histogenesis and mechanisms in the development of osteofluorosis. In: Simons JH, ed. Fluorine chemistry, Vol. 4. New York: Academic Press 1965: 424-41.

32. Jowsey J, Riggs BL. Effect of concurrent calcium ingestion on intestinal absorption of fluoride. Metabolism 1978; 27: 971-4.

33. Jowsey J, Riggs BL, Kelly PJ, Hoffman DL. Effect of combined therapy with sodium fluoride, vitamin D and calcium in osteoporosis. Am J Med 1972; 53: 43-9.

34. Jowsey J, Schenk RK, Reutter FW. Some results of the effect of fluoride on bone tissue in osteoporosis. J Clin Endocrinol Metab 1968; 28: 869-74.

35. Kanis JA, Meunier PJ. Should we use fluoride to treat osteoporosis? A review. Quart J Med 1984; 53: 145-64.

36. Kassem M, Mosekilde L, Eriksen EF. 1,25-dihydroxyvitamin D_3 potentiates fluoride-stimulated collagen type I production in cultures of human bone marrow stromal osteoblast-like cells. J Bone Miner Res 1993; 8: 1453-8.

37. Kassem M, Mosekilde L, Eriksen EF. Effects of fluoride on human bone cells in vitro: differences in responsiveness between stromal osteoblast precursors and mature osteoblasts. Eur J Endocrinol 1994; 130: 381-6.

38. Khokher MA, Dandona P. Fluoride stimulates 3Hthymidine incorporation and alkaline phosphatase production by hyman osteoblasts. Metabolism 1990; 39: 1118-21.

39. Kleerekoper M, Peterson E, Phillips E, Nelson D, Tilley B, Parfitt AM. Continuous sodium fluoride therapy does not reduce vertebral fracture rate in postmenopausal osteoporosis. Osteoporosis Int 1991; 1: 155-8.

40. Kopp JB, Robey PG. Sodium fluoride does not increase human bone cell proliferation or protein synthesis in vitro. Calcif Tissue Int 1990; 47: 221-9.

41. Kuntz D, Marie P, Naveau B, Maziere B, Tubiana M, Ryckewaert A. Extended treatment of primary osteoporosis by sodium fluoride combined with 25 hydroxycholecalciferol. Clin Rheumatol 1984; 3: 145-53.

42. Lane JM, Healey JH, Schwartz E, Vigorita VJ, Schneider R, Einhorn TA, Suda M, Robbins WC. Treatment of osteoporosis with sodium fluoride and calcium: effects on vertebral fracture incidence and bone histomorphometry. Orthop Clin North Am 1984; 15: 729-45.

43. Largent EJ.Metabolism of inorganic fluorides. In: Shaw JH, ed. Fluoridation as a public health measure. Washington D.C.: American Association for the Advancement of Science 1954: 49-78.

44. Leone NC. The effects of the absorption of fluoride. I. Outline and summary. Arch Indus Health 1960; 21: 324-5.

45. Lindemann G. Experimental chronic fluorosis in young rats receiving supplementary doses of vitamin D. Acta Odontol Scand 1965; 23: 575-92.

46. Mamelle N, Dusan R, Martin JL et al. Evaluation of risk-benefit ratio of sodium fluoride treatment in primary osteoporosis. A prospective controlled study in medical practice. Lancet 1988; 2: 361-3.

47. Mosekilde Li, Kragstrup J, Richards A. Compressive strength, ash weight and volume of vertebral trabecular bone in experimental fluorosis in pigs. Calcif Tissue Int 1987; 40: 318-22.

48. Møller PF, Gudjonsson SU. Massive fluorosis of bones and ligaments. Acta Radiol 1932; 13: 269-94.

49. O'Duffy JD, Wahner HW, O'Fallon WM, Johnson KA, Muhs JM, Beabout JW, Hodgson SF, Riggs BL. Mechanism of acute lower extremity pain syndrome in fluoride-treated osteoporotic patients. Am J Med 1986; 80: 561-6.

50. Olah AJ, Reutter FW, Dambacher MA. Effects of combined therapy with sodium fluoride and high doses of Vitamin D in osteoporosis. A histomorphometric study in the iliac crest. In: Courvoisier B, Donath A, Baud CA, eds. Fluoride and bone. Bern: Hans Huber 1978: 242-8.

51. Parfitt AM. Morphologic basis of bone mineral measurements: transient and steady state effects of treatment in osteoporosis (editorial). Miner Electrolyte Metab 1980; 4: 273-87.

52. Parfitt AM. Age-related structural changes in trabecular and cortical bone; cellular mechanisms and biomechanical consequences. Calcif Tissue Int 1984; 3: 123-8.

53. Parsons V, Mitchell CJ, Reeve J, Hesp R. The use of sodium fluoride, vitamin D and calcium supplements in the treatment of patients with axial osteoporosis. Calcif Tissue Res (Suppl.) 1977; 22: 236-40.

54. Power GRI, Gay JDL. Sodium fluoride in the treatment of osteoporosis. Clin Invest Med 1986; 9: 41-3.

55. Reutter FW, Olah AJ. Bone biopsy findings and clinical observations in longterm treatment of osteoporosis with sodium fluoride and vitamin D_3. In: Courvoisier B, Donath,A, Baud CA, eds. Fluoride and bone. Bern: Hans Huber 1978: 249-55.

56. Riggs BL. Treatment of osteoporosis with sodium fluoride: an appraisal. Bone Miner Res 1984; 2: 366-93.

57. Riggs BL, Baylink DJ, Kleerekoper M, Lane JM, Melton LJ, III, Meunier PJ. Incidence of hip fractures in osteoporotic women treated with sodium fluoride 1987. J Bone Miner Res 1987; 2(2): 123-6.

58. Riggs BL, Hodgson SF, Hoffmann DL, Kelly PJ, Johnson KA, Taves D. Treatment of primary osteoporosis with fluoride and calcium: clinical tolerance and fracture occurrence. JAMA 1980; 243: 446-9.

59. Riggs BL, Hodgson SF, O'Fallon WM, Chao, EYS, Wahner HW, Muhs JM, Cedel SL, Melton LJ. Effect of fluoride treatment on fracture rate in postmenopausal women with osteoporosis. N Engl J Med 1990; 322: 802-6.

60. Riggs BL, Melton LJ, eds. Osteoporosis, etiology, diagnosis and management. New York: Raven Press 1988.

61. Riggs BL, Seeman E, Hodgson SF, Taves DR, O'-Fallon WM. Effect of the fluoride/calcium regimen on vertebral fracture occurrence in postmenopausal osteoporosis: comparison with conventional therapy. N Engl J Med 1982; 306: 446-50.

62. Ringe JD, Kruse HP, Kuhlencordt F. Long term treatment of primary osteoporosis by sodium fluoride. In: Courvoisier B, Donath A, Baud CA, eds. Fluoride and bone. Bern: Hans Huber 1978: 228-32.

63. Ryckwaert A, Kuntz D, Teyssedou JP, Tun Chot S, Bordier P, Hioco D. Étude histologique de l'os chez des sujets ostéoporotiques en traitement prolongé par le fluorure de sodium. Rev Rhum Mal Osteoartic 1972; 39: 627-34.

64. Schenk RK, Merz WA, Reutter FW. Fluoride in osteoporosis: quantitative histological studies on bone structure and bone remodelling in serial biopsies of the iliac crest. In: Vischer TL, ed. Fluoride in medicine. Bern: Hans Huber 1970: 153-68.

65. Schnizler CM. Stress-fractures in fluoride therapy for osteoporosis. In: Christiansen C, Arnaud CD, Nordin BEC, Parfitt AM, Peck WA, Riggs BL, eds. Osteoporosis. Aalborg: Aalborg Stiftsbogtrykkeri 1984: 629-34.

66. Schlatter CH. Metabolism and toxicology of fluorides. In: Courvoisier B, Donath A, Baud CA, eds. Fluoride and bone. Bern: Hans Huber 1978: 1-21.

67. Schnizler CM, Solomon L. Histomorphometric analysis of a calcaneal stress fracture: a possible complication of fluoride therapy for osteoporosis. Bone 1986; 7: 193-8.

68. Schulz EE, Engstrom H, Sauser DD, Baylink DJ. Osteoporosis: radiographic detection of fluoride-induced extra-axial bone formation. Radiology 1986; 159: 457-62.

69. Schulz EE, Libanati CR, Farley SM, Kirk GA, Baylink DJ. Skeletal scintigraphic changes in osteoporosis treated with sodium fluoride: concise communication. J Nucl Med 1984; 25: 651-5.

70. Susheela AK, Jha M. Cellular and histochemical characteristics of osteoid formed in experimental fluoride poisoning. Toxicol Lett 1983; 16: 35-40.

71. Søgaard CH, Mosekilde L, Richards A, Mosekilde L. Marked decreases in trabecular bone quality after five years of sodium fluoride therapy - assessed by biomechanical testing of iliac crest bone biopsies in osteoporotic patients. Bone 1994; 15: 393-9.

72. Taves DR. New approach to the treatment of bone disease with fluoride. Fed Proc 1970; 29: 1185-7.

73. Teotia M, Teotia SPS, Kunwar KB. Endemic skeletal fluorosis. Arch Dis Child, 1971; 46: 686-91.

74. Thiébaud M, Zender R, Courvoisier B, Baud CA, Jacot C. The action of fluoride on diffuse bone atrophies. In: Vischer TL, ed. Fluoride in medicine. Bern: Hans Huber 1970: 136-42.

75. Vesterby A, Gundersen HJG, Melsen F, Mosekilde L. Marrow space star volume in iliac crest decreases in osteoporotic patients after continuous treatment with fluoride, calcium and vitamin D_2 for five years. Bone 1991; 12: 33-7.

76. Vose GP, Keele DK, Milner AM, Rawley R, Roach TL, Sprinkle EE. Effect of sodium fluoride, inorganic phosphate, and oxymetholone, therapies

in osteoporosis: a six-year progress report. J Gerontol 1978; 33: 204-12.

77. Waterhouse C, Taves D, Munzer A. Serum inorganic fluoride: changes related to previous fluoride intake, renal function and bone resorption. Clin Sci 1980; 58: 145-52.

78. Wergedal JE, Lau KHW, Baylink DJ. Fluoride and bovine bone extract influence cell prolifera-

tion and phosphatase activities in human bone cell cultures. Clin Orthop 1988; 233: 274-82.

79. Whitford GM, Pashley DH. Fluoride absorption: the influence of gastric acidity. Calcif Tiss Int 1984; 36: 302-7.

CHAPTER 8

THE EFFECT OF FLUORIDE ON TOOTH MINERALIZATION

O. Fejerskov • A. Richards • P. DenBesten

Introduction

Dental fluorosis is as old as mankind. It can be observed in ancient skulls from areas in the "Near East", and Galén (131-201 AD) reported on the peculiar features of teeth which most likely had been developmentally disturbed/affected by fluoride (for Greek text see Koch et al.[58]).

In modern dentistry, however, we usually acknowledge that tooth changes caused by fluoride were first systematically reported on in 1916 when Black & McKay[11] described mottled enamel. They demonstrated the endemic nature of these enamel changes and suggested that mottled enamel could be related to the water supply in the endemic areas. Fluoride was later proved to be the cause in both man and experimental animals.

During the 1930s, Dean and coworkers con-ducted extensive epidemiologic surveys to establish the relationship between mottled enamel, or "chronic endemic dental fluorosis" as it was thereafter designated, and the level of fluoride in the water supplies. Dean suggested a classification of each person into one of seven categories depending on the degree of enamel changes (see p. 120). Although his proposals were later modified, it is remarkable that Dean's method of classification, even today, influences concepts of how fluoride affects dental enamel during formation.

When it became evident that low concentrations of fluoride in the water supplies were also associated with lower-than-expected caries experience, Dean's method of scoring dental fluorosis became an important tool in reductions of caries experience without causing "unacceptable" dental fluorosis. This led to an ongoing discussion of how to define what was seen at the time as an "optimal" dose of fluoride. Because the early research on the health effects of waterborne fluoride showed no general health problems associated with the mildest forms of fluorosis (Chapter 15), dental fluorosis came to be considered a public health problem only if it was esthetically unacceptable. Interpretation of subsequent fluorosis research has at times been confused because some researchers see any fluorosis as a problem whereas others view only "unesthetic" fluorosis that way. These philosophical differences are not always explicitly stated, and yet the clinical differences represent quite different levels of fluoride intake during tooth development. To fully appreciate how fluoride affects the forming tissues, the gradient of early changes in the enamel, indicating a biological effect of fluoride, needs to be examined.

To do this, a clinical classification system (the TF-index) has been developed, based on the histopathology of dental fluorosis in human teeth. In this chapter, our present knowledge of human dental fluorosis in its various aspects is presented, and by combining human data with recent information from animal studies, we will discuss possible mechanisms of action of fluoride on amelogenesis.

Clinical features of dental fluorosis

Long-term intake of fluoride during enamel formation results in a continuum of clinical changes of the enamel varying from fine white lines in the enamel to severely chalky, opaque, enamel which breaks apart soon after tooth eruption. The severity of changes depends on the amount of fluoride ingested during the long period of tooth formation. In the following, the principal characteristics of dental fluorosis will be described as they appear on the single tooth surface from the mildest to the most severe forms.

Clinical features of increasing severity

The first signs of dental fluorosis are thin white striae across the enamel surface. The fine, opaque lines follow the perikymata pattern and can best be distinguished after drying the surface of the tooth (Fig. 8-1). If the surface is covered with plaque, it must be cleaned, for example with a cotton wool roll. Even at this stage of dental fluorosis, the cusp tips, incisal edge or marginal ridges may appear opaque white, the "snow cap phenomenon" (Fig. 8-2).

In slightly more affected teeth, the fine white lines are broader and more pronounced. Occasional merging of several lines occurs to produce smaller, irregular, cloudy or paper-white areas scattered over the surface (Fig. 8-3). These changes may be recorded without drying the teeth, but they become more evident after wiping and drying the tooth surface.

In these early manifestations of dental fluorosis it should be appreciated that the enamel changes may vary somewhat along the surface. This is a reflection of i) the structural composition of the enamel and ii) the variation in enamel thickness, combined with iii) the presence and variation in thickness of the underlying dentin. Along incisal edges, cusp tips and marginal ridges the arrangement of enamel rods is very irregular and there is no underlying dentin. Hence, these parts will exhibit signs of fluorosis more easily. Moreover, crystal and prism arrangement varies in the outermost enamel between individuals and within the single tooth[52] so a slight increase in tissue porosity (opacities) of the same degree may manifest itself differently on different parts of the tooth surface.

With increasing severity, the entire tooth surface exhibits distinct, irregular, opaque or cloudy white areas. Between these irregular opacities, accentuated perikymata lines are often visible (Fig. 8-4). Certain variations may occur at this stage of severity, as a result of the above-mentioned variations in tooth structure.

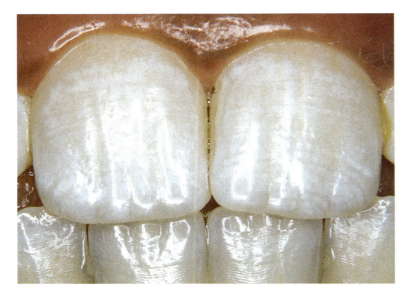

Fig. 8-1. The earliest clinical sign of dental fluorosis appears as thin white opaque lines running across the tooth surface corresponding to the position of the perikymata. An example of TF score 1, from a child born and raised in East Africa in an area with 0.7-0.8 ppm fluoride in the water supply.

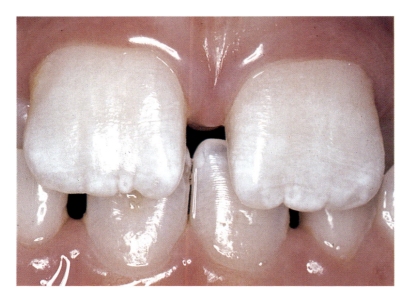

Fig. 8-2. In addition to the thin white opaque lines, the earliest signs of dental fluorosis may also include small opaque white areas along cusp tips, incisal edges or marginal ridges. From a Danish child living in an area with 0.2 ppm fluoride in the water supplies who has daily, since the age of about 1 year, swallowed toothpaste after toothbrushing (a toothpaste containing 1000 ppm fluoride).

Frequently the cervical enamel appears more homogeneously opaque, and the mesio-incisal part of the maxillary incisors may exhibit various degrees of brownish discoloration (Fig. 8-5). Such brown stains are a result of posteruptive staining. In rare cases, the patchy, cloudy areas may exhibit small surface enamel defects because of damage to the surface layer covering particularly pronounced subsurface porosity of the tissue.

The next degree of severity manifests as irregular opaque areas which merge so that the

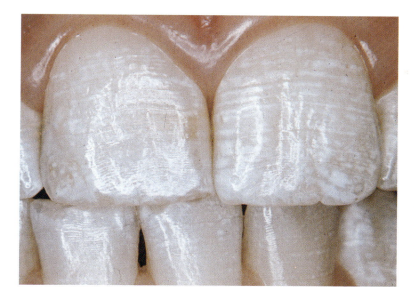

Fig. 8-3. In TF score 2 the opaque white lines are more pronounced and frequently merge to form wider bands. From a Danish child born and raised in an area with 1.4 ppm fluoride in the water supplies.

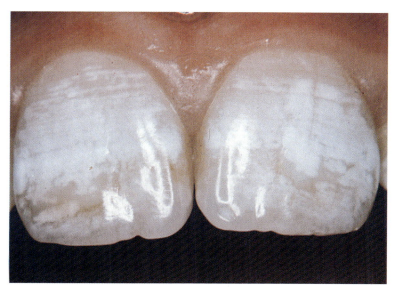

Fig. 8-4. An example of TF score 3. The entire tooth surface exhibits cloudy, white opaque areas between which accentuated perikymata lines are evident. From a child born and raised in Denmark with 2.1 ppm in the water supply.

entire tooth surface appears chalky white (Figs. 8-6, 8-7). At the time of eruption, this stage may vary clinically from a white opaque tooth which feels relatively hard on probing, to a totally chalky tooth which immediately following eruption exhibits surface damage. When such surfaces are probed vigorously, part of the surface enamel may flake off.

In even more severe stages, the tooth surface is entirely opaque with focal loss of the outermost enamel. Such small enamel defects are usually designated "pits" (Figs. 8-6, 8-8). The

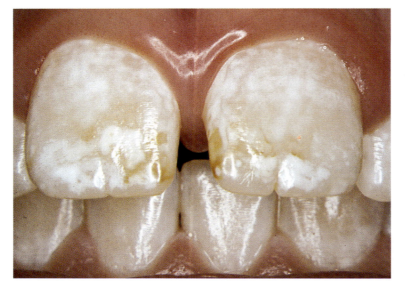

Fig. 8-5. A case classified as TF score 3 exhibiting a brownish discoloration at the mesio-incisal part of the maxillary incisors in addition to an overall cloudy opaque appearance of the surface of the tooth. From a child living in a low fluoride area in Switzerland but having followed the local fluoride supplement scheme from 1½ years until 6 years of age.

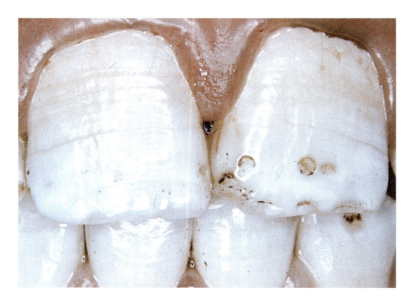

Fig. 8-6. An example of TF score 4 (maxillary right incisor) and score 5 with distinct pitting (maxillary left incisor). The entire tooth surface appears opaque white. An adolescent born and raised in Tanzania in an area with 2.8-3.0 ppm in the water supply.

pits may vary in diameter and occur scattered over the surface, although most frequently they occur along the incisal/occlusal half of the tooth. With increasing severity these pits merge to form horizontal bands. In more severely affected teeth, confluence of the pitted areas produces larger "corroded" areas (Figs. 8-8, 8-9, 8-10). Along the incisal edges and cusps, the surface enamel often flakes off. The pits and other damaged areas frequently appear discolored.

Ultimately, the most severely fluorotic teeth

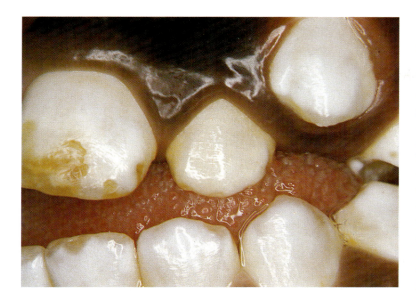

Fig. 8-7. Examples of teeth classified as TF score 4 (maxillary left lateral and canine, mandibular left canine and first premolar). The maxillary left central incisor represents an example of TF score 7. Notice that at time of eruption, even in severely fluorosed areas, teeth erupt entirely chalky white, but immediately following eruption, surface damage occurs. From an East African child born and raised in an area with 5.0-5.4 ppm fluoride in water supplies.

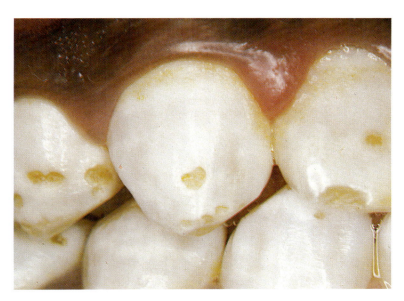

Fig. 8-8. Examples of tooth surfaces classified as TF score 7 (maxillary right premolar), TF score 5 (maxillary right canine) and TF score 6 (maxillary lateral incisor). Notice that in addition to the posteruptive damage, the entire tooth crown appears chalky white. From an East African child born and raised in an area with 6.0-6.2 ppm fluoride in the water supply.

exhibit an almost total loss of surface enamel whereby the normal tooth morphology is severely affected (Fig. 8-11). The loss of surface enamel may be so extensive that only a cervical rim of intact, markedly opaque enamel is left. The remaining part of the tooth often exhibits a dark brownish discoloration. The discoloration is entirely dependent on such posteruptive environmental conditions as dietary habits, and the degree of discoloration should, therefore, not be used as an indication of severity of fluorosis as such.

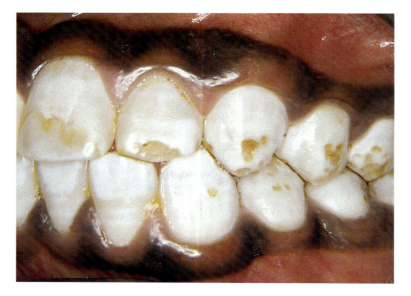

Figs. 8-9, 8-10. Examples of tooth surfaces exhibiting posteruptive damage classified as TF score 7. Notice the irregular loss of the outermost enamel where the exposed areas take up brownish stain. From children born and raised in East Africa in an area with about 6.0 ppm fluoride in the water supply.

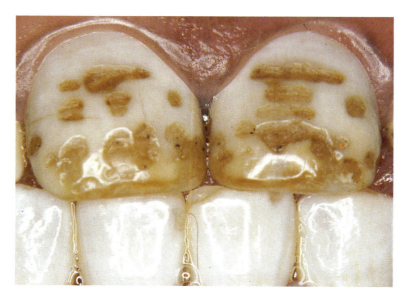

Fig 8-10.

When the teeth are highly opaque at the time of eruption, they are very susceptible to attrition and extensive occlusal abrasion is often observed in high fluoride areas even in young individuals (Fig. 8-12).

It is important to emphasize that the loss of enamel in dental fluorosis, whether focal or extensive, involves only the surface enamel and not the full thickness of the enamel.

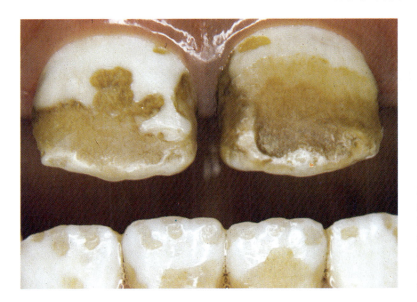

Fig. 8-11. Maxillary central incisors exhibiting TF scores 8 (maxillary right incisor) and TF score 9 (maxillary left incisor). From an East African child living in an area with 6.4 ppm fluoride in the water supply.

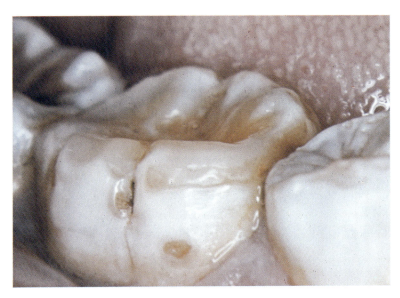

Fig. 8-12. In areas where the teeth are highly porous and opaque at time of eruption, extensive occlusal abrasion occurs shortly after eruption. Note pitting of white opaque buccal surface. From an East African child born and raised in an area with about 5.0 ppm fluoride in the water supply.

Table 8-1

Score	
0.	The normal translucency of the glossy creamy-white enamel remains after wiping and drying of the surface.
1.	Thin white opaque lines are seen running across the tooth surface. Such lines are found on all parts of the surface. The lines correspond to the position of the perikymata. In some cases, a slight "snowcapping" of cusps/incisal edges may also be seen.
2.	The opaque white lines are more pronounced and frequently merge to form small cloudy areas scattered over the whole surface. "Snowcapping" of incisal edges and cusp tips is common.
3.	Merging of the white lines occurs, and cloudy areas of opacity occur spread over many parts of the surface. In between the cloudy areas, white lines can also be seen.
4.	The entire surface exhibits a marked opacity, or appears chalky white. Parts of the surface exposed to attrition or wear may appear to be less affected.
5.	The entire surface is opaque, and there are round pits (focal loss of outermost enamel) that are *less than* 2 mm in diameter.
6.	The small pits may frequently be seen merging in the opaque enamel to form bands that are less than 2 mm in vertical height. In this class are included also surfaces where the cuspal rim of facial enamel has been chipped off, and the vertical dimension of the resulting damage is *less than* 2 mm.
7.	There is a loss of the outermost enamel in irregular areas, and *less than* half the surface is so involved. The remaining intact enamel is opaque.
8.	The loss of the outermost enamel involves more than half the enamel. The remaining intact enamel is opaque.
9.	The loss of the major part of the outer enamel results in a change of the anatomic shape of the surface/tooth. A cervical rim of opaque enamel is often noted.

From Fejerskov et al.[41] As modified from the original work by Thylstrup, Fejerskov 1978.[100]

Classification systems

The TF classification

Based on this description of various degrees of severity of dental fluorosis, the enamel changes as observed on the single tooth surface can be arranged into 10 classes (Table 8-1) where a score ranging from 0 (normal) to 9 is assigned to each degree of enamel change (compare also with schematic drawings in Fig. 8-13).[41,100] The single score represents a measurement on an ordinal scale and should, therefore, only be regarded as an arbitrary point along the continuum of macroscopic changes. The usefulness and limitations of such a scoring system will be discussed later in this chapter. This classification system will be referred to as the TF-index.

Dean's classification

Dean originally classified mottled enamel ranging from 0 ("normal") to 7 ("severe").[28] The scores in between comprised the stages "questionable", "very mild", "mild", "moderate", and "moderately severe". Later, Dean combined "moderately severe" and "severe" into one score, now designated "severe".[27] This latter category includes all enamel surfaces exhibiting any type of surface destructions, irrespective of their degree and is, thus, unable to

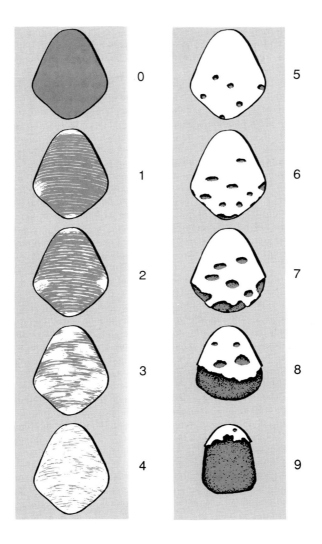

Fig. 8-13. Diagrammatic illustration of the clinical features of dental fluorosis from its mildest form –
TF score 1 to the most severe score – TF score 9. Compare with the description in Table 8-1.

distinguish between scores 5-9 of the TF-index. In the milder forms of fluorosis, Dean apparently did not realize that the entire tooth surface is affected (see also the histopathology of the early stage, p. 124) and, therefore, he distin-guished between "very mild" and "moderate", depending on the amount of tooth surface involved.

Dean's score "questionable" continues to cause considerable confusion. This score was

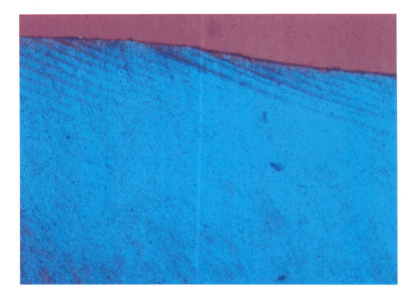

Fig. 8-14. Microphotograph of a tooth scored TF 1. The bluish color indicates normal enamel porosity (≤ 0.1% pore volume). Notice the reddish color along the lines of Retzius running towards the surface. The color indicates a pore volume in this area of about 5% or less. The section examined in polarized light after imbibition of the section in water.

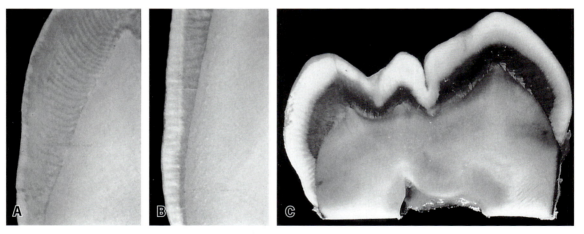

Fig. 8-15. Ground sections of teeth examined in transmitted light. Notice how the early stages of dental fluorosis (A) exhibit a porous zone in the outermost enamel. With increasing severity this zone of porosity extends deeper into the enamel (B) and in very severe cases the porosity extends deep into the enamel tissue along the entire tooth crown (C) and in cervical areas extends to the enamel dentin junction.

utilized where a definite diagnosis of the mildest form of fluorosis was not warranted and the classification of "normal" not justified. There is no doubt that the score also included enamel opacities of non-fluoride cause in addition to fluoride-induced enamel changes. As an example, Dean drew attention to the fact that the white opaque cusps in his earlier studies were classified as "questionable" whereas they were later invariably listed under the category

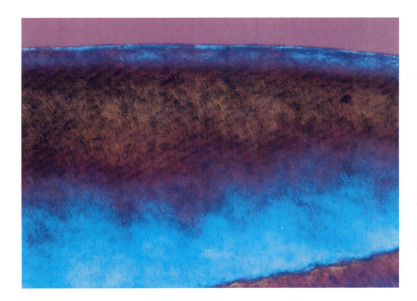

Fig. 8-16. Microphotograph of a tooth scored TF 4. The ground section is examined in polarized light after imbibition in water. The brownish red areas deep to the surface represent areas of 10% pore volume or more.

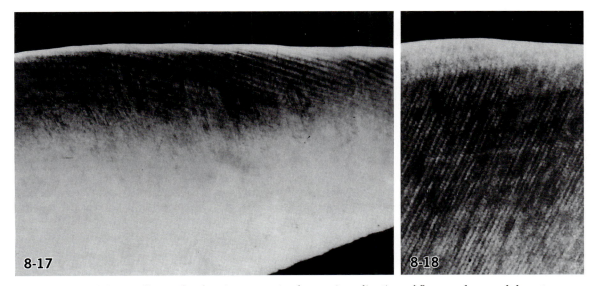

8-17

8-18

Figs. 8-17, 8-18. Microradiographs showing extensive hypomineralization of fluorosed enamel deep to a well-mineralized surface zone. Notice the classical rod pattern in the enamel with cross-striation as well as the incremental lines of Retzius.

"very mild". Wenzel & Thylstrup,[107] who used Dean's index, as well as the TF-index, observed a number of teeth which were assigned the score "questionable" according to Dean's classification whereas they were classified as normal in the TF-index, i.e. the opacities present were considered non-fluorotic.

In a subsequent analysis of data from a number of studies in which Dean's index was used, Myers[71] showed that the prevalence of the "questionable" category of Dean's index is positively associated with fluoride levels in water supplies. These findings further support that former doubts about the nature of the "questionable" category are no longer justified.

Other fluorosis indexes

Other classification systems such as the Tooth Surface Fluorosis Index (TSFI)[51] and Fluorosis Risk Index (FRI)[73] have been developed. The TSFI, which combines elements from Dean's and the TF classifications, emphasizes cosmetic appearance by examining the teeth without drying them. This index may be relevant to studies of the cosmetic appearance of fluorosis. The FRI relates the risk of dental fluorosis to the timing of tooth development and may be used to address the time at which fluoride exposure occurred. As such it may be appropriate for epidemiologic studies to identify risk factors.

Histopathology of dental fluorosis

The changes in fluorotic human enamel have been described using light and electron microscopy. However, the numbers of teeth examined in most of the reports are very limited and unfortunately most authors have not assigned a clinical degree of fluorosis to the teeth examined. So far, the TF-index represents the only attempt to correlate the clinical appearance of various degrees of fluorosis to the pathologic changes in the tissue.

In principle, increased ingestion of fluoride during tooth formation leads to an increase in enamel porosity. TF-score 1 is a result of increased porosity along the striae of Retzius in the outer enamel surface as seen in ground sections examined in the polarized light microscope (Fig. 8-14). In specimens assigned TF-score 2, the striae of Retzius are even more pronounced, and a continuous narrow zone of po-

rosity is seen along the surface enamel (Fig. 8-15). The pore volume in the striae of Retzius in such cases amounts to about 5%. Of particular interest in teeth scored TF 1 and 2 is the fact that the thin cervical enamel and cusp tips/incisal edges, due to their structural characteristics, often exhibit a more uniform porosity. This may explain why this part of the crown occasionally appears clinically more homogeneously opaque. Ground sections from teeth exhibiting TF-score 3 show a 80-100 μm broad, porous subsurface zone exhibiting a pore volume which exceeds 5%. These porous areas are observed as a continuous zone varying in degree of porosity, but running over the entire surface of the tooth from the cervical edge to the cusps and occlusal surfaces (Fig. 8-15).

The changes that are clinically assigned to TF-score 4 represent very extensive porous enamel lesions (10% or more pore volume) located deep to a well-mineralized surface layer about 50 μm in thickness (Fig. 8-16). The degree of porosity and the depth of the lesions vary, depending on the fluoride exposure. The chalky appearance of the teeth thus affected at time of eruption reflects the degree of porosity.

In very severely affected teeth the subsurface pore volume exceeds 25% at time of eruption and the lesions extend almost to the enamel-dentin junction in the cervical region. In the occlusal part of the teeth, the degree of porosity decreases towards the inner half of the enamel (Fig. 8-15).

The porous areas are highly hypomineralized, as seen on microradiographs (Figs. 8-17, 8-18). When enamel from these areas is examined in the transmission electron microscope it is apparent that the hypomineralization, or increased porosity, is a result of an increase in intercrystalline spaces both in rod and interrod enamel, but is particularly pronounced along the arcade-shaped rod boundaries (Fig. 8-19). The width, thickness and cross-sectional shape of the individual enamel crystals are within the normal range (Fig. 8-21).

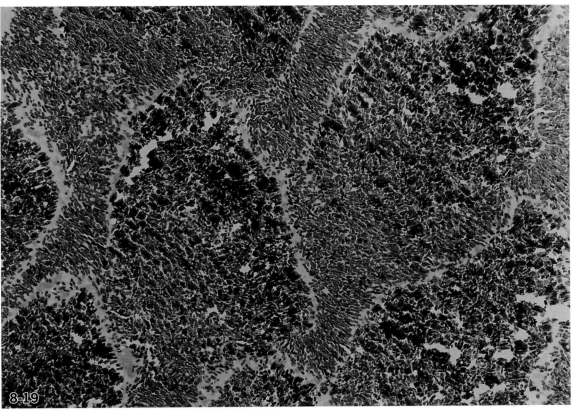

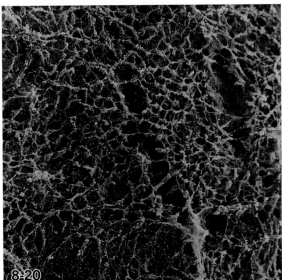

Fig. 8-19. Transmission electron micrograph of severely fluorotic enamel. In both rod and interrod enamel the individual crystals are clearly visible separated by extensive intercrystalline spaces. The rods are separated from interrod enamel by arcade-shaped boundaries.

Fig. 8-20. Scanning electron micrograph of demineralized human fluorotic enamel showing the network of insoluble protein of highly porous enamel. From Thylstrup 1979.[99]

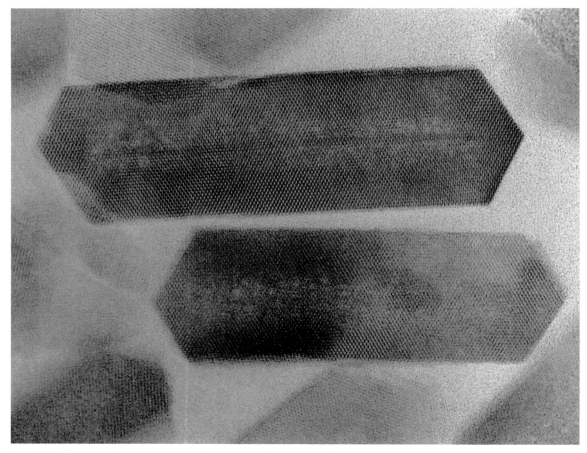

Fig. 8-21. High resolution electron micrograph of two enamel crystals sectioned perpendicular to the C-axis from human fluorotic enamel. Notice the distinct lattice pattern. A central dark line can be observed in the largest crystal. Courtesy of Dr. H. Tohda, Tokyo.

The intercrystalline spaces are occupied by water and protein, the insoluble part of which may be visualized even in the scanning electron microscope as a fine network after demineralization of the enamel (Fig. 8-20).

It is evident that the more extensive the zone of hypomineralization, deep to a mineralized thin surface layer, the more susceptible the enamel will be to posteruptive damage. Histologically, the pits in TF-scores 5 and 6 represent "punched out" areas in the enamel surface when observed in microradiographs and in the scanning electron microscope (Figs. 8-22, 8-23). In the microradiographs, significant changes are observed in the porous enamel which has been exposed to the oral environment. Thus, it seems as if a considerable mineral acquisition takes place when the intact enamel surface is removed. In TF-scores 7-9 virtually all the porous enamel has become exposed to the oral environment due to breakdown of the surface layer and this results in highly irregular mine-

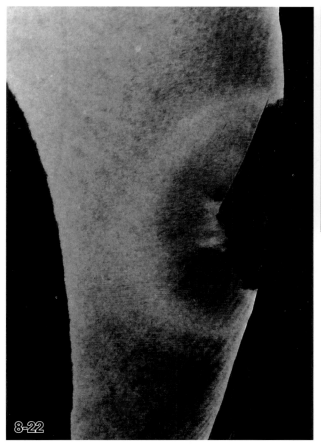

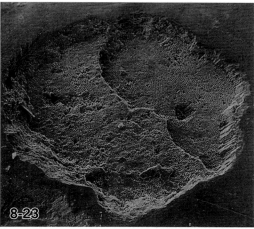

Fig. 8-22. Microradiograph of fluorotic human tooth with large pitted area. Deep within the enamel the subsurface porous enamel at the bottom of the pit exhibits a half-moonshaped zone of higher mineral content.

Fig. 8-23. Scanning electron micrograph of fluorotic pit, which appears as a punched out area. At the bottom of the pit the layering within the enamel is reflected, corresponding to the opening of a line of Retzius. From Thylstrup, Fejerskov 1979.[101]

ral distribution in the remaining enamel (Figs. 8-24, 8-25) as well as pronounced irregularity in crystal size and shape (Figs. 8-26, 8-27).

In the milder forms of dental fluorosis, it is only possible to record histologic changes in the enamel, but the dentin is also affected in the more severe cases (Fig. 8-28). These changes are reflected in an enhancement of the lines of von Ebner and are particularly evident in the pulpal part of the dentin, which is obviously hypomineralized.

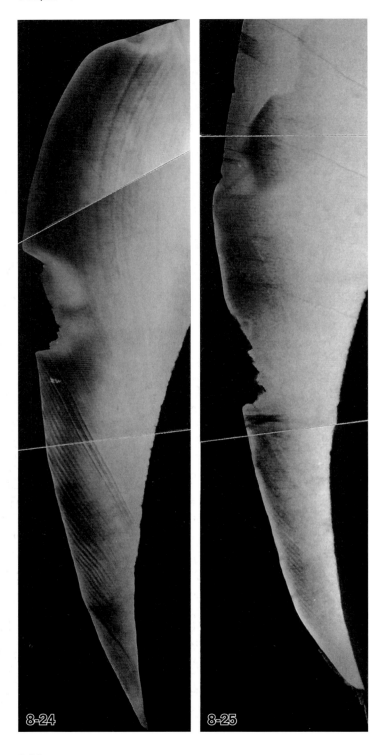

Figs. 8-24, 8-25. Two micrographs from severely fluorotic teeth (TF score 7). Notice the extensive subsurface hypomineralized areas which are exposed corresponding to larger pitted areas. At the bottom of these exposed areas, the enamel exhibits a higher mineral content indicative of a posteruptive mineral uptake subsequent to surface damage. From Fejerskov *et al.* 1991.[46]

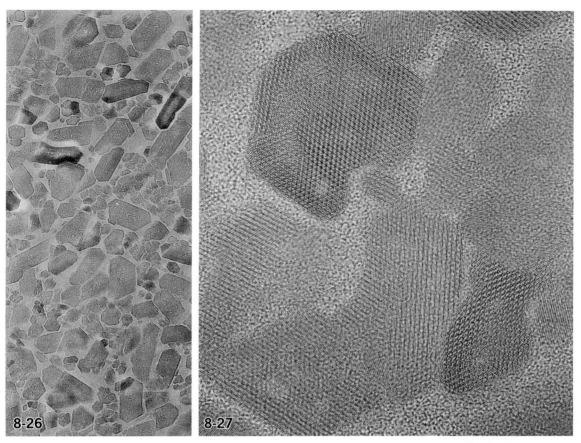

Figs. 8-26, 8-27. Transmission electron micrographs from the surface zone of severely fluorotic human enamel showing enamel crystals varying extensively in shape and size indicative of a substantial posteruptive transformation. From Yanagisawa *et al*. 1989.[110]

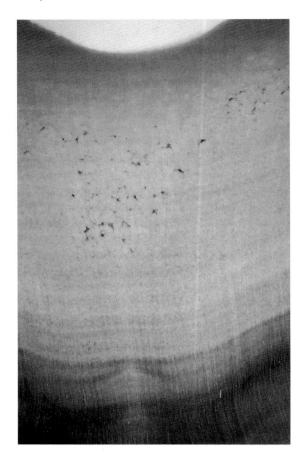

Fig. 8-28. Microradiograph of severely fluorotic human molar demonstrating an extensive enhancement of incremental pattern in the dentin which is particularly enhanced as a result of bands of hypomineralization towards the pulp. From Fejerskov *et al.* 1977.[44]

Chemical and biochemical aspects of dental fluorosis

The distribution of fluoride in teeth is dealt with in great detail in Chapter 5. However, a few additional data will be given with special emphasis on dental fluorosis. In teeth with fluorosis of increasing clinical severity, a distinct increase in fluoride concentrations is found not only in the superficial enamel layers, but also deeper in the enamel (Figs. 8-29, 8-30). It is not surprising that when dealing with teeth exhibiting severe posteruptive surface destruction a highly irregular fluoride concentration is

found, which most likely reflects a posteruptive uptake of fluoride from the oral environment by the exposed porous tissue.

Some recent results of the fluoride content in the outermost surface enamel in mild forms of dental fluorosis are of interest. In a study where children born and reared in a fluoride area with 1.5-2.0 ppm fluoride in the water supplies were compared with children born and reared in areas with less than 0.7 ppm water fluoride, enamel biopsies were taken from all buccal surfaces in the maxilla and the buccal surfaces were scored according to the TF-index.[63] For each tooth type there was an increase in fluoride content of the surface enamel with an

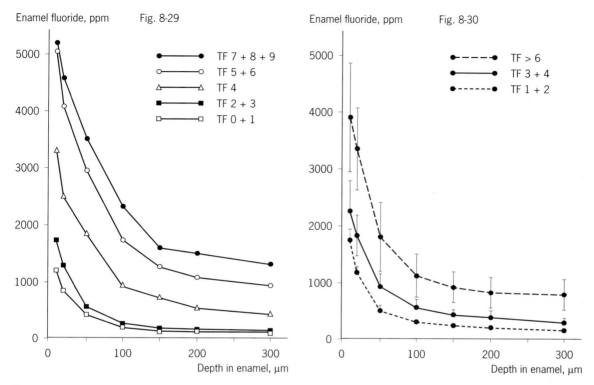

Figs. 8-29, 8-30. Enamel fluoride concentrations measured from the surface of the enamel into a depth of 300 microns into the enamel in erupted (Fig. 8-29) and unerupted (Fig. 8-30) fluorotic teeth of different severity. Notice that with increasing severity the fluoride concentrations in the outermost layers increase substantially. Moreover, even in the inner bulk of the enamel, there is a significant increase in fluoride content with increasing severity of fluorosis. From Richards *et al.* 1989[74], Richards *et al.* 1992.[79]

increase in TF-scores 1-3. When studying all tooth types in the maxilla, it was evident that the pattern of surface fluoride concentration did not differ for any tooth type, but the fluoride levels in the maxillary first molars were constantly higher than those observed in premolars exhibiting the same degree of fluorosis. These data indicate that there is an association between increasing degrees of fluorosis and an increase in both surface and total enamel fluoride content.

Fluorosed enamel contains more protein in the porous tissue than does normal, non-fluorosed enamel. During maturation, relatively fewer amelogenins than enamelins are lost by the fluorosed enamel. The resulting fluorosed enamel retains a relatively high proportion of immature matrix proteins, i.e. it appears that the amelogenins may not be degraded to the same extent as in the normal mature enamel.[36]

No studies are available which allow definite conclusions concerning biochemical changes in fluorosed dentin as compared to normal dentin. Some studies have suggested changes in the proteoglycan structure and composition of fluorosed rat and human dentin[88,95,103], although the relative significance of these findings is obscure.

131

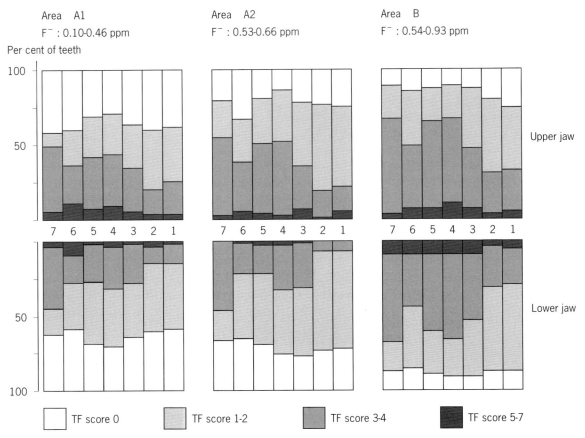

Fig. 8-31. Diagram of distribution of fluorosis scores according to the TF index within the dentition in three Kenyan populations born and raised in areas with only slight differences in water fluoride concentrations. From Manji *et al.* 1986.[69]

Assessment of dental fluorosis within individuals and populations

Distribution within the permanent dentition

Because dental fluorosis is of developmental origin it is expected that homologous tooth surfaces will display the same degree of enamel changes. Moreover, all surfaces of a given tooth exposed preeruptively for the same time period exhibit the same degree of dental fluorosis at the time of eruption. However, as the different surfaces will inevitably be exposed to various types of posteruptive challenge (attrition etc.), it is not to be expected that exactly the same score will be assigned to all surfaces in teeth which have been exposed to the oral environment for the same period.

The posterior teeth, in severely affected populations, are more affected than are the anterior teeth in both the maxilla and mandible.[100] In low-fluoride areas, however, this pattern is slightly different. Fig. 8-31 shows for

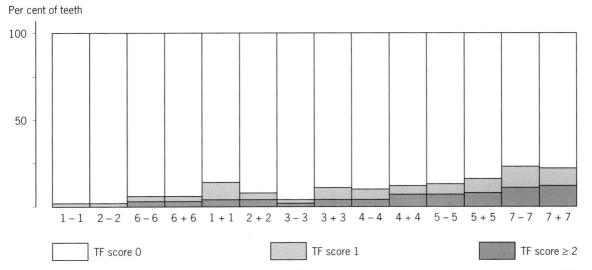

Per cent of teeth

TF score 0   TF score 1   TF score ≥ 2

Fig. 8-32. Diagram showing the percentage of teeth exhibiting dental fluorosis as scored according to the TF classification. The tooth types are ranked from left to right in the order of mineralization. The data originate from children born and raised in an area of Denmark with less than 0.1 ppm fluoride in the drinking water. From Larsen *et al.* 1985.[62]

every tooth type the proportion of teeth according to severity of fluorosis from three very low-fluoride areas in Eastern Africa. In all three areas, it is apparent that the incisors and the first molars are the least affected, and the second molars and the premolars the most affected. A similar trend is known from low-fluoride areas in industrialized countries. In Fig. 8-32 the percentage prevalence of dental fluorosis within each tooth type of the dentition in a very low fluoride area in Denmark (0.1 ppm) is illustrated. It is apparent that the teeth which mineralize early in life develop less dental fluorosis. This means that the later any given tooth undergoes mineralization, the greater will be the prevalence and severity of dental fluorosis of that particular tooth type. These observations are in strict accordance with the observation already presented in 1936 by Dean & El-vove[28] who demonstrated that premolars and second molars even in low fluoride areas show manifestations of mild dental fluorosis. These

teeth are "calcified at a somewhat later state" and these authors indicated that the findings are "suggestive of accumulative action of fluorine".

Distribution within the primary dentition

Given the above statement of an association between period of mineralization of the individual teeth and severity of fluorosis, and assuming a constant exposure to fluoride , it is not surprising that dental fluorosis has seldom been reported in primary teeth. In Fig. 8-33 the degree of fluorosis in permanent first molars and primary second molars in the mandible of children 4-5 and 7-10 years old from a high fluoride area in Eastern Africa is seen. Among the oldest children a relatively invariable pattern is noted, in contrast to the observations in the younger children. Four children in the younger age group showed an apparent inverse pattern between the permanent and primary teeth with the permanent molar being the

133

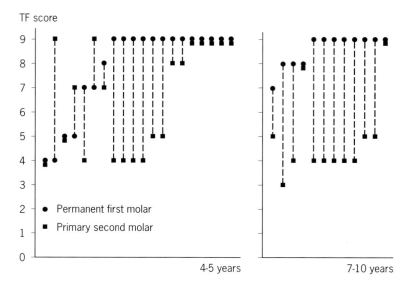

Fig. 8-33. Dental fluorosis scored according to the TF index in the first permanent molar (dark circle), and in primary second molars (dark square) within the same child in the right half of the mandible. The children were 4-5 and 7-10 years old living in a high fluoride area of Tanzania. From Thylstrup 1978.[98]

least affected. However, this pattern was only found with newly erupted permanent molars. This is an excellent example of the effect of posteruptive damage to severely hypomineralized fluorotic teeth. Even in areas with severe fluorosis, erupting permanent molars do not exhibit any sign of pit formation, in contrast to the primary molars, which have been in functional occlusion for a period of time.

It can thus be concluded that the primary teeth exhibit less dental fluorosis than their permanent successors, but the distribution within the dentition follows a very similar pattern. From a diagnostic point of view, it is important that while the more severe grades are easy to diagnose, the assessment of mild dental fluorosis in primary teeth is more difficult because of the thinner enamel, which normally has a more whitish appearance than that of permanent teeth. In addition, as the incremental pattern of Retzius is often lacking or much less pronounced than in permanent teeth, the milder degrees of fluorosis are not as characteristic in primary teeth as in their permanent successors.

Posteruptive changes in dental fluorosis

Posteruptive challenges will modify the appearance of the porous enamel tissue. As already described, the tooth erupts with an intact enamel surface, but the degree of subsurface porosity determines the subsequent posteruptive clinical features of that particular tooth. Thus, if the degree of porosity is so extensive at the time of eruption that the hypomineralized fluorotic enamel is covered only by a relatively thin, but well-mineralized surface layer, the tooth will be very susceptible to mechanical trauma. Pitting occurs shortly after eruption, often leading to more extensive surface destruction depending on the initial degree of hypomineralization. As seen from Fig. 8-7, this damage may occur shortly after the tooth merges into the oral cavity, but in populations with a certain severity of fluorosis within the dentition, the posteruptive breakdown of the outer enamel may continue gradually over several years.

If the degree of subsurface porosity at the time of eruption is not so severe that the surface enamel flakes off, the tooth may nevertheless

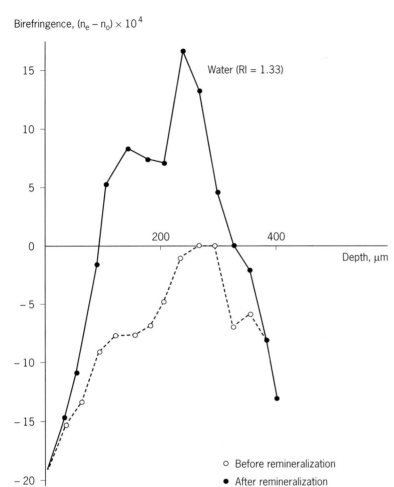

Birefringence, $(n_e - n_o) \times 10^4$

Water (RI = 1.33)

Depth, μm

○ Before remineralization
● After remineralization

Fig. 8-34. Imbibition graphs through the porous fluorotic enamel from the surface to a depth of 400 microns into the enamel. Birefringence is measured after immersion in water with a refractive index (RI) of 1.33 before (dark dot) and after (open dot) remineralization *in vitro*. Positive birefringence indicates 5% porevolume or more of the tissue. From Christensen *et al.* 1979.[19]

be very susceptible to enhanced attrition, as previously pointed out by Dean. In particular, the occlusal surfaces and the cusps may readily be worn down, whereby the whitish appearance of the enamel disappears at these sites. The porosity in the enamel of the anterior maxillary incisors gives rise to a particular cosmetic problem because even with an intact enamel surface the superficial part of the porous enamel may take up stains (Fig. 8-5). The shape of the discolored areas of the tooth usually follows the position of the border of the upper lip,

and it is likely that the continuous drying out of the incisal part of the maxillary incisors in combination with the immediate exposure of these teeth to any sort of staining from food makes them particularly susceptible to discoloration.

It should be remembered that in the milder forms of dental fluorosis the porosity is located in the outermost part of the enamel and even buccal surfaces exhibit with time a certain amount of wear which may be enough to diminish the opaque appearance of the tooth over time. This may give the impression of a de-

135

crease in severity of the milder degrees of fluorosis over time. This has also been suggested to be a result of "remineralization", but whether a mineral uptake into the porous enamel covered by a relatively well-mineralized surface layer is of any clinical significance, remains to be shown. In laboratory experiments, it has been shown that it is difficult even when using sections of severely fluorotic enamel to obtain any major mineral uptake, although a certain "remineralization" was demonstrated under these extreme conditions (Fig. 8-34).[19] The significant clinical change which may be obtained when slightly fluorotic and discolored teeth are exposed to intensive acid etching, polishing and topical fluoride treatments, is most likely a result of abrasion of the outer enamel (see treatment below).

Community index of dental fluorosis, F_{ci}

The occurrence of dental fluorosis in populations is still often recorded using Dean's classification, and usually expressed as the community index of dental fluorosis, F_{ci}. This community index was developed to facilitate a comparison of the degree of dental fluorosis in different populations and is calculated as the sum of individual scores (based on the most severely affected tooth group of an individual) divided by the number of individuals examined.

The basic problem with the F_{ci} is that the ordinal scale has a ratio scale tacked onto it, and that ratio scale is quite arbitrary. A ratio scale is defined as one which includes a true zero and in which the numbers on the scale purport to have a mathematical relation to each other. Score 1, for example, implies a condition that is twice as bad as 0.5, score 3 is three times as bad as 1, and so on. It is not clear whether Dean had this in mind when he assigned his F_{ci} numbers.

Dean was the first to emphasize that his proposed index should be validated by histologic studies of the effect of fluoride on the enamel.

As should now be apparent from the previous discussion, subsequent studies have shown that to some extent Dean's classification does coincide with histopathologic changes in the enamel. The inclusion of stained enamel in the severe category of Dean's index means that the index is not strictly a scale of increasing rank of severity. Thus, the use of the arithmetic mean may sometimes be misleading. It should also be appreciated that the arithmetic mean, being a summary number representing a central tendency, provides little information on the actual nature of the distribution of severity in a population, and F_{ci} should be referred to only as a broad indicator of relative group severity of fluorosis. By treating data such that each category of the index (whether Dean's or the TF-index) is descriptive, a much better appreciation of the effect of fluoride on enamel can be gained.

Frequency distribution and cumulative distribution of severity

A more accurate and reliable way of characterizing the severity of fluorosis in a population is, therefore, simply to present the frequency distribution of the various scores assigned to the buccal surface of the teeth known to be most severely affected in the population. An example of this is seen in Fig. 8-31 where the frequency distribution of children is presented in relation to scores of dental fluorosis on the buccal surface of the maxillary first premolar in three areas. Of course, a similar distribution can be made using the scores of the maxillary central incisor. It is evident, however, that if presenting the scores for the buccal surface of that tooth, only, an underestimation of the severity of fluorosis within the entire dentition will take place, unless the intraoral distribution of dental fluorosis is appreciated. *Therefore, when using frequency distributions it may be more useful to show the scores on both the maxillary central incisor and one of the premolars*, thereby demonstrating the severity of fluorosis in the popu-

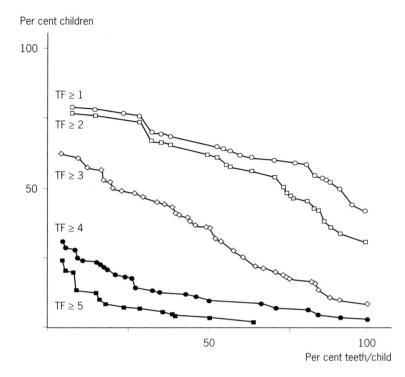

Fig. 8-35. Cumulative frequency distribution curves of the proportion of teeth per child exhibiting TF scores ≥ 1, 2, 3, 4 and 5, respectively in an area of East Africa. From Manji *et al.* 1986.[69]

lation and also recording the magnitude of cosmetic problems in that particular population.

Recently, a much more useful way of characterizing dental fluorosis in any population has been presented. As seen in Fig. 8-35 the idea is to show the *cumulative distribution of severity of scores* in any population. In this figure, data from the population in a 0.5-0.9 ppm fluoride area of Kenya is used and this way of presenting data allows an immediate estimation of the prevalence of the "disease" (percentage of individuals exhibiting fluorosis, irrespective of severity). At the same time, the percentage of individuals in relation to the percentage of teeth affected by any given severity of fluorosis can be read immediately. Thus, Fig. 8-35 shows that 78% of the children examined had at least one tooth with TF ≥ 1 (the prevalence of fluorosis). TF score 4 or higher was found in 31% of the children while teeth with TF ≥ 5 was seen in

about 25% of the children. Conversely, about 65% of the children had at least 50% of their teeth exhibiting TF ≥ 1, about 35% had at least 50% of their teeth exhibiting TF ≥ 3, and about 10% of the children had at least 15% of their teeth scored TF ≥ 5.

It can be concluded therefore that, at present, *the best way to assess the effect that fluoride has on tooth development in an individual or in a population is to use as sensitive a clinical scoring system as possible.* The TF-index records very initial stages of enamel changes and is the only index developed on known pathology of the tissue changes. By using either frequency distribution of TF scores of individual teeth and/or the cumulative distribution of severity as mode of presentation, it will be possible to produce exact and comparable estimates of severity of dental fluorosis in various populations.

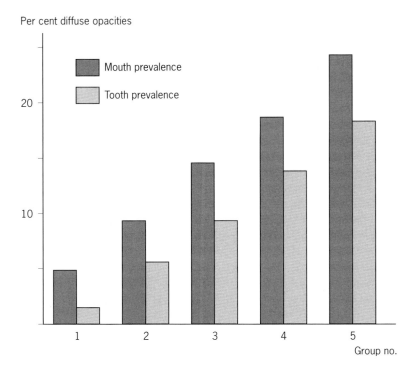

Per cent diffuse opacities

Group no.

Fig. 8-36. Prevalence of so-called diffuse types of enamel defects of permanent maxillary incisor teeth of 9-year-old children exposed since birth to various amounts of fluoride. Group 1 refers to naturally fluoridated drinking water with a fluoride concentration of less than 0.3 ppm; Group 2: same as Group 1, but also with a history of occasionally ingestion of F-tablets; Group 3: same as Group 1, but with regular F-tablet ingestion; Group 4: refers to drinking water artificially fluoridated to 1 ppm and Group 5 refers to 1 ppm fluoridated drinking water combined with ingestion of fluoride tablets (1 mg fluoride). From Cuttress *et al.* 1985.[25]

Variables affecting prevalence and severity of dental fluorosis

The prevalence and severity of dental fluorosis have been shown unequivocally to be directly related to the fluoride concentration in the drinking water as previously demonstrated.

However, it is the total amount of fluoride ingested, and in particular the amount which has become bioavailable, that is of importance. Therefore, the fluoride content of air, water, food and various caries preventive products determines the human intake of fluoride. In this context, it is relevant that the introduction of fluoride supplements in the form of tablets was based on the assumption that the "dose" should mimic what an average child was expected to ingest from so-called "optimally" fluoridated water. However, as stressed earlier in this chapter, the definition of the optimal con-

centration was based purely on empiricism, and it is therefore not surprising that several reports have shown a close association between fluoride tablet consumption and prevalence and severity of dental fluorosis[1,56,102] (for further discussion see Chapter 9). In a recent study of 9-year-old children in New Zealand,[25] it is apparent that the prevalence of what the authors designate "diffuse types of enamel defects" increases with fluoride exposure, irrespective of whether the fluoride originates mainly from water or from fluoride supplements (Fig. 8-36).

As this is not surprising, it is to be expected that the widespread use of fluoridated toothpaste in the industrialized countries may increase prevalence and severity of dental fluorosis in these countries. The use of toothpaste, however, varies from child to child, and based on available data it is difficult to get an exact idea of the magnitude of the problem (see

Chapter 9). In general, it should be remembered that it is the daily total fluoride intake over a prolonged period during the developmental phase of the teeth which determines the risk for developing dental fluorosis.

It is generally held that water requirements increase in hot climates and a number of studies have demonstrated more dental fluorosis in tropical than in temperate climates given the same level of waterborne fluoride. A formula has been suggested which could be used for calculation of the "optimal fluoride concentration" based on studies of fluid intake amongst children in California (see Chapter 9). It is, however, apparent that increased temperature and, thereby, expected increased water consumption, do not alone explain high prevalence and severity of fluorosis in very low-fluoride areas in developing countries.[67-69] As shown previously, a higher prevalence and severity of fluorosis has been found in Kenya than would be anticipated even when taking maximum annual temperature into account. Similar data have been published from other areas.[15] Recent studies in Tanzania suggest that this in some parts may be explained by certain dietary habits which result in much more fluoride ingested than what would be anticipated from the water content.[66]

It is important therefore to seek other explanations for this unexpectedly high susceptibility to rather low fluoride concentrations. The most commonly stated variable is that the nutritional status of the individuals plays a role. Although there are indications of an association between distinct malnutrition and increased susceptibility to dental fluorosis, no systematic studies in humans are available which clarify the exact mechanisms. As an example, in the East African studies, it is not possible to find any association at present between a group of children who may be characterized as malnourished and their degree of enamel changes in relation to fluoride. In all populations in developing countries, however,

it seems evident that the composition of the diet and daily eating habits are rather simple, with few meals. There is a severe lack of scientific data on the possible association of dietary habits, nutritional status and bioavailability of fluoride in children living in any country.

It has even been argued that the enamel changes observed in these populations may not be fluoride-induced. As will be discussed in the next section, however, *no other single etiologic factor has been identified so far which is associated with enamel changes identical to those of dental fluorosis.* It seems more likely that certain variables may modify the susceptibility of individuals to low concentrations of fluoride. There is no doubt that even in these populations there exists a strict association between an increased, although very low, fluoride concentration in the water supplies and an increase in enamel changes.

These observations show that the use of a so-called "optimal dose" of fluoride no longer seems relevant as far as the previous ways of estimating this concentration is concerned. In particular, it seems as if extrapolation from data mainly obtained in a few industrialized countries in the northern hemisphere cannot be justified when dealing with a decision as to the amount of fluoride to be considered "optimal" for caries prevention in most developing countries.

Differential diagnosis of dental fluorosis

It is frequently claimed that it is very difficult or almost impossible to discriminate between dental fluorosis and other enamel disturbances. The generalized nature of dental fluorosis within the dentition and over the entire tooth surface in fact makes it rather easy to distinguish fluoride-induced enamel changes from other defects which may be symmetrically dis-

Table 8-2
Differential diagnosis: Milder forms of dental fluorosis (TF scores 1-3) and enamel opacities of non-fluoride origin

Characteristics	Dental fluorosis	Enamel opacities
Area affected	The entire tooth surfaces (all surfaces) often enhanced on or near tips of cusps/incisal edges.	Usually centered in smooth surface of limited extent.
Lesion shape	Resemble line shading in pencil sketch which follow incremental lines in enamel (perikymata). Lines merging, and in score 3, a cloudy appearance. At cusps/incisal edges formation of irregular white caps ("snow cap").	Round or oval.
Demarcation	Diffuse distribution over the surface of varying intensity.	Clearly differentiated from adjacent normal enamel.
Colour	Opaque white lines or cludes; even a chalky appearance! "Snow caps" at cusps/incisal edges. Score 3 may become brownish discoloured at mesio-incisal part of central upper incisors after eruption.	White opaque or creamy-yellow to dark reddish-orange at time of eruption.
Teeth affected	Always on homologous teeth. Early erupting teeth (incisors/1st molars) least affected. Premolars and second molars (and third molars) most severely affected.	Most common on labial surfaces of single or occasionally homologous teeth. Any tooth may be affected but mostly incisors.

tributed in the oral cavity, but of non-fluoride origin (Table 8-2). Some authors have confused the matter by stating that it is extremely difficult to decide just how many cases of enamel fluorosis occurring in endemic areas are due to etiologic factors other than fluoride. However, up to now, no other single etiologic factor has been identified which is capable of causing diffuse symmetrically distributed opacities in man. To list the numerous etiologic factors which are able to produce localized opacities or other enamel defects in man is of course interesting, but from a differential diagnostic point of view this information is of limited use as certainly nobody trained in dentistry will risk mistaking enamel defects caused by medical or local infectious traumas for fluoride-induced enamel changes.

As a consequence of the concept that the nonspecific appearance of various mild degrees of dental fluorosis makes it impossible to associate these changes with fluoride, a descriptive classification system of developmental defects of dental enamel has been proposed for use in epidemiologic surveys.[20] When this classification system was used recently the only etiologic factor which could be identified as associated with any of the enamel changes recorded was fluoride. The fluoride history is positively associated with what in that classification system is defined as "diffuse types of enamel defects".

It can be concluded that although it is frequently claimed as difficult or even impossible to diagnose the early stages of dental fluorosis, this does not seem to be justified if a sensitive scoring system is used.

Finally, it has been claimed that in particular the TF-index is "oversensitive", identifying more enamel changes as fluoride-induced than do other indices because it requires cleaning and some drying of the tooth. It is important to

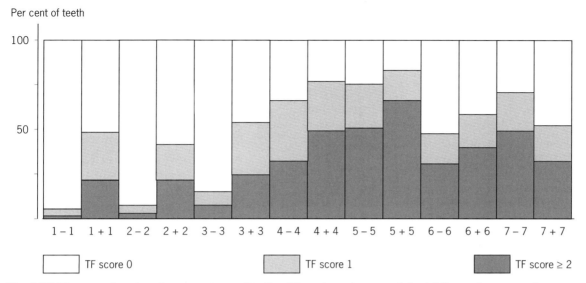

Fig. 8-37. Diagram showing the percentage of teeth with various degrees of dental fluorosis as scored according to the TF index in a Danish population living in an area with 1.5-2.0 ppm fluoride in the water supply. From Larsen *et al.* 1986.[63]

realize that although the initial changes induced by fluoride in the enamel may not be immediately visible without drying (just as with early carious lesions), they still represent the first biologic sign of an elevated intake of fluoride. Therefore, any index which is able to distinctively diagnose these will be of great public health importance. In this context, it is of interest to compare the prevalence of enamel changes using the TF-index in a Danish population living in an area with 1.5-2.0 ppm fluoride in the water supply with the prevalence of "diffuse types of enamel defects" observed in permanent maxillary incisor teeth of 9-year-old children in New Zealand living in a 1.0 ppm fluoridated area and in addition ingesting 1 mg of fluoride per day during tooth development. In the latter case, the percentage prevalence of diffuse opacities is about 25% (Fig. 8-36), which is indeed not very different from the prevalence of TF-score 2 in maxillary central incisors in the Danish population (Fig. 8-37). However, it should be stressed that this comparison can only be made between incisors. In the Danish study, it is apparent that if incisors are considered only, there is a rather strong underestimation of the actual prevalence and severity of fluorosis in the population when the most severely affected teeth in the dentition are taken into account. This emphasizes the statement already put forward by Dean that examination of age groups under 12 years of age (with few permanent teeth erupted) in areas where the fluoride content is relatively low introduces an error of considerable magnitude.

Possible mechanisms of action of fluoride on tooth formation

The major effects of fluoride throughout the body appear to occur in mineralizing tissues.

141

The fact that human dentin also exhibits hypo-mineralization in human fluorotic teeth[44] indicates that fluoride exerts its effect on very basic processes involved in biomineralization in general, irrespective of whether crystal formation and growth occurs in mesenchymally or ectodermally derived mineralized tissues. However, relatively little work has been done to identify the mechanisms by which low serum levels of fluoride which result in dental fluorosis affect the development of mineralizing tissues.

Mechanisms which have been proposed to explain the formation of fluorosed enamel include a systemic effect of fluoride on calcium homeostasis, altered matrix biosynthesis (protein secretion, synthesis or mineral composition), a direct or indirect effect on matrix proteinases affecting protein removal, and specific effects on cell metabolism and function. Most available evidence indicates that fluoride has an effect on cell function, either directly through interactions with the developing ameloblasts or more indirectly by interacting with the extracellular matrix. Although studies of humans consuming water with fluoride levels high enough to result in skeletal fluorosis show elevated levels of parathyroid hormone (PTH),[92,97] well-controlled animal studies investigating the effects of chronic ingestion of high levels of fluoride found no effects of fluoride on serum calcium and PTH.[3,59,87] These studies indicate that disturbances in calcium homeostasis which may occur at chronic exposure to high levels of fluoride are not an essential mechanism by which fluorosis occurs.[34]

Plasma fluoride in relation to oral dose and fluoride in the enamel
A number of reviewers have stressed the importance of use of doses of fluoride in animal experiments which are relevant to the human situation.[42,75,84] Relevant doses in this context should be assessed in terms of the fluoride exposure at the target organ, i.e. plasma fluoride

levels, because factors such as bioavailability and renal clearance may have a considerable effect on the oral dose given[37,108] (see Chapter 4).

In several recent animal experiments[4,5,32,33,77,93] the fasting plasma fluoride levels, when reported, were up to 12 µM F/L or when not measured may be estimated to have been below this level. Plasma levels of 10 or even 20 µM F/L have been reported in humans exposed to extremely high concentrations of 10 ppm or more of fluoride in the drinking water,[38,96] and it has been suggested[5,75] that plasma fluoride concentrations causing dental fluorosis in man and various animals may in fact be rather similar despite very different amounts of fluoride being ingested.

In contrast to enamel, the mineralizing bone tissue will not only gradually take up and accumulate fluoride, but also release fluoride during the processes of bone remodeling. Plasma fluoride concentrations will steadily increase even when the fluoride dose per kg body weight is kept constant.[37,78] This is important when extrapolating to the human situation because it indicates that the earlier in life the body is exposed to elevated fluoride levels (from water, infant formulas, supplements, etc.), the greater the risk of developing dental fluorosis.

This would also imply that the later in life enamel mineralization occurs, the more severe enamel fluorosis might be, even assuming a constant dose of fluoride from birth. The intraoral distribution of severity of fluorosis seems to support this hypothesis.[62,63]

The important implication is that the same amount of fluoride ingested daily by, for example children of 4-6 years of age and of the same weight may result in a very different risk of development of dental fluorosis depending on these children's previous (and not necessarily present!) fluoride exposure from birth from fluoridated water, infant F-tablet programs, etc.

The concentrations of fluoride may be higher in secretory enamel than in mature enamel, suggesting that a redistribution of fluoride takes place during enamel development.[91,105] Another explanation for the apparent loss of fluoride from the secretory enamel has been presented by Aoba et al.[6], who suggested that the rate of mineral uptake is slow at the beginning of the secretory phase. As the rate of mineral deposition subsequently increases, the amount of fluoride per unit mass of mineral deposited will decrease, provided the fluoride available for incorporation is constant. The apparent lowering of the fluoride content is then explained by dilution with low-F mineral. Chemically, this explanation is acceptable. A redistribution would require fluoride to be loosely bound to the crystals or even "leave" the apatite lattice without dissolution of mineral, contrary to the observations of only marginal fractions of the total fluoride in the tissue being present in either free ionic form or in labile forms.[9]

Single dose experiments

Acute single dose experiments in animals and man result in a hypermineralized band in enamel and dentin followed by a band of hypomineralization.[45] As the mechanisms of action of fluoride in such studies may be different from those associated with chronic exposure to low fluoride levels – as is the case when human fluorosis develops – the present discussion will focus on new knowledge obtained from studies in which animals have been exposed for longer periods of time to known levels of fluoride.

Protein synthesis and secretion

As long as the single pits and more severe defects observed in human dental fluorosis were interpreted as true hypoplasias, it was thought that the secretory ameloblast was particularly sensitive to fluoride, and most experimental studies were focused on possible effects of fluoride on enamel matrix secretion and composition (for review see Fejerskov et al.[44]). Early studies showed that uptake of radioactively labeled serine and proline in rats injected with fluoride was reduced.[60,61] However, later studies of rats ingesting fluoride in drinking water (chronic rather than acute exposure) found no difference in either protein or amino acid composition of animals exposed to fluoride in drinking water as compared to controls.[9,29]

Although the protein composition of secretory enamel is not altered, several studies have shown that high levels of fluoride exposure do inhibit protein synthesis[109] and reduce the total amount of secretory enamel present. Cell culture studies using fibroblasts[50] have indicated that fluoride has an effect on amino-acid transport, perhaps via coupled ATPase activity. There is some controversy, however, about the minimal levels of fluoride required to produce this effect. Such inhibition of amino-acid uptake could be responsible for the reported inhibition of protein synthesis.[109] In vitro studies by Bronckers & Wöltgens[14] have shown that fluoride levels up to 0.5 µM/L in the culture medium had little effect on ^{3}H proline incorporation into enamel proteins. Above this level, however, a reduction was observed. DenBesten & Crenshaw[31] also found that ingestion of high levels of fluoride in the drinking water by rats (100 ppm fluoride) reduced the total amount of secretory enamel. Therefore, it appears that at high levels of fluoride, the amount of protein secreted into the enamel matrix is reduced.

Mineral composition

The fluoride concentration of fluorotic human inner enamel is elevated compared to normal enamel. Recent studies by Richards et al.[76] using the pig model, showed that this inner enamel fluoride concentration is specifically raised when fluoride is administered during all phases of enamel development, even though fluorosis can occur with fluoride exposure during only the maturation stage of enamel development.[77] In this artificial situation, dental flu-

143

orosis may therefore be produced without this being reflected by increased fluoride accumulation in the bulk enamel.

Studies by Bronckers et al.[12,13] determined the effects of fluoride on mineralization in vitro using hamster molar tooth organ culture. They showed that fluoride in the media irreversibly affected the existing mineralizing matrix, producing a more rapid deposition and disruption of crystal growth. Secondly, fluoride in the media interfered with the deposition of crystal in the new matrix. However, when fluoride was removed, the matrix recovered and mineralized normally. These studies suggest that fluoride may interfere with initial nucleating sites in the matrix, perhaps by labile binding of the fluoride to the nucleating site in the matrix.[22]

Several investigators have suggested that the secretory enamel matrix proteins bind fluoride. The binding of fluoride by the secretory matrix may either alter enamel formation in the secretory stage or, as proposed by Crenshaw & Bawden,[21] may act as a reservoir for fluoride which is later released when proteins are hydrolyzed at the maturation stage. Later studies by the same investigators showed that with extensive dialysis, fluoride binding to the secretory matrix was eliminated,[64] challenging the hypothesis that secretory enamel matrix can act as a fluoride reservoir. However, recent studies of fluoride binding to rat secretory and maturation enamel following chronic ingestion of fluoride have suggested that fluoride is bound to enamel protein extracts, possibly related to calcium binding proteins. Aoba and co-workers[6] found that much of the fluoride associated with secretory enamel appears to be in labile form and it probably becomes available for incorporation into the mineral phase as amelogenins are lost and maturation proceeds.

The beginning of enamel maturation is defined by a secondary influx of mineral ions and is characterized by the white opaque zone first described in rat incisors by Hiller et al.[49]

and later shown to be present in most species.[82,83] However, recent studies[106] have shown that this opaque boundary is in fact located within the region of ameloblast modulation, i.e. is part of the area of enamel maturation. The white opaque zone and the preceding transitional enamel are also characterized by a selective uptake of fluoride,[105] possibly due to the high degree of hydration at this stage,[81,85] allowing free access to this tissue, or to some aspects of enamel organ permeability.[10] An increase in the influx of fluoride at this early-maturation stage may be partially responsible for the susceptibility of the early-maturation enamel to the effects of fluoride. The high concentrations of fluoride in the enamel matrix at the transition/early-maturation stage of enamel formation could reduce the available ionic calcium, resulting in reduced proteolytic activity at this critical stage.[21,34]

Fluorosed enamel has been shown to have an increased magnesium concentration,[82] and in bone mineral, fluoride has been shown to result in increased manganese[57] and decreased carbonate, citrate,[112] and zinc.[57] These changes in the mineral chemistry could affect mineral/matrix interactions and enzyme activity. For example, it has been suggested that enamel proteins produced in the presence of fluoride may be more tightly bound to fluorapatite, thereby making them less accessible to degradation by enamel proteinases.[26,84]

Protein removal from the matrix

Studies of human fluorosed enamel by both light and electron microscopy,[39,43] suggested that fluoride interferes with the complex process involved in protein removal and subsequent mineral acquisition during enamel maturation. Amelogenin (the major secreted enamel protein) is hydrolyzed and removed from the matrix beginning in the secretory stage, and at a more rapid rate during the transition/early maturation-stage of enamel formation.[47,48,80] Animal studies of the effect of high levels of chronic fluoride exposure in developing enamel have shown that fluoride does indeed cause a dose-dependent delay in the hydrolysis and removal of amelogenin protein at the maturation-stage of enamel development.[26,29,30] This delay in the removal of amelogenins during the maturation stage is most likely due to changes in the function or secretion of enamel matrix proteinases during enamel maturation.

A number of enamel matrix proteinases have been identified and include both metalloproteinases and serine proteinases. At the secretory stage of enamel formation, only metalloproteinases (proteinases which require a metal ion for activity) have been identified. Beginning at the early-maturation stage of enamel development, a serine proteinase (proteinases which contain a serine at the active site) which is highly active against amelogenin is present in the enamel matrix.[16,33,72,89] It has been suggested that fluoride may specifically alter the quantity and/or activity of the extracellular proteinases[22,33,34,94] needed to degrade enamel proteins during the maturation stage of amelogenesis.

It appears that removal of protein during maturation is a critical step for final enamel mineralization. Both amelogenins and non-amelogenins have been shown to inhibit crystal growth *in vitro*.[7,35] *In vitro* studies which used proteinases to hydrolyze enamel matrix protein resulted in increased crystal growth in the maturation enamel.[86] Therefore, a delayed withdrawal of amelogenin may be a critical mechanism in the formation of enamel fluorosis by delaying the growth of enamel crystals so that when the tooth erupts, the enamel remains incompletely mineralized.

Cell function

A number of studies have been carried out to determine the effects of fluoride on ameloblast cell proliferation and differentiation. These studies which have been done largely *in vitro*, do not support an effect of fluoride on cell proliferation or differentiation at fluoride levels to which the ameloblasts are likely to be exposed *in vivo*.[14,65,104]

A study by Fejerskov et al.[40] showed that a high dose of fluoride given in drinking water over prolonged periods reduces the length of the zone of ameloblast modulation and the number of modulation cycles in the maturation stage in the rat. Although this effect was only observed at very high dosages (113 ppm F in water), it was speculated that this could result in less protein being removed from the maturing enamel, since the two distinctly different types of maturation ameloblasts were thought to play a key role in protein removal and subsequent mineral deposition.[55] Hence, this disturbance in cell modulation might well result in a hypomineralized enamel (enamel fluorosis).

Subsequent studies on rats[32] confirmed this effect of fluoride on ameloblast modulation but, more important, these authors showed a complete recovery of the ameloblast modulation 9-12 days after fluoride exposure was discontinued. During this period of time the ameloblasts which had been exposed to high levels of fluoride while in the stage of matrix secretion were apparently able to enter the modulation process unaffected. A more recent study by Smith et al.[90] has shown that the rate at which ameloblasts modulate between smooth-ended and ruffle-ended cells is altered at high levels of fluoride ingestion in rats. Ameloblasts in fluoride-exposed rats initially showed a significantly slower modulation time earlier in maturation, and an increased rate of modulation as compared to controls later in maturation. Smith and co-workers[90] have suggested that fluoride reduces proteolytic activity in the enamel matrix, which indirectly lengthens the maturation ameloblast cell modulation time as the ameloblasts respond by remaining in the ruffle-ended phase longer.

Clinical signs of dental fluorosis – a result of an impaired enamel maturation only?

Definitive evidence that fluoride can induce

dental fluorosis solely by affecting the stage of enamel maturation, was provided by Richards et al.[77] in controlled studies on pigs, which showed that the start of fluoride exposure after completion of enamel secretion did cause a subsurface type of enamel hypomineralization similar to that seen in human fluorosis. Similar conclusions have recently been derived from studies in sheep[93] and are supported by human data.[53]

The question therefore arises whether the evidence provided by animal studies described above tends to suggest that the main clinical features of human enamel fluorosis may turn out to be the result of an effect of fluoride on the maturation phase of dental enamel. There is so far very little evidence which would contradict this hypothesis. Matrix removal and mineral deposition also occur during enamel secretion, and it would be logical to assume that fluoride could also have a retarding effect on these processes during enamel secretion. However, it is not certain whether this by itself would be sufficient to cause hypomineralization of the final enamel if the fluoride insult was removed prior to the maturation phase.

Suckling et al.,[93] reporting on a low dose fluoride experiment in sheep, described an increased severity of fluorosis in fully formed enamel when fluoride doses were given *prior to* as well as during the maturation stage compared to enamel exposed to fluoride during the maturation phase alone. However, this finding does not necessarily indicate an effect of fluoride on the secretory phase *per se*. This is because the levels of plasma fluoride will have increased constantly during this experiment due to skeletal accumulation of fluoride in these animals, as discussed above. As a result, the enamel which went through both secretory and maturation stages would have been exposed to higher fluoride concentrations when it was in the maturation phase than enamel which was already in the maturation phase at the start of fluoride exposure.

It would be interesting to know the outcome of fluoride exposure strictly limited to the secretory phase. It is, however, difficult to envisage how this could be tested adequately as the long biological half-life of fluoride inevitably would lead to elevated plasma fluoride levels long after termination of fluoride administration. Such elevated plasma fluoride levels should be borne in mind when studying intermittent exposure to high doses of fluoride in children. For example, the severity of fluorosis was greater in children who had been exposed to high fluoride doses in early childhood, which then ceased abruptly, than in others who were first exposed to high concentrations of fluoride in drinking water at a later age.[53] Rather than indicating an effect of fluoride on early enamel formation as suggested by these authors, this phenomenon appears more convincingly explained by the "carry over" effect described above.

The most likely explanation for the pathogenesis of enamel fluorosis as it appears clinically in man may therefore lie in an effect on processes occurring predominantly during enamel maturation. A review of the possible effects of fluoride on proteolysis of enamel matrix has been published by DenBesten & Crenshaw,[31] and the role of enamel matrix proteins for crystal growth has recently been covered extensively by Aoba and coworkers (for review see[8])

Cosmetic treatments of enamel fluorosis

Various forms of treatments have been suggested to deal with discolorations such as moderately to severely fluorosed enamel. The most obvious alternative is prosthetically replacing all discolored tooth-material. In addition, a number of empirically derived treatments have been described. These have in-

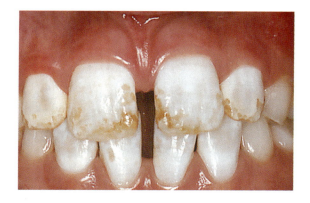

Figs. 8-38 and 8-39. A case of dental fluorosis before and after several treatments with acid etching followed by polishing.

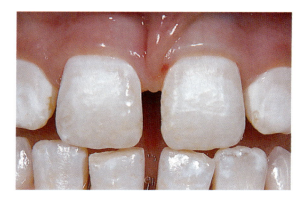

Fig. 8-39.

cluded rubbing the teeth with 18% hydrochloric acid both with and without heat[24,70] and treatment with hydrogen peroxide with or without heat.[2,17,18,111] Croll[23] suggested that all these techniques could be enhanced by microabrasion or grinding off the surface layer of enamel. In addition, several studies have suggested that mild fluorotic lesions "repair" with time. An example of treatment is shown in Figs. 8-38 & 8-39.

In fact, treatments of fluorosis can be more simply understood if the basic fluorotic lesion, a subsurface porosity of the enamel is analyzed. This subsurface porosity results in a change in the light reflectance from the enamel surface, resulting in an altered (lighter) color,

which of course can be further altered by posteruptive staining. Therefore, the change in the appearance of mildly fluorotic lesions over time indicates a decrease in subsurface porosity, possibly by mineral deposition through long-term exposure to saliva.[19] Indeed, the above described empirical treatments may act to remove the outer enamel surface, and allow more rapid subsurface mineralization of the fluorotic lesion through exposure to saliva. However, due to the lack of carefully controlled studies, specific recommendations for any single treatment modality to improve the cosmetic appearance of fluorosed enamel cannot be made at this time.

147

Literature cited

1. Aasenden R, Peebles TC. Effects of fluoride supplementation from birth on human deciduous and permanent teeth. Arch Oral Biol 1974; 19: 321-6.

2. Ames JW. Removing stains from mottled enamel. J Am Dent Assoc 1937; 24: 1674-7.

3. Andersen L, Richards A, Care AD, Kerzel Andersen HM, Kragstrup J, Fejerskov O. Parathyroid glands, calcium, and vitamin D in experimental fluorosis in pigs. Calcif Tissue Int 1986; 38: 222-6.

4. Angmar-Månsson B, Whitford GM. Plasma fluoride levels and enamel fluorosis in the rat. Caries Res 1982; 16: 334-9.

5. Angmar-Månsson B, Whitford GM. Enamel fluorosis related to plasma F levels in the rat. Caries Res 1984; 18: 25-32.

6. Aoba T, Collins J, Moreno EC. Possible function of matrix proteins in fluoride incorporation into enamel mineral during porcine amelogenesis. J Dent Res 1989; 68: 1162-8.

7. Aoba T, Fukae M, Tanabe T, Shimizu M, Moreno EC. Selective adsorption of porcine amelogenins onto hydroxyapatite and their inhibitory activity on hydroxyapatite growth in supersaturated solutions. Calcif Tissue Int 1987; 41: 281-9.

8. Aoba T, Moreno EC. Structural relationship of amelogenin proteins to their regulatory function of enamel mineralization. In: Sikes CS, Wheeler AP, eds. Surface reactive peptides and polymers. Washington DC: American Chemical Society, 1991: 85-106.

9. Aoba T, Moreno EC, Tanabe T, Fukae M. Effects of fluoride on matrix proteins and their properties in rat secretory enamel. J Dent Res 1990; 69: 1248-50.

10. Bawden JW, Crenshaw MA, Takano Y, Hammarström L. Ion transport through the enamel organ - an update. J Dent Res 1982; 61: 1552-4.

11. Black GV, McKay FS. Mottled teeth: an endemic developmental imperfection of the enamel of the teeth, heretofore unknown in the literature in dentistry. Dent Cosmos 1916; 58: 129-56.

12. Bronckers ALJJ, Jansen LL, Wöltgens JHM. A histological study of the short-term effects of fluoride on enamel and dentin formation in hamster tooth-germs in organ culture *in vitro*. Arch Oral Biol 1984; 29: 803-10.

13. Bronckers ALJJ, Jansen LL, Wöltgens JHM. Long-term effects of exposure to low concentrations of fluoride on enamel formation in hamster tooth-germs in organ culture *in vitro*. Arch Oral Biol 1984; 29: 811-9.

14. Bronckers ALJJ, Wöltgens JHM. Short term effects of fluoride on biosynthesis of enamel-matrix proteins and dentin collagens and on mineralization during hamster tooth-germ development in organ culture. Arch Oral Biol 1985; 39: 181-91.

15. Brouwer ID, Backer Dirks O, De Bruin A, Hautvast JGAJ. Unsuitability of World Health Organisation guidelines for fluoride concentrations in drinking water in Senegal. Lancet 1988; 1: 223-5.

16. Carter J, Smillie AC, Sheperd MG. Purification and properties of a protease from developing porcine dental enamel. Arch Oral Biol 1989; 34: 195-202.

17. Chandra S, Chawla TN. Clinical evaluation of heat method for bleaching of discoloured mottled teeth. J Indian Dent Assoc 1974; 46: 313-8.

18. Chandra S, Chawla TN. Clinical evaluation of the sandpaper disc method for removing fluorosis stains from teeth. J Am Dent Assoc 1975: 90: 1273-6.

19. Christensen JL, Larsen MJ, Fejerskov O. Effect of a mineralizing solution on sections of fluorosed human dental enamel *in vitro*. Caries Res 1979; 13: 47-56.

20. Clarkson J, O'Mullane DM. Modified DDE index for use in epidemiological studies in enamel defects. J Dent Res 1989; 68: 445-50.

21. Crenshaw MA, Bawden JW. Fluoride binding by organic matrix from early and late developing bovine fetal enamel determined by flow rate dialysis. Arch Oral Biol 1981; 26: 437-76.

22. Crenshaw MA, Bawden JW. Proteolytic activity in embryonic bovine secretory enamel. In: Fearnhead RW, Suga S, eds. Tooth enamel IV. Amsterdam: Elsevier Science, 1984: 109-13.

23. Croll TP. Enamel microabrasion: the technique. Quintessence Int. 1989; 20: 395-400.

24. Croll TP, Cavanaugh RR. Enamel color modifications by controlled hydrochloric acid-pumice abrasion. I. Techniques and examples. Quintessence Int 1986; 17: 81-7.

25. Cuttress TW, Suckling GW, Pearce EIF, Ball ME. Defects of tooth enamel in children in fluoridated and non-fluoridated water areas of the Auckland Region. N Z Dent J 1985; 81: 12-9.

26. Dajean S, Menanteau J. A western-blotting study of enamel glycoproteins in rat experimental fluorosis. Arch Oral Biol 1989; 34: 413-8.

27. Dean HT. The investigation of physiological effects by the epidemiological methods. In: Moulton FR, ed. Fluorine and dental health. Washington D.C.: American Association for the Advancement of Science, 1942: 23-31.

28. Dean HT, Elvove E. Some epidemiological aspects of chronic endemic dental fluorosis. Am J Public Health 1936; 26: 567-75.

29. Den Besten PK. Effects of fluoride on protein secretion and removal during enamel development in the rat. J Dent Res 1986; 665: 1272-7.

30. DenBesten PK, Crenshaw MA. The effects of chronic high fluoride levels on forming enamel in the rat. Arch Oral Biol 1984; 29: 675-80.

31. DenBesten PK, Crenshaw MA. Studies on the changes in developing enamel caused by ingestion of high levels of fluoride in the rat. Adv Dent Res 1987; 1: 176-80.

32. DenBesten PK, Crenshaw MA, Wilson MH. Changes in the fluoride-induced modulation of maturation stage ameloblasts of rats. J Dent Res 1985; 64: 1365-70.

33. DenBesten PK, Heffernan LM. Enamel proteases in secretory and maturation incisor enamel of rats ingesting 0 and 100 ppm fluoride in drinking water. Adv Dent Res 1989; 3: 199-202.

34. DenBesten PK, Thariani H. Biological mechanisms of fluorosis and level and timing of systemic exposure to fluoride with respect to fluorosis. J Dent Res 1992; 71: 1238-43.

35. Doi Y, Eanes ED, Shimokawa H, Termine JD. Inhibition of seeded growth of enamel apatite crystals by amelogenin and enamel proteins *in vitro*. J Dent Res 1984; 63: 98-105.

36. Eastoe J, Fejerskov O. Composition of mature enamel proteins from fluorosed teeth. In: Fearnhead RW, Suga S, eds. Tooth enamel IV. Amsterdam: Elsevier, 1984: 326-30.

37. Ekstrand J, Spak C-J, Vogel G. Pharmacokinetics of fluoride in man and its clinical relevance. J Dent Res 1990; 69: 550-5.

38. Ericsson Y, Gydell K, Hammarskiöld T. Blood plasma fluoride. An indicator of skeletal fluoride content. J Int Res Communi 1973; 1: 33.

39. Fejerskov O, Johnson NW, Silverstone LM. The ultrastructure of fluorosed human dental enamel. Scand J Dent Res 1974; 82: 357-72.

40. Fejerskov O, Josephsen K, Joost Larsen M, Thylstrup A. Cytological feature of rat ameloblasts following long-term fluoride exposure. Caries Res 1980; 14: 181-2.

41. Fejerskov O, Manji F, Baelum V, Møller IJ. Dental fluorosis. A handbook for health workers. Copenhagen: Munksgaard, 1988.

42. Fejerskov O, Richards A, Josephsen K. Pathogenesis and biochemical findings of dental fluorosis in various species. In: Shupe JL, Peterson HB, Leone NC, eds. Fluorides. Effects on vegetation, animals and humans. Salt Lake City: Paragon Press, 1983: 305-17.

43. Fejerskov O, Silverstone LM, Melsen B, Möller IJ. Histological features of fluorosed human dental enamel. Caries Res 1975; 9: 190-210.

44. Fejerskov O, Thylstrup A, Joost Larsen M. Clinical and structural features and possible pathogenic mechanisms of dental fluorosis. Scand J Dent Res 1977; 85: 510-34.

45. Fejerskov O, Yaeger JA, Thylstrup A. Microradiography of acute and chronic administration of fluoride on human and rat dentin and enamel. Arch Oral Biol 1979; 24: 123-30.

46. Fejerskov O, Yanagisawa T, Tohda H, Larsen MJ, Josephsen K, Mosha HJ. Posteruptive changes in human dental fluorosis - a histological and ultrastructural study. Proc Finn Dent Soc 1991; 87: 607-19.

47. Fincham AG, Belcourt AB, Termine JD. Changing patterns of enamel matrix proteins in the developing bovine tooth. Caries Res 1982; 16: 64-71.

48. Fukae M, Shimizu M. Studies on the proteins of developing bovine enamel. Arch Oral Biol 1974; 19: 381-6.

49. Hiller CR, Robinson C, Weatherell JA. Variations in the composition of developing rat incisor enamel. Calcif Tissue Res 1975; 18: 1-12.

50. Holland RI, Hongslo JK. The effect of fluoride on the cellular uptake and pool of amino-acids. Acta Pharmacol Toxicol 1979; 44: 354-8.

51. Horowitz HS, Heifetz SB, Driscoll WS, Kingman A, Meyers RJ. A new method for assessing the prevalence of dental fluorosis - The tooth surface index of fluorosis. J Am Dent Assoc 1984; 109: 37-41.

52. Hörsted M, Fejerskov O, Joost Larsen M, Thylstrup A. The structure of surface enamel with special reference to occlusal surface of primary and permanent teeth. Caries Res 1976; 10: 287-96.

53. Ishii T, Nagaki H. Study of the correlation between the degree of dental fluorosis and the duration of fluoride present in drinking water. In: Fearnhead R, Suga S, eds. Tooth enamel IV. Amsterdam: Elsevier Science Publishers, 1984: 338-41.

54. Ishii T, Suckling G. The severity of dental fluorosis in children exposed to water with a high fluoride content for various periods of time. J Dent Res 1991; 70: 952-6.

55. Josephsen K, Fejerskov O. Ameloblast modulation in the maturation zone of the rat incisor enamel organ. A light and electron microscopic study. J Anat 1977; 124; 45-70.

56. Kalsbeek H, Verrips GH, Backer Dirks O. Use of fluoride tablets and effects on prevalence of dental caries and dental fluorosis. Community Dent Oral Epidemiol 1992; 20; 241-5.

57. Kanwar KC, Singh M. Zinc, copper and manganese levels in various tissues following fluoride administration. Experientia 1981: 37: 1328-9.

58. Koch G, Fejerskov O, Thylstrup A. Fluoride in caries treatment – clinical implications. In: Thylstrup A, Fejerskov O, eds. Textbook of clinical cariology. Copenhagen: Munksgaard, 1994: 259-81.

59. Kraintz L. The effect of fluoride ingestion on the response of the rat to parathormone and calcitonin. Can J Physiol Pharmacol 1969; 47: 477-81.

60. Kruger BJ. Autoradiographic assessment of the effect of fluoride on the uptake of ^{3}H-proline by ameloblasts in the rat. Arch Oral Biol 1970; 15: 103-8.

61. Kruger BJ. Utilization of ^{3}H-serine by ameloblasts of rats receiving sub-mottling doses of fluoride. Arch Oral Biol 1972; 17: 1389-94.

62. Larsen MJ, Kirkegaard E, Fejerskov O, Poulsen S. Prevalence of dental fluorosis after fluoride-gel treatments in a low-fluoride area. J Dent Res 1985; 64: 1076-9.

63. Larsen MJ, Kirkegaard E, Poulsen S, Fejerskov O. Enamel fluoride, dental fluorosis and dental caries among immigrants to and permanent residents of five Danish fluoride areas. Caries Res 1986; 20: 349-55.

64. Lussi A, Fridell RA, Crenshaw MA, Bawden JW. Absence of *in vitro* fluoride-binding by the organic matrix of developing bovine enamel. Arch Oral Biol 1988; 33: 531-3.

65. Lyaruu DM, DeJong M, Bronckers ALJJ, Wöltgens JM. Ultrastructural study of fluoride induced *in vitro* hypermineralization of enamel in hamster tooth germs explanted during the secretory phase of amelogenesis. Arch Oral Biol 1986; 31: 109-17.

66. Mabelya L, König KG, van Pelenstein Helderman WH. Dental fluorosis, altitude, and associated dietary factors. Caries Res 1992; 26: 65-7.

67. Manji F, Baelum V, Fejerskov O. Fluoride, altitude and dental fluorosis. Caries Res 1986a; 20: 473-80.

68. Manji F, Baelum V, Fejerskov O. Dental fluorosis in an area of Kenya with 2 ppm fluoride in the drinking water. J Dent Res 1986b; 65: 659-62.

69. Manji F, Baelum V, Fejerskov O, Gemert W. Enamel changes in two low-fluoride areas of Kenya. Caries Res 1986; 20: 371-80.

70. McCloskey RJ. A technique for removal of fluorosis stains. J Am Dent Assoc 1984; 109: 63-64.

71. Myers HM. Dose-response relationship between water fluoride levels and the category of questionable dental fluorosis. Community Dent Oral Epidemiol 1983; 11: 109-12.

72. Overall CM, Limeback H. Identification and characterization of enamel proteinases isolated from developing enamel. Biochem J 1988; 256: 965-72.

73. Pendrys DG, Katz RV. Risk of enamel fluorosis associated with fluoride supplementation, infant formula, and fluoride dentifrice use. Am J Epidemiol 1989; 103: 1199-208.

74. Richards A, Fejerskov O, Baelum V. Enamel fluoride in relation to severity of human dental fluorosis. Adv Dent Res 1989; 3: 147-53.

75. Richards A. Nature and mechanisms of dental fluorosis in animals. J Dent Res 1990; 69: 701-5.

76. Richards A, Fejerskov O. Enamel fluoride concentrations in relation to stage of enamel development. J Dent Res 1992; 72: 696.

77. Richards A, Kragstrup J, Josephsen K, Fejerskov O. Dental fluorosis developed in postsecretory enamel. J Dent Res 1986; 65: 1406-9.

78. Richards A, Kragstrup J, Nielsen-Kudsk F. Pharmacokinetics of chronic fluoride ingestion in growing pigs. J Dent Res 1985; 64: 425-30.

79. Richards A, Likimani S, Baelum V, Fejerskov O. Fluoride concentrations in unerupted fluorotic human enamel. Caries Res 1992; 26: 328-32.

80. Robinson C, Briggs HD, Atkinson PJ, Weatherell JA. Matrix and mineral changes in developing enamel. J Dent Res 1979; 58: 871-80.

81. Robinson C, Fuchs P, Deutsch D, Weatherell JA. Four chemically distinct stages in developing enamel from bovine incisor teeth. Caries Res 1978; 12: 1-11.

82. Robinson C, Kirkham J. Enamel matrix components, alterations during development and possible interactions with the mineral phase. In: Fearnhead RW, Suga S, eds. Tooth enamel IV. Amsterdam: Elsevier, 1984: 261-5.

83. Robinson C, Kirkham J. The dynamics of amelogenesis as revealed by protein compositional studies. In: Butler WT, ed. The chemistry and biology in mineralized tissues. Birmingham, Alabama: Ebsco Media, Inc, 1985: 248-63.

84. Robinson C, Kirkham J. The effect of fluoride on the developing mineralized tissues. J Dent Res 1990; 69: 685-91.

85. Robinson C, Kirkham J, Hallsworth AS. Volume distribution and concentration of protein mineral and water in developing dental enamel. Arch Oral Biol 1988; 33: 159-62.

86. Robinson C, Shore RC, Kirkham J, Stonehouse NJ. Extracellular processing of enamel matrix proteins and the control of crystal growth. J Biol Buccale 1990; 18: 355-61.

87. Rosenquist JB, Lorentzon PR, Boquist LV. Effect of fluoride on parathyroid activity of normal and calcium-deficient rats. Calcif Tissue Int 1983; 35: 533-7.

88. Smalley JW, Embery G. The influence of fluoride administration on the structure of proteoglycans in the developing rat incisor. Biochem J 1980; 190: 263-72.

89. Smith CE, Borenstein A, Fazek A, Nanci A. In vitro studies of the proteinases with which degrade amelogenins in developing rat incisor enamel. In: Fearnhead RW, ed. Tooth enamel V. Yokohama: Florence Publishers, 1989: 286-90.

90. Smith CE, Nanci A, DenBesten PK. Effects of chronic fluoride exposure on morphometric parameters defining the stages of amelogenesis and ameloblast modulation in rat incisors. Anat Rec 1993; 237: 243-58.

91. Speirs RL. Fluoride incorporation into developing enamel of permanent teeth in the domestic pig. Arch Oral Biol 1975; 20: 877-83.

92. Srivastava RN, Gill DS, Moudgil A, Menon RK, Thomas M, Dandona P. Normal ionized calcium, parathyroid hypersecretion, and elevated osteocalcin in a family with fluorosis. Metabolism 1989; 38: 120-4.

93. Suckling GW, Thurley DC, Nelson DGA. The macroscopic and scanning electron-microscopic appearance and microhardness of the enamel, and the related histological changes in the enamel organ of erupting sheep incisors resulting from a prolonged low daily dose of fluoride. Arch Oral Biol 1988; 33: 361-73.

94. Suga S. Histochemical observation of proteolytic enzyme activity in the developing dental hard tissue of the rat. Arch Oral Biol 1970; 15: 555-8.

95. Susheela AK, Sharma K, Rajan BP, Gnanasundaram N. The status of sulphated isomers of glycosaminoglycans in fluorosed human teeth. Arch Oral Biol 1988; 33: 765-7.

96. Teotia M, Teotia SPS, Singh RK. Metabolism of fluoride in pregnant women residing in endemic fluorosis areas. Fluoride 1976; 12: 58-64.

97. Teotia SPS, Teotia M. Secondary hyperparathyroidism in patients with endemic skeletal fluorosis. Br Med J 1973; 1: 637-40.

151

98. Thylstrup A. Distribution of dental fluorosis in the primary dentition. Community Dent Oral Epidemiol 1978; 6: 329-37.

99. Thylstrup A. A scaning electron microscopical study of normal and fluorotic enamel demineralized by EDTA. Acta Odontol Scand 1979; 37: 127-35.

100. Thylstrup A, Fejerskov O. Clinical appearance of dental fluorosis in permanent teeth in relation to histological changes. Community Dent Oral Epidemiol 1978; 6: 315-28.

101. Thylstrup A, Fejerskov O. A scanning electron microscopic and microradiographic study of pits in fluorosed human enamel. Scand J Dent Res 1979; 87: 105-14.

102. Thylstrup A, Fejerskov O, Bruun C, Kann J. Enamel changes and dental caries in 7 year old children given fluoride tablets from shortly after birth. Caries Res 1979; 13: 265-76.

103. Waddington RJ, Embery G, Hall RC. The influence of fluoride on proteoglycan structure using a rat odontoblast in vitro system. Calcif Tissue Int 1992; 52: 392-8.

104. Walton RE, Eisenmann DR. Ultrastructural examination of various stages of amelogenesis in the rat following parenteral fluoride administration. Arch Oral Biol 1974; 19: 171-82.

105. Weatherell JA, Deutsch D, Robinson C, Hallsworth AS. Fluoride concentrations in developing enamel. Nature (London) 1975; 256: 230-2.

106. Weile V, Josephsen K, Fejerskov O. Scanning electron microscopy of final enamel formation in rat mandibular incisors following single injections of 1-hydroxyethylidene-1,1-bisphosphonate. Calcif Tissue Int 1993; 52: 318-24.

107. Wenzel A, Thylstrup A. Dental fluorosis and localized enamel opacities in fluoride and non-fluoride Danish communities. Caries Res 1982; 16: 340-8.

108. Whitford GM, Birdsong-Whitford NL, Augeri JM. Fluoride balance and tissue concentrations: effect of dose frequency. Proc. Finn Dent Soc 1991; 87: 561-9.

109. Wiseman A. Effect of fluoride on enzymes. In: Smith FA, ed. Pharmacology of fluorides. Berlin: Springer Verlag, 1970: 48-97.

110. Yanagisawa T, Takuma S, Tohda H, Fejerskov O, Fearnhead RW. High resolution electron microscopy of enamel crystals in cases of human dental fluorosis. J Electron Microsc 1989; 38: 441-8.

111. Younger HB. Bleaching fluoride stain from mottled enamel. Tex Dent J 1939; 57: 380-2.

112. Zipkin I, McClure FJ, Lee WA. Relation of the fluoride content of human bone to its chemical composition. Arch Oral Biol 1960; 2: 190-5.

DOSE-RESPONSE AND DENTAL FLUOROSIS

O. Fejerskov • V. Baelum • A. Richards

Introduction – Daily fluoride intake (dose) versus dental fluorosis (response)
Daily fluoride dose from dentifrices

Introduction

Epidemiologic studies conducted around the 1940s by Dean and coworkers demonstrated a positive association between the fluoride concentration in drinking water and the prevalence and severity of dental fluorosis (see Chapter 15). Table 9-1 shows the prevalence and the F_{ci} values for different water fluoride concentrations according to the data presented by Dean.[4,5] Since then, numerous studies have established that the more fluoride which is ingested during the periods of tooth formation and mineralization, the greater the risk of severe manifestations of dental fluorosis at the time of tooth eruption (see Chapter 8).

However, Dean's studies also demonstrated a negative association between water fluoride concentrations and the caries experience of 12-14-year-old children. In the 1940's and 50's there was little doubt in the scientific community that fluoride exerted this caries-preventive effect solely through the systemic route. The concept was that ingestion of fluoride caused fluoride to be incorporated into the enamel during tooth development and that this was a prerequisite for obtaining the cariostatic effect of fluoride.

Since it was clearly desirable to mimic the caries preventive effect of fluoride which was observed by Dean and coworkers in their studies of naturally fluoridated communities (see Chapter 15), numerous water supplies with low concentrations of naturally occurring fluoride in the USA were artificially adjusted with respect to fluoride. It was also clear, however, that the water fluoride concentration had to be determined by balancing the caries-preventive beneficial effect against the risk of development of dental fluorosis, which was now considered a side effect of artificial water fluoridation.

This problem of determining the so-called "optimum" water fluoride concentration was apparently solved by Hodge.[15] Hodge first plotted the average index values of dental fluorosis (the F_{ci}-values) of 21 communities examined by Dean against – on a logarithmic scale – the water fluoride contents of these communities (Fig. 9-1). This logarithmic transfor-

Table 9-1

Prevalence of dental fluorosis (the category "Questionable" is included) and F_{ci} values in 12 Illinois communities and 5 Ohio communities in the USA examined by Dean et al.[4,5]

Water fluoride concentration (ppm)	Prevalence of dental fluorosis (%)	F_{ci} value
0.0	2.1	0.012
0.0	9.4	0.050
0.0	8.2	0.049
0.1	7.0	0.037
0.1	11.1	0.062
0.2	14.6	0.081
0.2	15.7	0.084
0.3	15.9	0.091
0.4	42.6	0.252
0.5	39.5	0.226
0.9	47.2	0.313
1.2	46.8	0.320
1.2	60.8	0.512
1.2	63.2	0.494
1.3	59.5	0.457
1.8	71.8	0.671
1.9	74.7	0.696

mation resulted in two straight lines intersecting at a water fluoride concentration of about 1 ppm. The line for fluoride concentrations below 1 ppm was almost horizontal, indicating that an increase in water fluoride concentration from 0.3 ppm to 1.0 ppm would only increase the F_{ci} from 0.03 to 0.47, which was considered of "negligible biologic (esthetic) significance".[15] Having thus established that no significant dental fluorosis occurred with water fluoride concentrations below 1 ppm, Hodge[15] added the average caries experience (the DMFT) of each of the communities to the graph (Fig. 9-2). This resulted in a third straight line which incidentally also intersected the two lines representing dental fluorosis at a water fluoride concentration of about 1 ppm. This intersection was for many years described as the "optimum" water fluoride concentration. This estimate of the "optimal" water fluoride concentration has subsequently been used to determine the amount of fluoride which should be given in other systemic fluoride regimens, such as tablets and vitamin drops.

As described in Chapter 15, about 50% of the USA population is now served by artificially fluoridated water supplies. In recent years many have claimed that the prevalence of dental fluorosis is increasing in the USA, and a review of the available data did indeed support this conclusion.[31] Dental fluorosis is the undesirable effect of fluoride ingestion, and it is therefore not surprising that this increase continues to be questioned and debated. Those who consider systemic ingestion of fluoride a prerequisite for obtaining the caries-preventive effect would clearly be interested in questioning the evidence for an increase. Indeed, it is possible that the interpretation of criteria for recording fluorosis has changed since the 1930s such that today more attention is perhaps paid to the milder forms of dental fluorosis. Different examiners apply criteria differently, and in Chapter 8 we have already pointed out the confusion created by Dean's classification category "Questionable", which has often been neglected in epidemiologic studies. In Dean's studies, natural light was the source of illumination, whereas today's studies are usually carried out under artificial light, which undoubtedly leads to increased detection of the milder forms of dental fluorosis. Although many such arguments have been put forward, it remains a fact that the potential fluoride exposure has increased substantially during the same time period. Dean's data were collected around 1940 in populations whose only sources

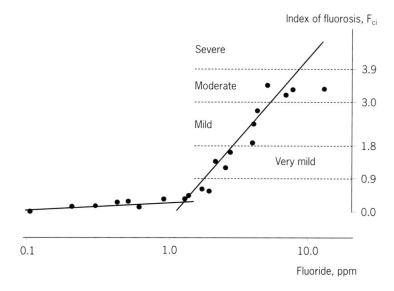

Fig. 9-1. Graph illustrating the relationship between community index of dental fluorosis (F_{ci}) and water fluoride concentration presented on a logarithmic scale.[15]

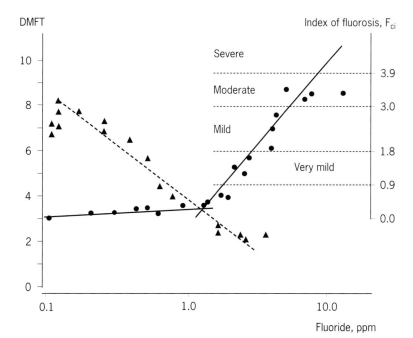

Fig. 9-2. The relationship between caries prevalence, dental fluorosis presented as F_{ci}, and water fluoride concentration. Note that the fluoride concentration is presented on a logarithmic scale.[15]

of fluoride were food and water.[3] Much has changed since then and the extensive use of other systemic (tablets, drops, salt, etc.) and topical (toothpastes, rinses, varnishes) fluoride measures in caries prevention has introduced a large number of additional fluoride sources. Dietary habits have changed extensively in the last half of this century among children - for example, today's extensive consumption of soft drinks rather than drinking water. All these re-

155

flections should be borne in mind when discussing the evidence for an increase in the prevalence (and severity) of dental fluorosis among children.

No one questions the early manifestations of dental fluorosis as being the undesirable but unavoidable effects of systemic ingestion of fluoride. Nevertheless, it has long been common to play down the early signs of enamel fluorosis and only to regard manifestations which are thought to be of cosmetic concern to children or parents as relevant diagnostic thresholds for dental fluorosis.

There is little doubt that increased awareness and knowledge about dental fluorosis results in more cases being diagnosed, but it is reasonable to expect that children in contemporary industrialized societies are ingesting increased quantities of fluoride. Much effort is therefore presently being directed towards estimating fluoride intake among small children and infants. Our knowledge about the actual dose-response relationship is rather limited, but as this chapter will show, we do in fact have information available which allows USA to develop dose-response curves to predict prevalence and severity of dental fluorosis in a population where we know the predominant sources of fluoride.

In the following, we will present these dose-response considerations. At the end of the chapter it will be shown why, for example, fluoride-containing dentifrices will add to the risk of developing dental fluorosis if used in a child population already exposed to fluoride supplements or living in "optimally" fluoridated areas (water F concentration ranging from 0.7 to 1.2 mg F/L).

Daily fluoride intake (dose) versus dental fluorosis (response)

Water fluoride studies

Although it has been known for decades that chronic exposure to small amounts of fluorides may produce toxic effects in humans, fluorides have seldom been considered in the same context as other drugs. While drugs are ordinarily prescribed in relation to body weight of the individual, this is quite uncommon with fluoride.

However, there are many difficulties inherent in attempts to produce valid estimates of the dose-response relationship. Firstly, precise estimates of the effects of fluoride on the human dentition can only be obtained when the premolars and the second molars have erupted around the age of 12-14 years (see Chapter 8). This means that there may be a considerable time-lapse between the fluoride exposure and the effect. Secondly, the period that the permanent dentition is susceptible to the effects of fluoride spans about 10-12 years, during which time the child grows extensively and is subject to considerable changes in dietary patterns and practices (from weaning, bottle-feeding, etc.). Thirdly, the relative contribution of food-borne fluoride to the development of dental fluorosis is still debatable, and no firm agreement exists as to how much fluoride is actually ingested from foods[29,32] (see Chapter 3). Fourthly, the bioavailability of fluoride once ingested is as yet uncertain since the fluoride compound in question and the contents of the stomach will determine the amount of fluoride absorbed by the organism (see Chapter 4).

Despite these difficulties, use can be made of the fact that epidemiologic studies throughout the world have shown a positive relationship between the water fluoride concentration and the occurrence of dental fluorosis.[3,18,21,22,23,28,33] Based on the concept that air temperature

Table 9-2

Formula provided by Galagan & Vermillion[11] for
the average water intake as a function of
the mean maximum air temperature

Water intake (fl.oz/lb)
   = − 0.038 + 0.0062 × mean max. temperature (°F)

Since
   1 fl.oz = 0.0296 liters and
   1 lb.   = 0.4536 kg,
   the formula may be transformed:

Water intake (l/kg)
   = − 0.0025 + 0.0004 × mean max. temperature (°F)

Table 9-3

Daily dose of fluoride from drinking water associated with
different levels of dental fluorosis in the 17 Illinois and Ohio
communities studied by Dean et al.[4,5]. The mean maximum
air temperature for these communities were reported by
Galagan & Vermillion[11] to be 61.6 and 61.8 °F, respectively.
r is the correlation coefficient between prevalence of
dental fluorosis and daily fluoride dose

Daily dose of fluoride from drinking water (mg F/kg)	Prevalence of dental fluorosis		F_{ci} value
	Quest. incl. (%)	Quest. excl. (%)	
0.0000	2.1	0.2	0.012
0.0000	9.4	0.6	0.050
0.0000	8.2	1.6	0.049
0.0023	7.0	0.3	0.037
0.0023	11.1	1.3	0.062
0.0045	14.6	1.5	0.081
0.0045	15.7	1.1	0.084
0.0068	15.9	2.2	0.091
0.0090	42.6	6.1	0.252
0.0113	39.5	4.2	0.226
0.0203	47.2	12.2	0.313
0.0271	46.8	15.0	0.320
0.0271	60.8	33.3	0.512
0.0271	63.2	31.6	0.494
0.0294	59.5	25.3	0.457
0.0406	71.8	40.0	0.671
0.0429	74.7	47.6	0.696
r	0.96	0.96	0.98

affects the daily consumption of water, Galagan et al. [11,12] formulated an equation describing the average water intake in relation to body weight in children as a function of air temperature (Table 9-2). Using this equation, it is possible to calculate the average daily dose of fluoride from drinking water, expressed as mg F/kg body weight, provided that the water fluoride concentration and the air temperature are known parameters. When this formula is applied to Dean's data from Illinois and Ohio,[4,5] it is possible to associate the dose of fluoride ingested from drinking water (mg F/kg body weight) with the prevalence and severity of dental fluorosis in these communities at that time (Table 9-3).

It is apparent from Table 9-3 that a fluoride intake from drinking water equivalent to 0.02 mg F/kg body weight is associated with a dental fluorosis prevalence of about 40-50% (15-25% when the category "Questionable" is excluded). Irrespective of whether the "Questionable" category of the Dean index is included or not, there is a strong positive association between the prevalence of dental fluorosis and the daily dose of fluoride from drinking water (r = 0.96).

The data in Table 9-3 also indicate that the community index values, F_{ci}, at an intake of 0.02 mg F/kg body weight range between 0.3

Table 9-4

Daily dose of fluoride from drinking waters, prevalence of dental fluorosis (Questionables included), and the Community Index of Dental Fluorosis, F_{ci} for 18 communities examined by Richards et al.[28]

Daily dose of fluoride from drinking water (mg F/kg)	Prevalence of dental fluorosis (%)	F_{ci} value
0.0018	2.7	0.015
0.0020	3.9	0.022
0.0022	47.4	0.240
0.0071	28.4	0.154
0.0080	25.8	0.162
0.0090	67.8	0.484
0.0143	55.3	0.358
0.0161	73.4	0.539
0.0179	81.9	0.618
0.0214	60.0	0.432
0.0241	77.2	0.619
0.0269	81.7	0.896
0.0286	66.9	0.497
0.0322	73.4	0.729
0.0358	91.6	1.102
0.0428	88.9	1.385
0.0483	85.2	1.386
0.0537	91.7	1.566
r	0.80	0.95

Originally, water fluoride contents were given as intervals: ≤ 0.15 ppm; 0.2-0.4 ppm; 0.5-0.7 ppm; 0.8-1.0 ppm; 1.1-1.3 ppm; and ≥ 1.8 ppm. The water fluoride concentration used for calculating the daily dose was the midpoints of these intervals, i.e. 0.075; 0.3; 0.6; 0.9; 1.2; and 1.8.

Similarly, mean annual air temperatures were given as intervals: ≤ 65 °F; 66-79°F; and ≥ 80 °F. The temperatures used for calculating the daily fluoride dose were 65 °F; 72.5 °F; and 80 °F.

Table 9-5

Daily dose of fluoride from drinking waters and the Community Index of Dental Fluorosis (F_{ci}) for 16 Texas communities examined by Butler et al.[2]

Daily dose of fluoride from drinking water (mg F/kg)	F_{ci} value
0.0058	0.14
0.0059	0.24
0.0088	0.05
0.0217	0.53
0.0285	0.47
0.0285	0.59
0.0316	0.33
0.0509	1.41
0.0512	1.36
0.0560	1.06
0.0591	1.33
0.0600	1.37
0.0607	1.35
0.0651	2.02
0.0668	1.20
0.0964	1.89
r	0.92

and 0.4. Even if it is assumed that fluoride from food would double this dose in small children,[24] these estimates are considerably lower than the estimates provided by Forsman,[10] who stated that dental fluorosis is unlikely to occur at a dosage below 0.1 mg F/kg body weight. This figure is often referred to in the literature, but the present calculations clearly demonstrate that dental fluorosis may occur at much lower dose values.

About 25 years after Dean's important studies, another large study of the relationship between waterborne fluoride, dental fluorosis and dental caries was performed in the USA by Richards and coworkers,[28] who examined over

7000 children from 18 areas with different water fluoride concentrations and different mean annual air temperatures. Based on the frequency distributions of Dean's fluorosis index presented by Richards et al.,[28] the F_{ci} values were calculated for each of the 18 communities and, using the formula presented in Table 9-2, the daily dose of fluoride from drinking waters in the different areas was estimated (Table 9-4). Table 9-4 shows that the estimated daily dose of fluoride was strongly and positively associated with both the prevalence of dental fluorosis (r = 0.80) and the F_{ci} (r = 0.95).

In 1985, Butler et al.[2] presented their data describing water fluoride concentrations, mean maximum air temperatures and community fluorosis index (F_{ci}) among 2,500 children from 16 Texas communities. These data are interesting from the point of view that they are collected in children who have been exposed to other sources of fluoride than drinking water and food, predominantly topical fluorides in the form of fluoridated dentifrices or (to a much lesser extent) other fluoride treatments. Table 9-5 presents the estimates of the daily dose of fluoride from drinking water and the associated F_{ci} values in these Texas communities. Again, the daily dose of fluoride from drinking water is strongly and positively associated with the F_{ci} values.

When the data of Dean et al.,[4,5] Richards et al.[28] and Butler et al.[2] are presented graphically, three regression lines appear (respectively Fig. 9-3A to C). In Fig. 9-3D all three data sets have been pooled. Three features of these Figures are strikingly apparent. First, regardless of the source of the data, the regression of the F_{ci} values on the daily dose of fluoride from drinking water clearly demonstrates that even with very low fluoride intake from water, a certain level of dental fluorosis will be found. Second, the dose-response relationship is clearly linear, and the data indicate that for every increase of the dose of 0.01 mg F/kg body weight, an increase in the F_{ci} of 0.2 can be anticipated. The implication of this observation is that there exists no "critical" value for the fluoride intake below which the effect on dental enamel will not be manifest. The conclusion reached by Hodge[15] that dental fluorosis will not occur at a water fluoride content below 1 ppm is therefore not tenable. Third, a comparison between the data presented by Richards et al.[28] and Butler et al.[2] does not indicate that the additional sources of fluoride (mainly topical fluorides) have led to an upward shift of the dose-response curve. Had such an upward shift occurred, it would be indicative of an increased fluoride ingestion.

As mentioned in the beginning of this chapter, Hodge[15] used a logarithmic scale for the x-axis (dose) when estimating the relationship between water fluoride contents and the resulting dental fluorosis (Fig. 9-1). Given the data presented in Fig. 9-3, one may wonder why a logarithmic transformation was used in the first place. The reason is that the increase in F_{ci} values with increasing water fluoride contents seemed to level off at extremely high water fluoride contents (> 7 ppm). This gave rise to an S-shaped (sigmoidal) dose-response curve, for which a logarithmic transformation should result in a straight line. However, the fact that Hodge[15] needed two lines (Fig. 9-1) to describe the transformed data ought perhaps to have challenged appropriateness of the logarithmic transformation. As already indicated in Chapter 8, the leveling-off of the F_{ci} at very high water fluoride levels is not an intrinsic feature of dental fluorosis but rather an illustration of the inability of Dean's index to sensitively record the most severe degrees of dental fluorosis.

Based on the above considerations, it is to be expected that prescription of additional (systemic) fluorides will result in an increase in the prevalence and severity of dental fluorosis. Evidence that such increases have indeed occurred has been reported from the USA.[20,31] In a number of countries, systemic fluorides, mainly in the form of tablets or drops, are recommended for use in infants and children as a specific

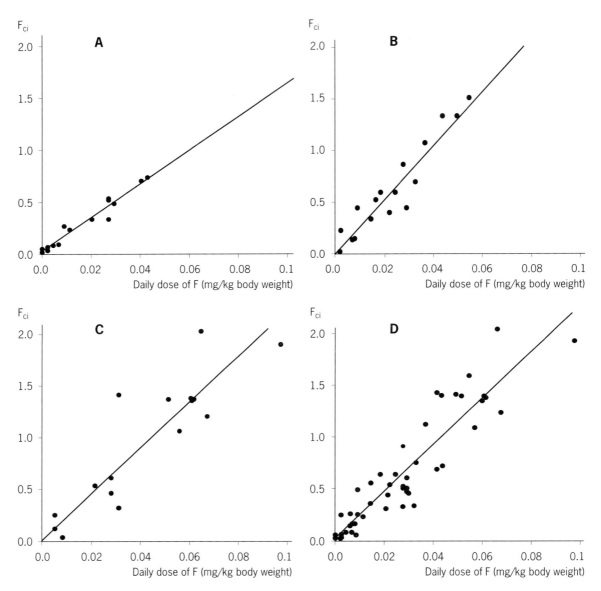

Fig. 9-3. Regression lines obtained between Fci and daily fluoride dose as calculated from the data of Dean *et al.*[4,5] (**A**), Richards *et al.*[28] (**B**) and Butler *et al.*[2] (**C**). In **D** all tree data sets are pooled.

measure in areas with low (< 0.70 ppm F) water fluoride contents. In the following section we will therefore consider to what extent fluoride tablets may in fact cause dental fluorosis.

Fluoride tablet studies

The prescription of systemic fluoride supplements is based on the belief that fluorides have to be incorporated into the developing enamel

Table 9-6

Prevalence of dental fluorosis according to Dean's classification in USA[1] and Swedish[13] child populations living in areas with 1.0-1.2 ppm fluoride in drinking waters or receiving fluoride tablet supplementation

Category	Aasenden & Peebles[1]		Granath et al.[13]	
	1 ppm water	F tablets	1-1.2 ppm water	F tablets
Normal	37.0%	16.0%	32.5%	71.4%
Questionable	30.0%	17.0%	31.0%	4.1%
Very mild	21.7%	34.0%	24.0%	14.3%
Mild	8.7%	19.0%	8.0%	10.2%
Moderate	2.2%	14.0%	4.4%	
Total prevalence	62.6%	84.0%	67.4%	28.6%

in order to obtain the caries-preventive effect. As described previously, it is commonly held that 1.0-1.2 ppm F in drinking waters is an "optimal" concentration, and fluoride supplementation is therefore given to compensate for not living in areas with "optimal" water fluoride levels. However, the recommended tablet dose schedules are quite crude, as exemplified by the USA schedule where 0.25 mg F/day is recommended from birth to the age of 2 years.[14] During this period the infant gains weight from an average weight of about 3.5 kg at birth to about 12 kg at age 2 years, and the dietary pattern changes dramatically from breast-feeding or use of infant formulas to a diet which approaches that of adults. The actual fluoride dose, measured as mg F/kg body weight, is therefore likely to fluctuate considerably and may during some periods be substantially higher than actually intended. During first 2 years of life, mineralization has begun of all permanent teeth except second premolars, and second and third molars, and most permanent teeth will therefore be affected by the fluoride ingested during the first 2 years of life.

In order to estimate the daily dose of fluoride from tablets that may result in dental fluorosis, we can compare the results of controlled studies from the USA and Sweden. In these studies, children were given fluoride tablets beginning at the age of 1 week to 4 months;[1] or beginning at the age of 6 months;[13] or they consumed drinking water containing about 1 ppm of fluoride.[1,13] The recommended fluoride supplement regimen in the USA population was at the time 0.5 mg F daily from birth to the age of 3 years and thereafter 1 mg F daily. In the Swedish population the recommended daily dose for children aged between 6 and 18 months was 0.25 mg F and thereafter 0.5 mg F until 6 years of age.

It is apparent from Table 9-6 that there is a strong similarity in the prevalence and severity of dental fluorosis of the two populations living in areas where the drinking water sources contained 1-1.2 ppm fluoride. However, the different tablet regimens resulted in quite different prevalences of dental fluorosis, with 84% affected in the USA and 28.6% in Sweden. This substantial difference may have several explanations. First, the fluoride tablet dose was higher in the USA group. Secondly, fluoride supplementation commenced at an earlier age in the USA group than in the Swedish group and this is known to lead to a higher prevalence of dental fluorosis.[16] Thirdly, as previously indicated, premolars will be more severely affected than incisors. In the Swedish study[13] only incisors were recorded, whereas in the USA group the recordings were occasionally

Table 9-7

The 2.5-, 50-, and 97.5-percentiles for the weight (kg) of children aged 6 months to 6 years.

Figures in ( ) denote the 5- and 95-percentiles, respectively.

Data from Documenta Geigy[6]

Age	Weight (kg)		
	2.5%	50%	97.5%
6 months	(6.3)	7.5	(8.6)
12 months	(8.2)	9.5	(11.3)
2 yr	9.1	11.9	14.7
3 yr	10.3	14.3	18.3
4 yr	11.7	16.3	23.1
5 yr	13.5	18.3	23.1
6 yr	14.9	20.6	26.3

based on erupted premolars. This may have added to the differences between the two groups.

In order to calculate the actual daily dose of fluoride (mg F/kg body weight) ingested in the form of tablets by the children in the two studies referred to above, we have used data on weights of children aged 0-6 years presented in Documenta Geigy.[6] As these data do not originate from the populations studied for dental fluorosis they cannot be used with absolute certainty, but they constitute the best available material. Table 9-7 shows the data for weight used in the subsequent calculations. Using these values, the median daily fluoride intake from tablets varied with age from 0.042 to 0.070 mg F/kg in the US group (Table 9-8) and from 0.020 to 0.042 mg/kg in the Swedish group (Table 9-9). The children in the Swedish fluoride tablet group lived in an area with 0.2 ppm fluoride in the drinking water and this would at most add 0.01 mg F/kg to the calculated intake. The background water fluoride levels of the US tablet group were not reported, but it is quite clear from the fluorosis prevalence data in

Table 9-6 that the daily fluoride dose received in the tablet group has been substantially higher than in the "optimal" (1 ppm) water fluoride group.

Unfortunately, calculation of the daily dose of fluoride from drinking waters in the 1 ppm area is subject to some uncertainty. Firstly, it was noted that the water fluoride levels in the area fluctuated considerably.[1] Secondly, use must be made of the Galagan et al.[12] formula for the daily intake of water as a function of temperature but there may be a big difference in fluoride intake depending on whether the infant is breast-fed or bottle-fed.[12,34] The average 1-month-old to 12-month-old bottle-fed child consumes 22-77 mL/kg[34,] which yields a daily fluoride intake of 0.015-0.077 mg. However, using a mean maximum air temperature for Boston, where the USA study was performed, of 59° Fahrenheit (15 °C),[30] it may be calculated that the children in the 1 ppm water fluoride group ingested about 0.025 mg F/kg body weight per day.

What consequences will this now have when considering the contribution of fluoride from daily use of fluoridated toothpastes?

Daily fluoride dose from dentifrices

There is no doubt that fluoride toothpastes contribute to total fluoride intake as this has been demonstrated by measurements of elevated fluoride concentrations in plasma and urine after toothpaste use.[7,8,9,27]

In order to compare the degree of fluoride exposure from toothpaste with the calculations presented for fluoride tablets, we may consider a population of children whose toothbrushing is supervised twice daily from 2 years of age. Assuming that the toothpaste contains 1000 ppm fluoride and using the mean values for amounts of toothpaste used per brushing and the mean percentages of these amounts which are ingested (shown in Tables 18-6 and 18-7 in

Table 9-8
The 2.5-, 50-, and 97.5-percentiles for the daily intake of fluoride (mg F/kg) according to age of the children in the USA F-tablet group[1].
Figures in ( ) denote the 5- and 95-percentiles, respectively

Age	Fluoride intake (mg F/kg)		
	2.5%	50%	97.5%
6 months	(0.079)	0.067	(0.058)
12 months	(0.061)	0.053	(0.044)
2 yr	0.055	0.042	0.034
3 yr	0.097	0.070	0.055
4 yr	0.085	0.061	0.048
5 yr	0.074	0.055	0.043
6 yr	0.067	0.049	0.038

Table 9-9
The 2.5-, 50-, and 97.5-percentiles for the daily intake of fluoride (mg F/kg) according to age of the children in the Swedish F-tablet group[13].
Figures in ( ) denote the 5- and 95-percentiles, respectively

Age	Fluoride intake (mg F/kg)		
	2.5%	50%	97.5%
6 months	(0.039)	0.033	(0.029)
12 months	(0.030)	0.026	(0.022)
2 yr	0.055	0.042	0.034
3 yr	0.049	0.035	0.027
4 yr	0.043	0.031	0.024
5 yr	0.037	0.027	0.022
6 yr	0.034	0.024	0.019

Table 9-10
Fluoride intake according to age from twice daily use of a 1000 ppm fluoride toothpaste compared with median fluoride intake calculated for the Swedish tablet study shown in Table 9-9

Age (years)	Toothpaste use per day (g)	Toothpaste ingested (%)	Fluoride intake mg F/kg	
			1000 ppm F toothpaste	Swedish tablet study
2	1.16	48	0.047	0.042
3	1.16	48	0.039	0.035
4	1.12	42	0.029	0.031
5	1.00	34	0.019	0.027
6	1.32	25	0.013	0.024

Chapter 18), fluoride exposure from toothpaste in relation to age may be calculated. These calculations are shown in Table 9-10, where the fluoride values calculated for toothpaste are compared with the median fluoride intake calculated for the Swedish tablet study. As this table shows, fluoride intake from toothpaste is similar to intake in the tablet study until age 4 years, after which it is less. As use of fluoride toothpaste was not recommended for children under 6 years at the time of the Swedish tablet study, the calculations presented here suggest that our theoretical population of supervised toothpaste users would be expected to develop a similar prevalence of dental fluorosis i.e. up to 28%.

Two factors may explain why much lower prevalences may be expected in normal populations. First of all, frequency of toothbrushing may not be as high as assumed in this theoretical population. Secondly, absorption of fluoride from toothpaste may be lower than for tablets due to the timing of toothbrushing in relation to mealtimes and composition of meals. Thus, toothbrushing after meals may result in lower fluoride exposure than would occur from a tablet given before or between meals (see Chapter 4).

On the other hand, the calculations presented here clearly demonstrate that increases in prevalence of dental fluorosis due to fluoride toothpaste may be expected, especially in areas with more than 0.2-0.3 ppm F in the drinking water. Obviously, this risk will be increased if high concentration toothpastes are used, if children use larger amounts of toothpaste than recommended, and if children are not discouraged from eating toothpaste. These conclusions are in keeping with results of studies which have reported increased prevalences of fluorosis related to toothpaste use. A *case study investigation* in a fluoridated area in Canada reported a statistically significant association between early use of fluoride dentifrices and increased risk of dental fluorosis.[25] A similar trend has been reported from a low fluoride area[26] and Leverett and coworkers[20] reported that severity of fluorosis was related to continuous use of fluoride toothpaste in both a fluoridated and a non-fluoridated community.

When considering the above comparison between fluoride tablet-induced dental fluorosis and risk of dental fluorosis from use of fluoride toothpaste, their effects are expected to be additive. Therefore, it is interesting to consider the results of a detailed study of fluoride tablets, dental fluorosis and dental caries prevalences in Tiel, Holland.[17] The most important predicting factor for the caries experience of a child in that study was the mother's motivation to engage in preventive dental behavior. In those cases where this motivation resulted in use of fluoride tablets, a statistically significant bivariate relation was found between the use of fluoride tablets and the prevalence of dental fluorosis. However, most important was the finding that when taking account of the motivation of the mother as a confounding factor an effect of fluoride tablets on caries experience could not be demonstrated, i.e. tablets *per se* are not necessary – the crucial thing is to engage mothers in preventive behavior.

The use of fluoridated toothpaste alone in children living in low water fluoride areas (< 0.3 mg F/L) is unlikely to cause significant dental fluorosis assuming a "normal pattern" of use.[19] It should be remembered, however, that many children are not normal users, as they eat the toothpaste. We can therefore conclude that both water fluoride studies and fluoride tablet studies indicate that a daily intake of fluoride as low as 0.020 mg F/kg body weight may result in dental fluorosis in the permanent dentition. Moreover, the data originating in water fluoride studies indicate that for each increase in dose of 0.01 mg F/kg body weight, an increase in Dean's Community Fluorosis Index, F_{ci}, of 0.2 can be expected. Moreover, any other source of fluoride which results in ingestion of fluorides will add to the risk of increasing prevalence and severity of dental fluorosis in a population.

Literature cited

1. Aasenden R, Peebles TC. Effects of fluoride supplementation from birth on human primary and permanent teeth. Arch Oral Biol 1974; 19: 321-6.

2. Butler WJ, Segreto V, Collins E. Prevalence of dental mottling in school-aged lifetime residents of 16 Texas communities. Am J Public Health 1985; 75: 1408-12.

3. Dean HT. The investigation of physiological effects by the epidemiological method. In: Moulton FR, ed. Fluorine and dental health. Washington DC: American Association for the Advancement of Science 1942: 23-31.

4. Dean HT, Jay P, Arnold FA, Elvove E. Domestic waters and dental caries. II. A study of 2832 white children ages 12-14 years of eight suburban Chicago communities, including Lactobacillus acidophilus studies of 1761 children. Public Health Rep 1941; 56: 761-92.

5. Dean HT, Arnold FA, Elvove E. Domestic water and dental caries. V. Additional studies of the relation of fluoride domestic waters to dental caries in 4425 white children, age 12-14 years, of 13 cities in 4 states. Public Health Rep 1942; 57: 1155-79.

6. Documenta Geigy. Scientific tables. 7th ed. Basel: Ciba-Geigy Ltd 1975: 693-8.

7. Dooland MB, Wylie A. Urinary fluoride levels in pre-school children in relation to the use of fluoride toothpaste. Aust Dent J 1988; 33: 101-3.

8. Ekstrand J, Ehrnebo M. Absorption of fluoride from fluoride dentifrice. Caries Res 1980; 14: 96-102.

9. Ekstrand J, Koch G, Petersson L. Plasma fluoride concentration in preschool children after ingestion of fluoride tablets and toothpaste. Caries Res 1983; 17: 379-84.

10. Forsman B. Early supply of fluoride and enamel fluorosis. Scand J Dent Res 1977; 85: 22-30.

11. Galagan DJ, Vermillion JR. Determining optimum fluoride concentrations. Public Health Rep 1957; 72: 491-3.

12. Galagan DJ, Vermillion JR, Nevitt GA, Stadt ZM, Dart RE. Climate and fluid intake. Public Health Rep 1957; 72: 484-90.

13. Granath L, Widenheim J, Birkhed D. Diagnosis of mild enamel fluorosis in permanent maxillary incisors using two scoring systems. Community Dent Oral Epidemiol 1985; 13: 273-6.

14. Heifetz SB, Horowitz HS. Amounts of fluoride in self-administered dental products: safety considerations for children. Pediatrics 1986; 77: 876-82.

15. Hodge HC. The concentration of fluorides in the drinking water to give the point of minimum caries with maximum safety. J Am Dent Assoc 1950; 40: 436-9.

16. Holm AK, Andersson R. Enamel mineralization disturbances in 12-year-old children with known early exposure to fluorides. Community Dent Oral Epidemiol 1982; 10: 335-9.

17. Kalsbeek H, Verrips GH, Backer Dirks O. Use of fluoride tablets and effect on prevalence of dental caries and dental fluorosis. Community Dent Oral Epidemiol 1992; 20: 241-5.

18. Larsen MJ, Kirkegaard E, Poulsen S. Patterns of dental fluorosis in a European country in relation to fluoride concentrations in drinking water. J Dent Res 1989; 66: 10-2.

19. Larsen MJ, Kirkegaard E, Fejerskov O, Poulsen S. Prevalence of dental fluorosis after fluoride gel treatments in a low fluoride area. J Dent Res 1985; 64: 1076-9.

20. Leverett DB, Adair SM, Proskin HM. Dental fluorosis among children in fluoridated and non-fluoridated communities [abstr.]. J Dent Res 1988; 67: 230.

21. Manji F, Baelum V, Fejerskov O, Gemert W. Enamel changes in two low fluoride areas of Kenya. Caries Res 1986; 20: 371-80.

22. Myers HM. Fluorides and dental fluorosis. Basel: Karger 1978.

23. Møller IJ. Dental fluorose og caries. Thesis. Copenhagen: Rhodos 1965.

24. Ophaug RH, Singer L, Harland BF. Dietary fluoride intake of 6-month and 2-year-old children in four dietary regions of the United States. Am J Clin Nutr. 1985; 42: 701-7.

25. Osuji OO, Leake JL, Chipman ML, Nikiforuk G, Locker D, Levine L. Risk factors for dental fluorosis in a fluoridated community. J Dent Res 1988; 67: 1488-92.

26. Pendrys DG, Katz RV. Risk of enamel fluorosis

associated with fluoride supplementation, infant formula, and fluoride dentifrice use. Am J Epidemiol 1989; 130: 1199-208.

27. Rajan BP, Gnanasundaram N, Santhini R. Serum and urine fluoride levels in toothpaste users. J Indian Dent Assoc 1987; 59: 137-42.

28. Richards LF, Westmoreland WW, Tashiro M, McKay CH, Morrison JT. Determining optimum fluoride levels for community water supplies in relation to temperature. J Am Dent Assoc 1967; 74: 389-97.

29. Smith F, Ekstrand J. Fluoride in the environment and intake in man. In: Ekstrand J, Fejerskov O, Silverstone LM, eds. Fluoride in dentistry. Copenhagen: Munksgaard 1988: 13-27.

30. Statistical Abstract of the United States. 104th edn. US Department of Commerce, Bureau of the Census 1984.

31. Szpunar SM, Burt BA. Trends in the prevalence of dental fluorosis in the United States: a review. J Public Health Dent 1987; 47: 71-9.

32. Taves DR. Dietary intake of fluoride ashed (total fluoride) v. unashed (inorganic fluoride) analysis of individual foods. Br J Nutr 1983; 49: 295-301.

33. Thylstrup A, Fejerskov O. Clinical appearance of dental fluorosis in permanent teeth in relation to histological changes. Community Dent Oral Epidemiol 1978; 6: 315-28.

34. Walker JS, Margolis FJ, Teate HL, Weil ML, Wildon HL. Water intake of normal children. Science 1963; 140: 890-1.

CHAPTER 10

FLUORIDE TOXICOLOGY AND HEALTH EFFECTS

G.M. Whitford

Introduction – Historical perspective – Acute toxic dose – Fluoride in dental products
Factors affecting acute toxicity – Characteristics and treatment of acute fluoride toxicity
Sublethal toxic effects of fluoride

Introduction

The fluoridation of public water supplies represents one of the most successful public health measures ever undertaken. First added to public drinking water supplies at controlled concentrations in 1945, fluoride is now added to school water supplies, salt or milk in regions where the fluoridation of central water supplies is not possible. It is available in tablet form and in drops which are designed as dietary supplements for children. Fluoride is present in a variety of dental products which are intended for topical application to the teeth. The widespread use of these various vehicles for the systemic or topical delivery of fluoride is undoubtedly responsible in large part for the remarkable decline in the prevalence of dental caries that is currently being experienced in many countries of the Western world.

Fluoride is also a toxic substance. Its acute ingestion in large quantities may be followed by rapidly developing signs and symptoms which may result in death. When it is ingested in relatively small amounts during the period of tooth development, it may produce changes in the quality and appearance of the enamel known as dental fluorosis. When somewhat larger amounts are ingested over a period of years, changes in the quality and quantity of the skeleton may occur. This, in fact, is the basis of the use of fluoride for the treatment of osteoporosis. The skeletal changes, however, may become severe enough to be classified as crippling skeletal fluorosis. Discussions of dental fluorosis and skeletal fluorosis can be found in Chapters 7, 8 and 9.

It is the responsibility of health practitioners, especially those in dentistry, to be aware of the toxic potential of fluoride and to ensure that it is used in ways that enhance health with minimal risk of causing adverse effects. The purposes of this chapter are to acquaint the reader with the nature and treatment of fluoride toxicity, the doses that can produce unwanted effects and to provide guidelines for the safe use of fluorides.

167

Historical perspective

Prior to the introduction of water fluoridation as a public health measure, the principal use of fluoride known to the layman was that of a pesticide. Indeed, the most extraordinary case of mass poisoning due to the ingestion of fluoride was due to mistaking roach powder for powdered milk.[21] Approximately 17 pounds of sodium fluoride were added to a 10-gallon mixture of scrambled eggs at the Oregon State Hospital. There were 263 poisoning cases of which 47 terminated fatally. Prior to this incident, most of the cases of accidental fluoride poisoning were due to mistaking sodium fluoride for sodium bicarbonate, flour or magnesium sulfate (Epsom salt). In one case, sodium fluoride was added to pancakes at a Salvation Army center. Forty persons were affected, of whom 12 died.

In 1965, Hodge & Smith published their excellent treatise which deals extensively with the toxicity of fluoride.[18] They pointed out that there were 607 documented fatalities in the USA from 1933 to 1955. Nearly two-thirds of these were suicides. The number of deaths was probably considerably higher because data from 1937-43 and from 1945-48 were not given. Moreover, there was no uniform procedure for reporting poisonings to a central facility during those years.

While three recent deaths of young children due to the ingestion of fluoride-containing dental products have been documented (see Acute toxic dose section), the number of fluoride poisonings with fatal outcomes appears to have decreased sharply in recent years. In 1984, the American Association of Poison Control Centers published its findings from a pilot project designed to collect and process data from participating poison control centers.[32] Since then, the AAPCC has published its findings annually in the American Journal of Emergency Medicine. Table 10-1 contains a summary of the fluoride-related data for 1989-92. Approximately 75% of the USA population was represented in each year, so the data in Table 10-1 are underestimations by about 25%. About 90% of the cases involved children under the age of 6 years and nearly all were accidental rather than intentional exposures.

During the 4-year period, 44,174 reports expressing concern about the possibility of excessive fluoride ingestion were made to the participating poison control centers and 3090 cases were treated in health facilities. Of all the reports, approximately 39% were related to exposures from prescription tablets or solutions (electrolytes and minerals), 34% to vitamins, and 27% to over-the-counter toothpastes and mouthwashes. The Medical outcome (seriousness of effect) data of Table 10-1 show that 75% of the cases listed under this category were classified as "None", 5307 cases were classified as "Minor", 118 as "Moderate", 3 as "Major" and there was 1 fatality. A minor outcome means that the patient had some symptoms but they were minimal or no treatment was provided. A moderate outcome means that: the symptoms were more pronounced, more prolonged or more of a systemic nature than minor symptoms; the symptoms were not life-threatening but some form of treatment was indicated; and the patient had no residual disability. A major outcome means that the symptoms were life-threatening or resulted in residual disability or disfigurement.

The fatality in 1989 involved a 73-year-old man who was mistakenly given a stannous fluoride solution instead of distilled water to take with his medication.[23] After swallowing an unknown amount of the solution, he vomited and had explosive diarrhea. He was taken to an emergency department where he exhibited the signs and symptoms of severe acute fluoride poisoning. In spite of continuing intensive care during the next 6 days, his renal function deteriorated to the point where hemodialysis was

Table 10-1

Summary of fluoride-related reports made to U.S. poison control centers from 1989 to 1992

Year	F category	Total number of reports	Treated in health facility	Medical outcome				
				None	Minor	Moderate	Major	Death
1989	A	4028	375	1807	663	14	1	1
	B	289	39	144	27	0	0	0
	C	3477	254	1379	175	1	0	0
	D	1392	101	464	371	15	0	0
	E	1185	56	503	115	3	0	0
Totals		10371	825	4297	1351	33	1	1
1990	A	4437	338	1950	653	10	0	0
	B	254	22	126	12	0	0	0
	C	3421	189	1117	125	0	0	0
	D	1379	107	468	329	7	0	0
	E	1299	64	511	109	2	0	0
Totals		10790	720	4172	1228	19	0	0
1991	A	4350	368	1593	667	12	1	0
	B	334	36	129	19	1	0	0
	C	3431	194	946	140	4	0	0
	D	1623	120	497	403	15	0	0
	E	1418	72	556	112	0	0	0
Totals		11156	790	3721	1341	32	1	0
1992	A	4171	340	1579	624	12	0	0
	B	286	29	112	23	0	0	0
	C	3681	193	1027	151	4	0	0
	D	2331	141	700	497	17	1	0
	E	1388	52	545	92	1	0	0
Totals		11857	755	3963	1387	34	1	0
1989-92	A	16986	1421	6929	2607	48	2	1
	B	1163	126	511	81	1	0	0
	C	14010	830	4469	591	9	0	0
	D	6725	469	2129	1600	54	1	0
	E	5290	244	2115	428	6	0	0
Totals		44174	3090	16153	5307	118	3	1

A – Electrolytes and minerals
B – Adult vitamins
C – Pediatric vitamins
D – Toothpaste
E – Mouthwash

required. Other serious complications developed and the patient died in the hospital 26 days after the exposure.

While there are tens of millions of exposures to fluoride-containing products in the USA each day, the data in Table 10-1 indicate that only about 30 reports about possible or actual over-exposures are made to poison control centers each day, the vast majority of which require no treatment. The data also indicate, however, that the presence of these products in the home presents a hazard about which parents and health professionals should be aware. This subject is discussed more fully below.

Acute toxic dose

Because there are several variables that can affect the outcome of acute fluoride poisoning, it is not surprising that the fatal dose is uncertain. In cases of human poisonings the uncertainty is amplified because, in most instances, the exact doses involved is not precisely known. Dreisbach[9] stated that the acute lethal dose of fluoride for humans is 6-9 mg F/kg while the data of Lidbeck et al.[21] suggested that it is over 100 mg F/kg.

The most frequently cited range for the certainly lethal dose of sodium fluoride was offered by Hodge & Smith.[18] After reviewing case reports, they concluded that 5-10 g of sodium fluoride would certainly be fatal for a person with a body weight of 70 kg. Because sodium fluoride is 45.2% fluoride by weight, the dose range for adults would be 32-64 mg F/kg. It should be noted that this range is equivalent to an LD_{100}, i.e. any 70 kg adult who ingested that much fluoride would be expected to die. This is important information but values such as the LD_{10}, the LD_{50} or the upper limit for the certainly safe dose would be of more utility from the public health and clinical perspectives. Although these values for humans are not known, by reviewing the case reports of three

recent deaths of young children, it is possible to refine our understanding of the fluoride doses that may be life-threatening.

Table 10-2 summarizes the important features of four deaths resulting from the ingestion of fluoride-containing dental products. An unusual case of fluoride poisoning was reported by Dukes involving a low dose and a prolonged period between the exposure to fluoride and death.[11] In most cases, if death does not occur during the first 1 or 2 days then the victim usually survives. In this case, however, a 27-month-old boy experienced respiratory failure after ingesting about 100 0.5-mg fluoride tablets. When gastric lavage was performed, four tablets were recovered. The child died 5 days later. The body weight was not given but it was probably between 11 and 16 kg, the 3rd and 97th percentiles for USA male children of this age. The fluoride dose, therefore, would have been less than 5 mg F/kg. Another child, a 3-year-old boy, died 7 hours after ingesting 200 1.0-mg fluoride tablets.[13] The child vomited immediately and then seemed to recover completely but collapsed 4 hours later. The body weight was 12.5 kg so that the fluoride dose was 16.0 mg F/kg. Church[7] reported a case of poisoning that resulted in the death of a 3-year-old boy. The child swallowed about 45 mL of a 4% stannous fluoride mouthrinse solution (ca. 435 mg of fluoride) in a dental office. Five minutes later the child vomited and had a convulsive seizure. Three hours later the child died in a nearby medical center. The body weight was not reported but it was probably between 12.3 kg and 17.8 kg, the 3rd and 97th percentiles for 3-year-old males. Therefore, the fluoride dose was probably between 24 and 35 mg F/kg.

Based on these reports it may be concluded that if a child ingests a fluoride dose in excess of 15 mg F/kg, then death is likely to occur. A dose as low as 5 mg F/kg may be fatal for some children. Therefore, the probably toxic dose (PTD), defined as the threshold dose that could

Table 10-2
Summary of four deaths caused by ingestion of fluoride-containing dental products

Age	Sex	Body weight (kg)	Dose (mg F/kg)	Comment	Reference
27 month	M	Not reported	3.1-4.5*	Ingested ca. 100 F tablets; death occurred 5 days later.	11
3 years	M	12.5	16	Ingested ca. 200 F tablets; vomited; death occurred 7 hours later.	13
3 years	M	Not reported	24-35*	Swallowed stannous fluoride rinse solution; vomited; death occurred 3 hours later.	7

* The dose ranges were calculated by use of the 3rd and 97th percentile body weights for U.S. boys.

cause serious or life-threatening systemic signs and symptoms and that should trigger immediate emergency treatment and hospitalization, is 5 mg F/kg.

Fluoride in dental products

It is essential that the fluoride concentrations in dental products be known by the persons who use them. It is even more important to know the amounts of fluoride that are contained in the unit packages (bottles, tubes, etc.) as well as the amounts involved during routine usage and how these amounts relate to the PTD. The concentrations in USA dentifrices are approximately 1000 ppm (± 10%) with the exception of Extra Strength Aim, which contains 1500 ppm fluoride. In some European countries, dentifrices for young children contain lower fluoride levels (because of concerns about dental fluorosis), in others, dentifrice fluoride levels range up to 2500 ppm (see also Chapter 18).

Most fluoride-containing mouthrinses contain either stannous fluoride or sodium fluoride. The concentrations in the mouthrinses are usually expressed in terms of percent. This means the number of grams of stannous fluoride or sodium fluoride per 100 mL of rinse solution. Most of the over-the-counter (OTC)

mouthrinses sold in the USA contain 0.05% sodium fluoride or 0.0226% fluoride. Thus, there are 22.6 mg F/100 mL or 226 mg F/L (mg/L or mg/kg = ppm). Some mouthrinses, such as the 0.2% sodium fluoride rinses, are available only on prescription. They have a fluoride concentration of 910 mg F/L. Those that contain 0.4% stannous fluoride, which is 24.3% fluoride by weight, have a fluoride concentration of 970 mg F/L. Some dentists prepare their own rinses as in the fatal case involving 4% stannous fluoride described above. Such a solution has a fluoride concentration of 9700 mg F/L. One of the standard textbooks on dental drugs, Accepted Dental Therapeutics[8], which is published by the American Dental Association, states that the preferred stannous fluoride solution for topical application to the teeth contains 8% stannous fluoride. Such a solution has an extremely high fluoride level (19,400 mg F/L) (see also Chapter 18).

The APF (acidulated phosphate fluoride) gels generally contain 1.23% fluoride, added as sodium fluoride, and 1% phosphoric acid (ca. pH 3.5). Thus, they have a fluoride concentration of 12,300 mg F/L. In seven alginate impression materials tested, the fluoride concentrations ranged from 8,600 to 30,500 mg F/kg (ppm). In a study with human volunteers, however, it was determined that only about 1.0

Table 10-3

Fluoride in dental products

Product		Compound %	Concentration of fluoride		Amount of product and F usually used		Amount containing the PTD[a]	
			%	PPM	Product	Fluoride	10 kg child[b]	20 kg child[c]
Rinse	NaF	0.05	0.023	230	10 mL	2.3 mg	215 mL	430 mL
	NaF	0.20	0.091	910	10 mL	9.1 mg	55 mL	110 mL
	SnF$_2$	0.40	0.097	970	10 mL	9.7 mg	50 mL	100 mL
Dentifrice	NaF	0.22	0.10	1000	1 g	1.0 mg	50 g	100 g
	MFP	0.76	0.10	1000	1 g	1.0 mg	50 g	100 g
	MFP	1.14	0.15	1500	1 g	1.5 mg	33 g	66 g
Topical gel or solution	NaF (APF)	2.72	1.23	12300	5 mL	61.5 mg	4 mL	8 mL
	SnF$_2$	0.40	0.097	970	1 mL	0.97 mg	50 mL	100 mL
	SnF$_2$	8.0	1.94	19400	1 mL	19.4 mg	2.5 mL	5 mL
Tablet	0.25 mg F	–	–	–	1/day	0.25 mg	200 Tab	400 Tab
	0.50 mg F	–	–	–	1/day	0.50 mg	100 Tab	200 Tab
	1.00 mg F	–	–	–	1/day	1.00 mg	50 Tab	100 Tab

a: the PTD is the "probably toxic dose", 5 mg F/kg. If this amount or more is ingested, the individual should receive emergency treatment and be hospitalized.

b: 10 kg is the approximate average body weight of a 1-year-old child.

c: 20 kg is the approximate average body weight of a 5-to-6-year-old child.

mg of fluoride was swallowed and absorbed during routine impression procedures.[35]

Table 10-3 shows the fluoride concentrations of a variety of dental products, the amounts of product and of fluoride that are typically involved with each use and the amounts of the products that contain enough fluoride to reach the PTD for a 10-kg child (ca. 1 year old) or a 20-kg child (5-6 years old). One point of interest is that, as the products are typically used in the home or the dental office, only the 1.23% APF gels contain sufficient fluoride to reach the PTD. Of course, 1-year-old children do not normally receive APF gel treatments so the value given in the table for this age group has little practical meaning. However, 2-year-old children do receive such treatments in some dental offices. The average body weight of a 2-year-old is 12.3 kg. The PTD for this body weight is 61.5 mg of fluoride, an amount that is contained in 5.0 mL of a 1.23% APF gel. With this exception, it can be concluded that if the listed dental products are used as recommended they present no risk of life-threatening acute fluoride toxicity.

Young children, however, often do not use dental products according to the recommendations of manufacturers or dental professionals. Some children occasionally drink mouthrinses or eat dentifrices or too many fluoride tablets. The OTC fluoride mouthrinses are available in the USA in bottles containing up to 18 ounces or 532 mL. This quantity is 2.5 times the PTD for a 10-kg child and 1.2 times the PTD for a 20-kg child (see Table 10-2). Fluoride dentifrices contain up to 8.2 ounces or about 230 grams. This weight contains enough fluoride to exceed the PTD for each of the dentifrices listed by at least a factor of 2.3. The 1.23% gels and the 8% stannous fluoride solutions are clearly hazardous to the health of young children or even adults. One bottle of 0.25-mg fluoride tablets would not pose a lethal hazard, at least in the USA, because they are supplied in 100-tablet amounts. There is, however, a life-threatening hazard in the case of the 0.5- or 1.0-mg fluoride tablets, which are also supplied in 100-tablet amounts.

Based on the data in Table 10-3, the following recommendations should be followed for mouthrinses, dentifrices, 0.4% stannous fluoride gels and tablets:

- They should not be used by young children without the supervision and presence of an adult; and

- They should be kept out of the reach of young children.

For the 1.23% APF gels, the high-concentration stannous fluoride solutions and other products with similarly high fluoride concentrations, the following recommendations should be followed:

- They should be applied only by dental professionals;

- The patient should not be left unattended;

- The quantities used and, after the application, the quantities left in the mouth should be minimized.

Factors affecting acute toxicity

The compounds of fluoride differ widely with respect to fluoride bioavailability (absorbability) and, therefore, in their acute toxic potentials. The differences in toxic potential are related to the solubilities of the compounds and they are apparent even when they are given parenterally. For example, the 24-hour LD_{50} values in the rat of intraperitoneally administered NaF, CaF_2 and Na_3AlF_6 (cryolite) have been reported to be about 20-40 mg/kg, > 1500 mg/kg and > 2500 mg/kg, respectively.[18] In some cases, the cation of the compound may also exert a toxic effect. Thus, stannous fluoride is slightly more toxic than sodium fluoride apparently because high doses of the tin ion adversely affect the kidneys and other organs.

Disodium monofluorophosphate (Na_2PO_3F, or MFP) is commonly used in dentifrices. The fluoride in MFP is covalently bonded to the phosphorus. Two toxicity studies with rats have suggested that the acute LD_{50} of fluoride when given as sodium fluoride is only about one-half that when it is given as MFP[22,29] while two other studies could not detect a difference.[16,36] If there is a real difference, it might be due to the slower absorption of fluoride when it is given as MFP.[14,40] Unlike the fluoride of sodium fluoride, which is easily ionized and rapidly absorbed from the stomach and early small intestine, the fluoride of MFP must be hydrolyzed, chiefly by phosphatase, before appreciable absorption can occur. Because the stomach mucosa has little phosphatase activity, the molecule must pass into the intestine before quantitatively important amounts of fluoride can be absorbed. The delayed absorption re-

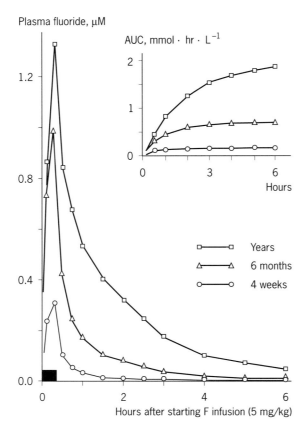

Fig. 10-1. The effect of age on the plasma fluoride levels in dogs. The dose to each dog was the same (5 mg F/kg) and it was given by constant iv infusion for 20 minutes (see black rectangle). The insert shows the cumulative areas under the time-plasma concentration curves (AUC).

sults in lower peak plasma levels than are achieved from the ingestion of sodium fluoride. The ultimate bioavailability of fluoride from MFP, however, is only slightly less than that from sodium fluoride.

A variety of other factors may also influence the toxicity of fluoride compounds, i.e. route of administration, age, rate of absorption and acid-base status. Results from animal studies have shown that younger animals are more resistant to the toxic effects of fluoride.[18,25] Mornstad[25] reported that the 24-hour LD_{50} of intraperitoneally injected sodium fluoride for rats declined sharply from about 50 mg F/kg at the age of 20 days to 20 mg F/kg at the age of 90 days.[25] That is, the younger animals were able to tolerate 2.5 times more fluoride than the older animals. A possible explanation for this is shown in Fig. 10-1. In this study with dogs of different ages, fluoride was administered intravenously at a constant rate for 20 min.[38] The dose, in terms of body weight, to each animal was the same (5 mg F/kg). The peak plasma level of the adult animal was 4.5 times higher than that of the 4-week-old puppy and the integrated area under the time-plasma concentration curve was nearly 10 times higher. Thus, fluoride was removed from the plasma and soft tissues much more rapidly by the younger animals, a phenomenon which is due mainly to the remarkable ability of the developing skeleton to rapidly take up the ion.

As stated above, it is generally believed (although without direct experimental verifica-

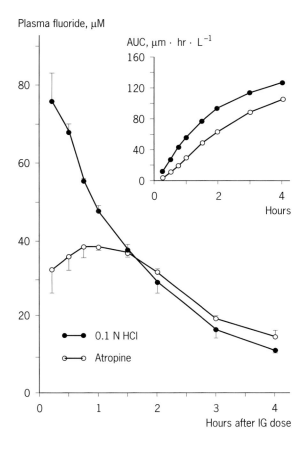

Plasma fluoride, μM

Fig. 10-2. The time courses of rat plasma fluoride levels and the cumulative areas under the time-plasma fluoride concentration curves (AUC) as affected by premedication with atropine or by administering the fluoride in an acidic solution.

tion) that one important determinant of the clinical outcome in fluoride poisoning is the magnitude of the peak plasma fluoride concentration that is achieved after ingestion. Fig. 10-2 shows the effect of gastric fluid pH on plasma fluoride in rats.[39] In this study, adult female rats were given 1.0 mg F/kg by gastric intubation. One group had been premedicated with atropine to diminish gastric acid secretion. The dosing solution contained 0.15 M NaCl with a pH of 6.7. The other group was not premedicated and received a dosing solution containing 0.1 N HCl with a pH of 1.4 so that nearly all the fluoride existed in the form of the undissociated acid, HF. The plasma fluoride curve of the atropine group failed to show a distinct peak: the average plasma levels during the first 2 hours after the dose did not differ with statistical significance. In contrast, the peak plasma level of the HCl group was observed in the samples taken 15 min after the intragastric dose, which indicated unusually rapid absorption. In a subsequent study with a similar design (Whitford, unpublished), the peak plasma levels were noted in the samples taken 5 min after the doses, which is akin to the time course observed when fluoride is given by intraperitoneal or subcutaneous injection. These findings strongly support the theory that the transepithelial and transmembrane transport of HF occurs much more rapidly than that of ionic fluoride, as discussed in Chapter 4 and below.

175

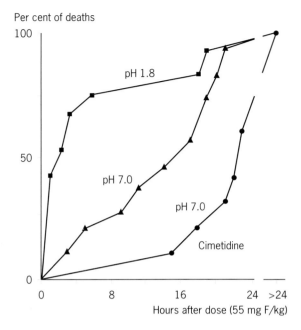

Fig. 10-3. The time course of death of rats after the intragastric administration of 55 mg F/kg as sodium fluoride. One group received its dose in HCl (pH 1.8), one in saline (pH 7.0), and one group had been premedicated with cimetidine before receiving its dose in saline (pH 7.0, cimetidine).

Table 10-4
Tissue-to-plasma (T/P) fluoride (^{18}F) concentration ratios of some soft tissues in the rat

Tissue	T/P ratio
Brain	0.08
Fat	0.11
Skin	0.43
Heart	0.46
Diaphragm	0.61
Salivary gland	0.63
Tongue	0.69
Lung	0.83
Liver	0.98
Kidney	4.16

If peak plasma fluoride concentrations are important in determing the clinical outcome, then the implication of these results for fluoride toxicity is that the acute toxic dose should be related to the pH of the administered solution or to the rate of gastric acid secretion. This hypothesis was tested in another study with rats that received 55 mg F/kg by gastric intubation.[37] The results of the study are shown in Fig. 10-3. The animals of the group that received fluoride in 0.1 N HCl (pH 1.8) died at the fastest rate; those that had been premedicated with cimetidine, a potent inhibitor of gastric acid secretion and had received their fluoride in saline died at the slowest rate;and those that were not premedicated but had received their fluoride in saline died at an intermediate rate. Ultimately, however, virtually the same number of animals died in each group (10-12 of 15). These results suggested that the magnitude of the peak plasma levels, which are shown in Fig. 10-4, did not affect the acute lethality of flu-

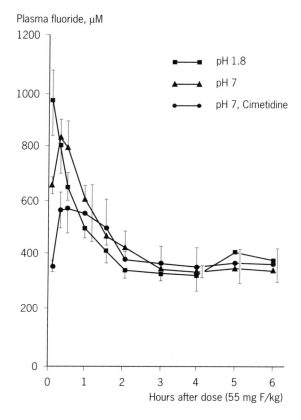

Plasma fluoride, μM

Hours after dose (55 mg F/kg)

Fig. 10-4. The time course of plasma fluoride levels of the groups described in Fig. 10-3. Ultimately, virtually the same number of animals died in each group, i.e. the outcome of the toxicity was not related to the peak plasma fluoride levels.

oride but did affect the elapsed time between giving the dose and death. Thus, the amount of time available for therapeutic intervention would be inversely proportional to the magnitude of the peak plasma fluoride levels.

Acid-base status and local pH gradients are important factors in the tissue distribution and renal clearance of fluoride.[34] Fluoride is present in the intracellular fluid of all cells. The tissue-to-plasma (T/P) fluoride concentration ratios for some tissues under steady-state and normal acid-base conditions are shown in Table 10-4.[41] The ratios for most tissues fall between 0.4 and 1.0, which indicates that intracellular fluoride concentrations are less than or approximately equal to plasma concentrations. Some notable exceptions to this range of T/P ratios include

kidney, brain and adipose tissue. Fluoride is concentrated to high levels in the renal tubular fluid so that when the entire organ is analyzed it has a higher concentration than that of plasma. The blood-brain barrier is effective in restricting the passage of fluoride into the central nervous system, where the fluoride concentration, like that of fat, is only about 20% of that in plasma.

The fact that the fluoride concentration in plasma and extracellular fluid is higher than in the intracellular fluids is consistent with the hypothesis that it is HF (a weak acid with a pH of 3.4), and not ionic fluoride, which is in diffusion equilibrium across cell membranes. This hypothesis has received support from a variety of experiments,[34] including studies using lipid

Alkaline urine

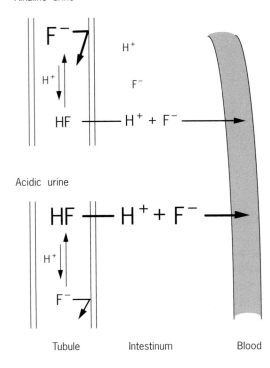

Acidic urine

Tubule	Intestinum	Blood

Fig. 10-5. The proposed mechanism to explain the pH dependence of the renal clearance of fluoride.

bilayer membranes where the permeability coefficient of HF was determined to be more than 10^6 times higher than that of ionic fluoride.[17] One consequence of this is that fluoride can be driven from plasma into cells or drawn from cells into plasma by changing the pH gradient across cell membranes, i.e. the difference between the pH values of the intracellular and extracellular fluid (for a full discussion of the mechanism see Whitford[34]). In general, the size of pH gradients can be reduced by acidifying the extracellular fluid, which would increase T/P ratios, and can be increased by alkalinizing the extracellular fluid, which would decrease T/P ratios. Thus, the T/P ratios shown in Table 10-4 are not absolute constants but vary with the size of the transmembrane pH gradient. This makes acid-base status a determining vari-

able in the susceptibility to acute fluoride toxicity, as will be demonstrated below.

Since the kidneys are the only significant route for removal of fluoride from the body, the adequacy of kidney function is also an important variable in cases of fluoride toxicity. The proposed mechanism for the pH dependence of the renal clearance of fluoride is shown in Fig. 10-5. The physiologic range for urinary pH is from 4.0 to 8.0. Because hydrogen fluoride is a weak acid ($pK_a = 3.4$), the fraction of fluoride in solution that exists as HF increases as the pH decreases. When the urine is alkaline, the concentration of HF is relatively low compared to that of ionic fluoride. As the urine becomes more acidic, the relative concentration of HF increases. In this way the diffusion gradient from the tubular lumen to the interstitial fluid

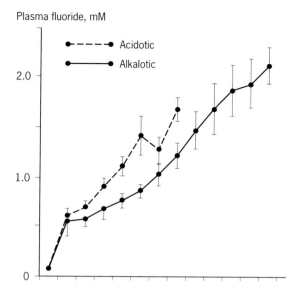

Plasma fluoride, mM

●----● Acidotic
●——● Alkalotic

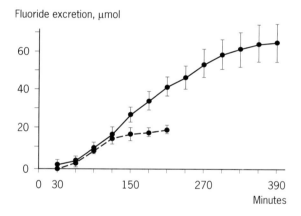

Fluoride excretion, μmol

Fig. 10-6. The time courses of plasma fluoride levels and the cumulative urinary excretions of fluoride in rats that were acidotic or alkalotic. Alkalosis enhanced fluoride excretion, caused the animals to tolerate more fluoride and delayed the time of death.

for HF, whose ability to permeate most types of epithelia or cell membranes is several orders of magnitude greater than that of ionic fluoride, varies inversely with the tubular fluid pH. Interstitial fluid pH always remains relatively constant near neutrality so HF molecules entering the interstitial fluid dissociate immediately to yield fluoride and hydrogen ions. Therefore, when the tubular fluid pH is relatively high, most of the fluoride remains within the tubule to be excreted, which means that the renal clearance is high. Conversely, when the tubular fluid is acidic, considerably more of the fluoride diffuses from the tubule as HF and is returned to the systemic circulation, which means that the renal clearance is low.

The effect of acid-base status on acute fluoride toxicity has been tested in two studies with rats.[28,42] Some of the results from these studies are shown in Fig. 10-6. In this experiment, rats received fluoride by constant intravenous infusion until death occurred. Metabolic acidosis was induced by administration of NH_4Cl and alkalosis by $NaHCO_3$. The alkalotic rats survived twice as long, died after higher fluoride doses (55 vs 25 mg F/kg) and with higher plasma fluoride concentrations, and they generally had higher systemic blood pressures, heart rates and glomerular filtration rates at any given plasma fluoride concentration. The cumulative fluoride excretion of the infused fluoride was nearly twice as high in the alkalotic group (12.3% vs 6.7%). Further, the tissue-to-plasma fluoride concentration ratios for heart and skeletal muscle were substantially lower in the alkalotic group compared to the acidotic group (0.63 vs 0.53 and 0.43 vs 0.28, respectively).

Characteristics and treatment of acute fluoride toxicity

After the ingestion of large amounts of fluoride, a toxic episode often develops with alarming rapidity. For example, in his discussion of the fatal case involving the 3-year-old who swallowed 4% stannous fluoride mouthrinse, Church[7] stated that approximately 5 minutes later the child vomited, followed by a convulsive seizure. A physical examination revealed the child was in shock. He died approximately 3 hours after accidental ingestion. It is for this reason that the PTD was defined earlier as the dose that should trigger immediate emergency treatment and hospitalization.

In nearly all cases of fluoride poisoning, the victims experience nausea, vomiting and abdominal pain within minutes after ingestion. There may or may not be a variety of non-specific symptoms such as excessive salivation, tearing, mucous discharges from the nose and mouth, diarrhea, headache, cold wet skin or convulsions. As the episode progresses, a generalized weakness, carpopedal spasms or spasm of the extremities and tetany often develop. These myopathologic signs accompany declining plasma calcium concentrations, which may fall to extraordinarily low values (< 5 mg%), and rising plasma potassium levels, which indicate a generalized toxic effect on cell membrane function. The pulse may be thready or not detectable. Blood pressure often falls precipitously to dangerously low levels. A respiratory acidosis, which diminishes the pH gradient across most cell membranes and results in a net migration of fluoride from extracellular fluid into the intracellular fluids, develops as the respiratory center is depressed. Cardiac arrhythmias may develop in association with the hypocalcemia and hyperkalemia. Extreme disorientation or coma usually precedes death, which may occur within the first few hours after the fluoride exposure.

The immediate treatment should be aimed at reducing the amount of fluoride available for absorption from the gastrointestinal tract. Thus, vomiting should be induced by administering an emetic, such as ipecac, followed by the oral administration of 1% calcium chloride or calcium gluconate. If the calcium-containing solutions are not available, then as much milk as can be ingested should be given. The hospital emergency department should be informed that a case of fluoride poisoning is in progress while these procedures are being carried out. The patient should be transported to the hospital at the earliest possible time. Vomiting should not be induced if the victim has no gag reflex or while unconscious or convulsing because of the danger of aspiration. In these cases, a cuffed endotracheal tube should be inserted followed by gastric lavage with a solution containing calcium or activated charcoal.

In the hospital, the medical treatment will depend on the severity of the signs and symptoms. If vomiting has not occurred already, then it should be induced. If the patient is symptomatic, immediate attention should be given to establishing a patent airway, an intravenous line and to monitoring and maintaining the cardiovascular circulation. If gastric lavage has not been performed, it should be done as described above. Blood samples should be taken hourly for the analysis of plasma fluoride concentrations. Fluid replacement may be required because of vomiting, diarrhea or gastrointestinal hemorrhage and to maintain urinary flow rate. The intravenous fluids should include sodium bicarbonate or lactated Ringer's to minimize the degree of acidosis and to elevate the urinary pH, which should increase the excretion rate of fluoride. Acetazolamide (Diamox) may be a useful adjunct for these purposes.[42] Continuous evaluation of evidence for hyperkalemia and hypocalcemia through serum chemistry analyses, ECG monitoring and testing for muscle excitability or tetany may be required. Intermittent intravenous calcium replacement, glucose administration, O_2 therapy, artificial respiration, electrocardioconversion, hemodialysis (against a solution made with fluoride-free water) or other supportive therapies should be given as required. If the patient shows signs of favorably responding to treatment, clinical monitoring and supportive therapy should nevertheless continue until the vital signs, serum chemistry profile and mental alertness are within normal ranges.

Sublethal toxic effects of fluoride

At the present time, the most common sources of fluoride intake are fluoridated drinking water or salt (e.g. in Switzerland and Hungary) and dental products. More rarely, fluoride exposure may come from fluorinated drugs such as certain steroids or analgesics, the fluorinated volatile anesthetics such as halothane, industrial exposure such as in phosphate fertilizer factories or aluminum processing plants, or the atmosphere downwind from such factories.

There is no possibility of serious acute toxicity from the ingestion of drinking water or salt with controlled fluoride levels (ca. 1 mg/L and 300 mg/kg, respectively). For example, to ingest the PTD (5 mg F/kg) with water, a 10-kg child would have to drink 50 liters of water. In the case of salt, a 10-kg child would have to ingest 167 g.

There have, however, been several acute poisonings due to the accidental over-fluoridation of community or school drinking water supplies.[1,5,15,19,33] In nearly all cases, the symptoms were relatively minor and of short duration. However, an accidental fluoride overfeed of water supply in Annapolis, Maryland, resulted in a water fluoride level of 50 ppm.[1] Several hemodialysis patients became ill and one died. More recently, a fluoride concentration of 15-25 ppm in the dialysate of a Chicago hemodialysis center resulted in several illnesses and three deaths.[5] At this time, the full report describing this accident has not been published but, according to the Centers for Disease Control in Atlanta, Georgia, the water supplied to the hospital from the city's central water supply did not have an elevated fluoride concentration. Apparently, excessive fluoride was somehow introduced into the water within the hospital. In 1992, the first death ever to occur from the ingestion of fluoride in drinking water was reported.[15] The drinking water in Hooper Bay, Alaska, reached 150 ppm due to equipment failure and/or operator error. It was estimated that 296 persons became ill but most cases were minor and of short duration. One man, however, continued to drink the water for several hours in an attempt to replace water losses due to vomiting and diarrhea. He was found dead the next morning. His fluoride dose during the episode was estimated to be 17.9 mg F/kg.

With the possible exception of osteocytes, the cells of the gastric mucosa and of the renal tubules, especially the loops of Henle and collecting ducts located in the renal medulla, are exposed to the highest fluoride concentrations in the body. Among healthy subjects living in

181

communities with fluoridated water, the usual plasma fluoride concentration is about 1 µmol/L while the urinary concentration is 30-50 times higher. The fluoride concentrations of the major anatomic sections of the kidney (i.e. cortex, outer medulla, inner medulla) describe a steep cortex-to-papilla fluoride concentration gradient is similar to that of sodium and chloride.[43] It is not surprising, therefore, that when plasma fluoride concentrations are elevated to about 30 µmol/L, as may occur after 1.23% APF gel treatments, after surgical anesthesia with the fluorinated anesthetic methoxyflurane (Penthrane), or exposure to other large amounts of fluoride, the ability of the kidney to appropriately concentrate the urine is diminished, resulting in a clinical condition that resembles diabetes insipidus.[24,43] In some postsurgical patients, the excessive output of dilute urine led to hemoconcentration and serious electrolyte imbalances.[24]

Due to inadvertent swallowing during and after the use of fluoride-containing rinses or dentifrices, or after the application of 1.23% APF gels, the cells of the gastric mucosa may be exposed to very high fluoride concentrations. For example, the millimolar concentration of a 1000 ppm dentifrice is 53; that of a 1.23% gel is 647. It is not surprising that some patients occasionally complain of nausea and vomiting after APF gel treatments[2,12,30]

The effects of fluoride on the structure and function of the gastric mucosa have been the subject of scientific investigations for over 30 years.[3,4,26,27] Studies with several species of laboratory animals have shown that fluoride concentrations of only 5 mM/L (95 ppm) adversely affect the normal secretory and absorptive functions of the gastric mucosa. In studies using light and electron microscopy, the structure of the gastric mucosa of rats was found to be damaged in a dose- and time-related manner starting with fluoride concentrations as low as 10 mM/L. The damage ranged from vascular engorgement, hemorrhage, loss of the mucus layer and patchy desquamation of mucous cells (10 mM/L F) to extensive loss of the mucosa, including parietal and chief cells, with exposure of the underlying lamina propria (50 mM/L F or more).

It is for these reasons that with products designed for topical application of the fluoride ion to the teeth, the systemic exposure to fluoride should be minimized. In the case of 1.23% APF gels, the following application technique should be used:

- The patient should be seated in an upright position with the head inclined slightly forward

- The gel should be placed in a tray (preferably a tray with an absorbent foam lining) and not wiped directly onto the teeth as with a cotton-tipped applicator

- The quantities of gel used should be minimized and in no case should they exceed 2.0 mL per tray

- The buccal vestibules and sublingual space should be evacuated by suction during and after the application procedure

- The patient should be required to expectorate multiple times after the procedure.

An important undesirable side effect associated with excessive fluoride intake is dental fluorosis (see Chapter 8). There is clear evidence that the prevalence and the severity of this developmental disorder of the teeth are increasing in the USA. Several studies have identified the sources of the additional fluoride intake and have attempted to determine their relative importance.[6,10,20,31] There are several possible ways to reduce the intake of non-dietary fluoride by young children. These include:

- Parental supervision of brushing or mouthrinsing
- The use of small amounts of toothpaste (pea-sized or smear layer amounts)
- The use of products with lower fluoride levels
- Placing a statement on dentifrice containers saying that they should not be used by children under the age of 6 years (as is done for US mouthrinses)
- Teaching children not to swallow toothpaste or mouthrinse;
- Strict adherence to current recommendations by professionals who prescribe fluoride dietary supplements.

Literature cited

1. Anonymous. Fatal fluoride intoxication in a dialysis unit, Annapolis. J Publ Health Dent 1980; 40: 360-2.

2. Beal JF, Rock WP. Fluoride gels: a laboratory and clinical investigation. Br Dent J 1976; 140: 307-10.

3. Bond AM, Hunt JN. The effect of sodium fluoride on the output of some electrolytes from the gastric mucosa of rats. J Physiol 1956; 133: 317-29.

4. Bowie JY, Darlow G, Murray MM. The effect of sodium fluoride on gastric acid secretion. J Physiol 1953; 122: 202-8.

5. Burlington DB. FDA safety alert: fluoride contamination of hemodialysis water supply. August 19, 1993.

6. Burt BA. The changing patterns of systemic fluoride intake. J Dent Res 1991; 71 (Spec Iss): 1228-37.

7. Church LE. Fluorides: use with caution. Maryland Dent Assoc J 1976; 19: 106.

8. Council on Dental Therapeutics of the American Dental Association. Fluoride compounds. In: Accepted dental therapeutics, 39th edn. Chicago: ADA 1982: 344-68.

9. Dreisbach RH. Handbook of poisoning: prevention, diagnosis and treatment. Los Altos, CA: Lange Medical Publishers 1980.

10. Driscoll WS, Heifetz SB, Horowitz HS, Kingman A, Meyers RJ, Zimmermann ER. Prevalence of dental caries and dental fluorosis in areas with optimal and above-optimal water fluoride concentrations. J Am Dent Assoc 1983; 107: 42-7.

11. Dukes MNG. Side effects of drugs. Annual 4. Oxford: Excerpta Medica 1980: 354.

12. Duxbury AJ, Leach FN, Duxbury JR. Acute fluoride toxicity. Br Dent J 1982; 153: 64-6.

13. Eichler HG, Lenz K, Fuhrmann M, Hruby K. Accidental ingestion of NaF tablets by children: report of a poison control center and one case. Int J Clin Pharmacol Ther Toxicol 1982; 20: 334-8.

14. Ericsson Y. Monofluorophosphate physiology: general considerations. Caries Res 1983; 17: 46-55.

15. Gessner BD, Beller M, Middaugh JP, Whitford GM. Acute fluoride poisoning from a public water system. N Eng J Med 1994; 330: 95-9.

16. Gruninger SE, Clayton R, Chang SB, Siew C. Acute oral toxicity of dentifrice fluorides in rats and mice. J Dent Res 1988; 67 (abstr): 334.

17. Gutknecht J, Walter A. Hydrofluoric and nitric acid transport through lipid bilayer membranes. Biochim Biophys Acta 1981; 644: 153-6.

18. Hodge HC, Smith FA. Biological properties of inorganic fluorides. In: Simons JH, ed. Fluoride Chemistry. New York: Academic Press 1965: 1-375.

19. Hoffman R, Mann J, Calderone J, Trumbull J, Burkhart M. Acute fluoride poisoning in a New Mexico elementary school. Pediatrics 1980; 65: 897-900.

20. Leverett DH. Fluorides and the changing prevalence of dental caries. Science 1982; 217: 26-30.

21. Lidbeck WL, Hill IB, Beeman JA. Acute sodium fluoride poisoning. J Am Med Assoc 1943; 121: 826-7.

22. Lim JK, Renaldo GJ, Chapman P. LD_{50} of SnF_2, NaF and Na_2PO_3F in the mouse compared to the rat. Caries Res 1978; 12: 177-9.

23. Litovitz TL, Schmitz BF, Bailey KM. 1989 annual report of the American Association of Poison Control Centers national data collection system. Am J Emerg Med 1990; 8: 394-442.

24. Mazze RI, Trudell JR, Cousins MJ. Methoxyflurane metabolism and renal dysfunction: clinical correlation in man. Anesthesiol 1971; 35: 247-52.

25. Mornstad H. Acute sodium fluoride toxicity in rats in relation to age and sex. Acta Pharmacol Toxicol 1975; 37: 425-8.

26. Pashley DH, Allison NB, Easmann RP, McKinney RV, Horner JA, Whitford GM. The effects of fluoride on the gastric mucosa of the rat. J Oral Pathol 1984; 13: 535-45.

27. Reed DJ, Smy JR. The effects of sodium fluoride on gastric acid and electrolyte output in anesthetized cats. J Physiol 1980; 301: 39-48.

28. Reynolds KE, Whitford GM, Pashley DH. Acute fluoride toxicity: the influence of acid-base status. Toxicol Appl Pharmacol 1978; 45: 415-27.

29. Shourie KL, Hein JW, Hodge HC. Preliminary studies of the caries inhibiting potential and acute toxicity of sodium monofluorophosphate. J Dent Res 1950; 29: 529-33.

30. Spoerke DG, Bennett DL, Gellekson DJK. Toxicity related to acute low dose sodium fluoride ingestion. J Family Pract 1980; 10: 139-40.

31. Szpunar SM, Burt BA. Trends in the prevalence of dental fluorosis in the United States: a review. J Publ Health Dent 1987; 47: 71-9.

32. Veltri JC, Litovitz TL. 1983 annual report of the American Association of Poison Control Centers national data collection system. Am J Emergency Med 1984; 2: 420-43.

33. Vogt RL, Witherell L, LaRue D, Klaucke DN. Acute fluoride poisoning associated with an on-site fluoridator in a Vermont elementary school. Am J Publ Health 1982; 72: 1168-71.

34. Whitford GM. The metabolism and toxicity of fluoride. Basel: Karger 1989: 31-87.

35. Whitford GM, Ekstrand J. Systemic absorption of fluoride from alginate impression material in humans. J Dent Res 1980; 59: 782-5.

36. Whitford GM, Birdsong-Whitford NL, Finidori C. Acute oral toxicity of sodium fluoride and monofluorophosphate separately or in combination in rats. Caries Res 1990; 24: 121-6.

37. Whitford GM, LeCompte EJ. Acute fluoride toxicity: influence of gastric acidity. J Dent Res 1983; 62 (abstr): 262.

38. Whitford GM, Pashley DH. Plasma fluoride levels in the dog as a function of age. Caries Res 1983; 17: 561.

39. Whitford GM, Pashley DH. Fluoride absorption: the influence of gastric acidity. Calcif Tissue Int 1984; 36: 302-7.

40. Whitford GM, Pashley DH, Allison NB. Monofluorophosphate physiology: discussion. Caries Res 1983; 17: 69-76.

41. Whitford GM, Pashley DH, Reynolds KE. Fluoride tissue distribution: short term kinetics. Am J Physiol 1979; 236: F141-8.

42. Whitford GM, Reynolds KE, Pashley DH. Acute fluoride toxicity: influence of metabolic acidosis. Toxicol Appl Pharmacol 1979; 50: 31-9.

43. Whitford GM, Taves DR. Fluoride-induced diuresis: renal tissue solute concentrations, functional, hemodynamic and histologic correlates in the rat. Anesthesiol 1973; 39: 416-27.

FLUORIDE AND THE ORAL ENVIRONMENT – THE EFFECT ON THE CARIES PROCESS

CHAPTER 11

DYNAMICS OF CARIES LESION FORMATION

O. Fejerskov • B.H. Clarkson

The enamel surface – Changes in surface enamel during early stages of lesion formation
The "white spot" lesion – Progression of the enamel lesion
Arrest of caries lesion progression – Occlusal caries – Root surface caries
Remineralization - demineralization

The enamel surface

When a tooth erupts into the oral cavity, the enamel is in principle fully mineralized. However, the surface enamel at the time of eruption is somewhat porous, and it has been suggested that it undergoes a period of "posteruptive maturation" subsequent to eruption. Nobody has fully explained the nature of such a maturation, but it is thought that during this period of time, mineral ions and fluoride in the oral environment diffuse into the surface enamel. Evidence for such a process is suggested by the fact that the fluoride concentration in surface enamel increases subsequent to eruption. However, from a chemical point of view it is difficult to appreciate how such a process is mediated as there does not seem to be a true driving force existing under neutral pH conditions.

There is no doubt, however, that the surface enamel is rather porous, as demonstrated by the openings of the striae of Retzius at the surface; the perikymata grooves acting as larger diffusion pathways. Similarly, the numerous

pits of the Tomes' processes are partly encircled by the openings of the arcade-shaped spaces that, throughout the enamel, partly separate the rod (or prism) from the interrod enamel.[8,20] Moreover, a varying number of developmental defects, designated focal holes, small irregular fissures and microholes less than 1 μm in diameter, are observed in the enamel.

Although these potential diffusion pathways may be visualized in the scanning electron microscope, it is important to appreciate that under *in vivo* conditions all spaces within the enamel, irrespective of their size, will contain protein of developmental origin, lipid and water. The presence of this organic component will naturally modify the diffusion processes into and out of enamel as well as modify the reaction of the mineral phase to the environmental factors in the oral cavity. When these structural features are appreciated, it is understandable why dental enamel should be considered a microporous solid.

Once the enamel has erupted into the oral cavity, its surface constantly undergoes modification and, therefore, it must be regarded as being in dynamic transformation at all times. Apart from the protein of developmental origin within the enamel, exogenous organic material from oral fluids will be adsorbed onto and possibly into the surface enamel. Moreover, as soon as any part of the enamel erupts into the oral environment, the enamel surface will be covered to a varying degree by microbial deposits (for review see.[41]) In these deposits, which when clinically detectable are designated dental plaque, there will be a continuous metabolic activity resulting in periods of demineralization and redeposition of mineral, depending on fluctuations in pH at the interface between the enamel and the microbial deposits. These processes represent the events which, if left undisturbed for prolonged periods of time, may result in a net loss of mineral from the enamel. It is therefore necessary from a clinical point of view – and not least from the point of view of understanding the possible mechanisms of actions of fluoride – to appreciate the fact that well before any clinical evidence of a change in surface enamel can be recorded, a variety of chemical reactions have occurred which modify the tissue.

Thus, what we commonly refer to in the clinic as "sound or normal enamel" is really enamel which, once the tooth is fully erupted into functional occlusion, has been subjected to substantial chemical and minor mechanical modifications. What is referred to as "secondary maturation" may more likely reflect the outcome of these chemical events, which have occurred at a subclinical level (for discussion see[16]) and have been described, perhaps incorrectly, as a period of "passive" mineral uptake.

In order to understand how fluoride may modify the caries lesion and the rate of progression of lesion formation, it should, therefore, be remembered that the entire enamel surface must be regarded as being in a dynamic equilibrium with its surrounding oral fluid at all times.

In this chapter, we shall briefly describe the changes which occur in surface enamel during very early lesion formation leading to the stage commonly referred to as the white spot lesion. Possible factors controlling further progression of enamel lesion development including its arrest will also be discussed. These events will be described for smooth surface enamel caries, and although the processes are in principle similar on all tooth surfaces, we will describe how the process is modified once lesions have developed in the occlusal or on root surfaces.

Finally, the chapter will review the results of *in vitro*, *in situ* and other *in vivo* experiments which have studied the possible effect of fluoride on enamel de- and remineralization during experimental caries lesion formation.

Changes in surface enamel during early stages of lesion formation

In order to fully appreciate what happens during early lesion formation, it should be remembered that the integrity of the enamel mineral phase in the oral environment will be totally dependent on the composition and chemical behavior of the surrounding fluids (saliva or the plaque fluid). The predominant factors controlling the stability of the enamel apatites will be the pH and the concentration of calcium, phosphate and fluoride in the surrounding solution. Under normal physiological conditions, mixed saliva will be supersaturated with respect to the tooth minerals (for recent review see,[55]) but this does not result in any significant mineral deposition into sound, plaque-free tooth surfaces. Likewise, saliva is not as promising a "remineralizing solution" as might be expected because saliva contains a variety of salivary macromolecules which inhibit precipitation of calcium and phosphate. In Fig. 11-1 the major chemical changes which are thought to occur in dental plaque and surface enamel

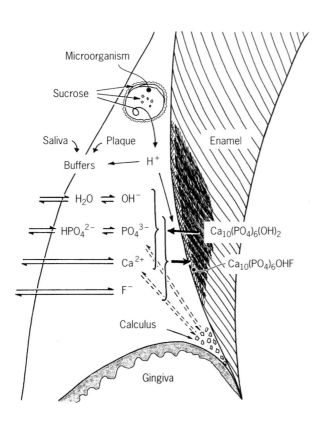

Fig. 11-1. Diagram of the major chemical changes occurring in plaque and enamel during bacterial fermentation of carbohydrates. Initially, H^+ will be taken up by buffers in plaque and saliva. Eventually, when the pH declines, the fluid medium will be depleted of OH^- and PO_4^{3-} which react with H^+ to form H_2O and HPO_4^{2-}. Below the "critical pH" of about 5.5 the aqueous phase becomes unsaturated with respect to hydroxyapatite. Most often, however, it remains supersaturated with respect to fluorapatite. This chemical condition leads to a dissolution of hydroxyapatite, preferentially from subsurface enamel, and a concurrent precipitation of fluorhydroxyapatite, preferentially in the enamel surface. Dissolution of mineral in the plaque, e.g. calculus, adds to the concentration of Ca^{2+} and PO_4^{3-} in the aqueous phase whereby the "critical pH" is lowered. From Larsen & Bruun 1986.[28]

during bacterial fermentation of carbohydrates are schematically illustrated.

A pH decrease in the oral fluids surrounding the teeth will result in a dramatic increase in the solubility of the enamel apatites. Thus, simple calculations have shown that a pH drop of one unit within the pH range pH 4-7 gives rise to a 7-fold increase in the solubility of the hydroxyapatite (for recent reviews see[28,29]).

The concentrations of calcium and phosphate already present in the oral fluids will determine the pH at which the aqueous phase will be exactly saturated with respect to the apatites in the enamel. It can be calculated that with the calcium and phosphate concentrations of normal mixed saliva,[35,55] between a pH of 5.2 and 5.5 saliva will be slightly undersaturated with respect to enamel hydroxyapatite. A drop below this pH level will then result in a rapid dissolution of the enamel hydroxyapatite; this pH value (or range) is often referred to as the "critical pH". It should be remembered, however, that while calcium and phosphate concentrations in saliva are fairly well known,[35] much less information is available concerning concentrations in the plaque fluid covering the enamel surface.[32,33] In other words, irrespective of the salivary pH, it will be the concentrations of calcium, phosphate and fluoride in the actual fluid at the tooth-plaque interface which will determine when the equilibrium between solid and liquid phase is disturbed.

Although the predominant mineral component of enamel is hydroxyapatite, it is far from a pure hydroxyapatite, and includes many different ions such as fluoride, which substitutes for hydroxyl ions (see Chapter 14). The more fluoride the apatite contains, the less soluble it will be at the same pH when compared with pure hydroxyapatite. This means that a range of pH occurs at the enamel-plaque interface where the biologic hydroxyapatite may dissolve because the oral fluid or plaque fluid is undersaturated with respect to this apatite, but where, because the solution (oral fluid) remains supersaturated with respect to fluorapatite (if the fluoride concentration is slightly increased), fluorhydroxyapatite can be deposited into the enamel. Therefore, conditions can occur in the oral environment when calcium and phosphate dissolve from the part of the enamel predominantly composed of hydroxyapatite (subsurface enamel), while at the same time fluorhydroxyapatite may be deposited in the surface enamel. This chemical condition can explain how the well-mineralized surface zone is maintained during subsurface enamel dissolution. This was originally proposed by Larsen[27] and has since gained substantial support. An interesting aspect of this theory is that it explains why a slight increase in fluoride ion concentration of 0.5-1.0 ppm at the actual site of dissolution can influence the demineralizing process by decreasing the rate of subsurface dissolution and enhancing the deposition of fluoridated apatite in the surface zone.

Now returning to Fig. 11-1. Initially, H^+ will be taken up by buffers in plaque and saliva, but when the pH continues to fall (H^+ increases), the fluid medium will be depleted of OH^- and PO_3^{4-}, which react with H^+ to form H_2O and HPO_2^{4-}. Once the depletion is complete, the pH can then fall below the critical value of 5.5 where the aqueous phase becomes undersaturated with respect to hydroxyapatite. Therefore whenever surface enamel is covered by a microbial deposit, the ongoing metabolic processes within this biomass result in pH fluctuations,[37,46] and occasional large pH drops, which may result in dissolution of the mineralized surface. The earliest sign of such dissolution in human enamel can be observed in the scanning electron microscope as an apparent "moth-eaten" appearance of the enamel surface (Fig.11-2). Because of variations in enamel structure, it may be difficult to distinguish the very early signs of surface dissolution from the spectrum of developmental defects observed at the ultrastructural level, but the following description reveals the basic principles.

The early signs of caries destruction appear as a dissolution of enamel crystals at the very outer surface whereby the intercrystalline spaces become widened (Fig. 11-3). The porosity of the surface increases significantly allowing more extensive diffusion of acid into the enamel, and resulting in diffusion out of the enamel of calcium and phosphate ions to a depth of several hundred μm. In addition to these surface reactions, it is apparent that after its initial dissolution, the outer 20-50 μm of enamel remains relatively well-mineralized compared with the increasing porosity of the underlying enamel, as long as the intermittent dissolution/redeposition phenomena can occur within the pH ranges available.

This highly characteristic subsurface type of dissolution in enamel caries was thought for a long time to be a result of the outer enamel surface being more resistant to acid attack because of either a specific chemical composition and/or its specialized ultrastructural configuration. More specifically, the fluoride content in this outermost part of the enamel was thought to be directly responsible for the relative resist-

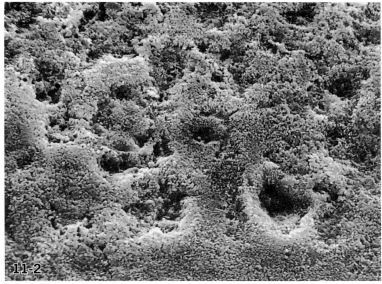

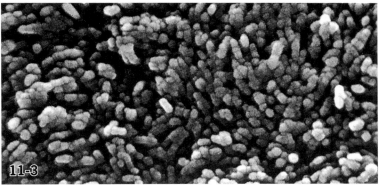

Figs. 11-2, 11-3. Scanning electron micrographs from surface enamel in early stages of natural caries lesion formation. The surface enamel appears motheaten and porous as a result of extensive widening of intercrystalline spaces (Fig. 11-3). In Fig. 11-2 impressions representing Tomes' processes pits are discernable, but the surface also exhibits several microholes.

ance of the surface enamel to caries dissolution. However, as a result of a variety of experimental *in vitro* and *in vivo* studies it has become apparent that this subsurface type of demineralization also occurs in surfaces where the outer fluoride-rich enamel surface has been removed. These observations, together with an improved understanding of the chemical behavior of dental enamel,[28,29] has led to the current concept that the relative "protection" of the outermost enamel, in direct contact with the acid-producing microbial plaque, is predominantly a result of the dynamic processes taking place at the interface between the liquid and mineral phases. Simplified, the maintenance of the relatively well-mineralized surface zone is the result of a remineralization process which leads to redeposition of calcium and phosphate, as well as fluoride ions, in the partly dissolved surface zone where the caries process is active (see Chapter 14). Thus, during the months following eruption into the oral cavity, enamel surfaces which are always partly plaque covered will tend to accumulate fluoride. In fact, this is exactly what was thought to be a "passive" accumulation of fluoride as a

191

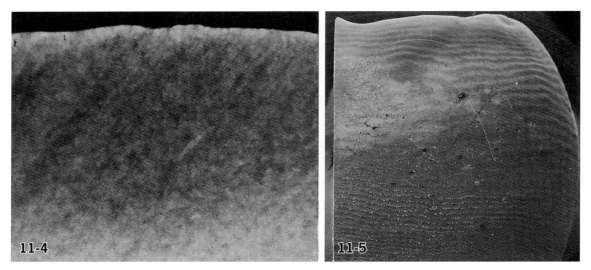

Figs. 11-4, 11-5. Microradiograph of a ground section through a white spot lesion on an approximal surface of an maxillary premolar shown by SEM in Fig. 11-5. Corresponding to the contact facet, the perikymata pattern has disappeared as a result of surface dissolution and abrasion. The microradiograph shows a sub-surface demineralization. Although the enamel surface appears rather well mineralized, numerous surface irregularities can be identified as well as minor radiolucent "channels" through the surface zone. Compare this picture with Fig. 11-2.

result of secondary maturation, but today we prefer to regard these chemical changes as evidence of the metabolic processes taking place in the plaque covering the tooth surface, i.e. the very early stages of caries lesion formation which are not manifested clinically!

The "white spot" lesion

It is essential to appreciate that in daily practice the terms dental caries and "the lesion" are used synonymously and are generally defined as the local destruction of the hard tissues. However, what we record clinically are the symptoms of the disease, not the disease itself.[21,58] Notwithstanding this dichotomy, we continue in this section to consider how the processes described above, further develop over time so as to gradually increase the tissue porosity. Once it reaches a level where the

drying of the enamel surface results in its increased opacity, it is common to refer to this stage of lesion development as a white spot lesion. This stage covers a wide range of changes from the very early whitish opaque spots on the enamel surface to extensive very chalky surfaces where small parts of the surface enamel may fracture.

On smooth accessible surfaces, it is possible to visualize early stages in lesion formation, but on such inaccessible surfaces as the approximal and fissure enamel surfaces, the subsurface loss of mineral may become extensive before the lesion is detectable clinically or even radiographically.[49]

The caries lesion progresses with time as a result of diffusion of acids into, and calcium and phosphate ions out of, the enamel. The range of structural changes in surface enamel during caries lesion formation can be demonstrated by scanning electron microscopy of a

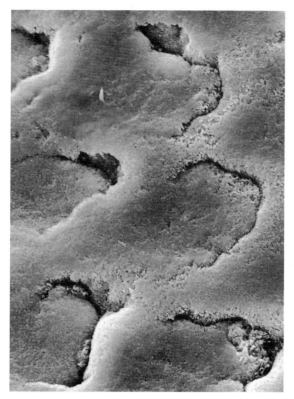

Fig. 11-6. Scanning electron micrograph showing the Tomes' processes pits, and the surrounding interrod enamel along the periphery of an active white spot lesion. Slight surface dissolution can be seen both at interrod enamel and corresponding to the pits.

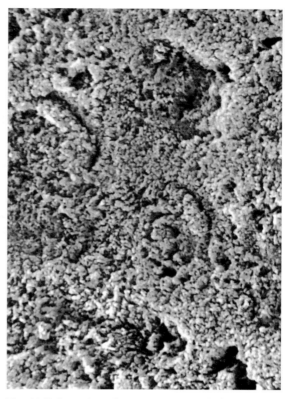

Fig. 11-7. Scanning electron micrograph from the central part of the lesion demonstrated in Figs. 11-4 and 11-5. Although the pattern of Tomes' processes pits can still be discerned with the openings of the periprismatic gaps, both rod and interrod enamel show sign of extensive demineralization.

"white spot", approximal enamel lesion (Fig. 11-5). At this stage a substantial mineral loss has already occurred, but clinically the surface is intact, although different from that of "normal sound enamel". Along the periphery of the lesion the perikymata pattern is still intact, but it is apparent that this pattern is blurred or even entirely absent in the central region of the lesion. The corresponding microradiograph (Fig. 11-4) shows a preferential subsurface loss of mineral. Although the enamel surface is apparently well mineralized, careful inspection shows the presence of numerous surface irregularities, as well as small radiopaque "channels" within the outer enamel surface.

The enamel changes at the periphery of such lesions reveal that the Tomes' processes pits and the surrounding interrod enamel appear "moth-eaten" as a result of enlargement of the intercrystalline spaces. Distinct, small surface defects with entire loss of outer enamel crystals are frequently seen (Fig. 11-6).

These early changes along the periphery of the white opaque surface lesion should be com-

193

pared with the more advanced changes in the central part of the same lesion (Fig. 11-7). A complete dissolution of the outer enamel surface has occurred producing extensive intercrystalline spaces. The normal structural entities of the enamel surface are difficult to discern, but the openings of the periprismatic gaps partly surrounding the rods are evident. Both rod and interrod enamel are equally severely demineralized. It is through this type of enamel surface that chemical diffusion takes place more easily causing further progression of the lesion towards the dentin.

Although clinical examination reveals an intact surface, this surface has undergone rather severe disintegration with formation of numerous microcavities. This pattern probably explains why a sharp probe or explorer gently moved across the enamel surface from the normal enamel into carious areas detects this as a roughening of the surface.

Progression of the enamel lesion

Depending on the severity of the cariogenic challenge of the plaque, enamel dissolution may progress in such a way that the entire thickness of enamel can be involved in the demineralization process – which may even reach the dentin – without the remaining outer enamel surface breaking down, as demonstrated in Fig. 11-8 and Fig. 11-9. The degree of subsurface demineralization in the body of the lesion shows a wide variation. No positive correlation has been found between the depth of a lesion and its degree of demineralization. It is common to find the most extensive subsurface demineralization in the outer part of the enamel with a gradual increase in mineral content towards the inner periphery of the lesion corresponding to the advancing front. Several workers[26,49] have described bands of high

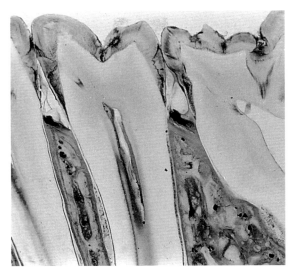

Fig. 11-8. Mesiodistal longitudinal undemineralized section through human mandible with two premolars and part of the first molar. Notice the approximal spaces with enamel caries lesions present, corresponding to the contact areas and extending in a triangular pattern towards the dentin. The enamel surface is intact, and it is apparent that prior to cavity formation distinct reactions occur in the underlying dentin and corresponding pulp tissue. From the Hanagawa collection with the kind permission of Professor Yanagisawa, Tokyo Dental College, Japan.

mineral content passing through the body of the lesion, giving such lesions a "laminated appearance" as demonstrated in Fig. 11-10. Explanation of this phenomenon is uncertain, but it has been suggested that these variations in mineral content of the body of the lesion are due to redeposition of mineral occurring during a transient phase of arrest of the carious process and persisting during further lesion progression. In this context, primary teeth exhibiting various but slight degrees of dental fluorosis, exhibit caries lesions with a surprisingly

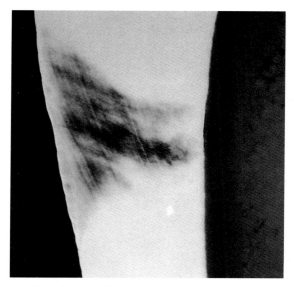

Fig. 11-9. Microradiograph of non-cavitated enamel caries lesion showing extensive demineralization throughout the enamel with early dissolution of the corresponding peripheral dentin. Notice the enamel surface zone of higher mineral content which varies in thickness.

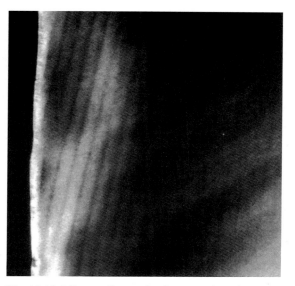

Fig. 11-10. Microradiograph of non-cavitated enamel lesion showing extensive subsurface demineralization. In addition to the highly mineralized surface zone, areas of higher mineral content are apparent within the subsurface body of the lesion.

high number of such "laminations".[25] These bands of differing mineral content are located most often at the contact facet of the approximal lesions where there has been abrasion of the outer enamel surface. It is tempting to interpret these observations as indicative of a certain degree of mineral redeposition in those parts of the lesion where the caries-inducing plaque gradually disappears as the contact facet widens. As the fluoride content in saliva in children living in these areas of endemic dental fluorosis is significantly higher than that occurring in a low fluoride area, these laminations may reflect the "remineralizing" potential of even low concentrations of fluoride in the oral environment.

The caries process in the enamel spreads as a result of a preferential dissolution of mineral along rod boundaries, possibly because these arcade-shaped periprismatic spaces, with their more irregular crystal packing and larger content of developmental protein, act as diffusion pathways in enamel (Figs. 11-11 and 11-12). The most pronounced demineralization – and the deepest penetration of dissolution into the inner enamel – will occur underneath the thickest part of the plaque. Therefore, the demineralization in the center of the lesion can reach the dentin, causing a significant response in the pulpo-dentinal organ without cavity formation.

At an early stage of enamel caries demineralization, crystal changes take place within both the rod and interrod enamel, resulting in

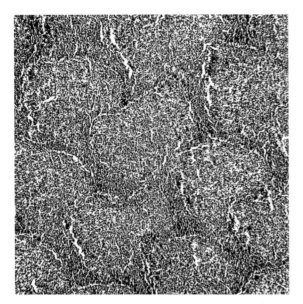

Fig. 11-11. Transmission electron micrograph of the body of the lesion shown in the previous figure. Despite extensive demineralization, as shown in the previous microradiograph, the rod and interrod enamel structure is clearly discernable.

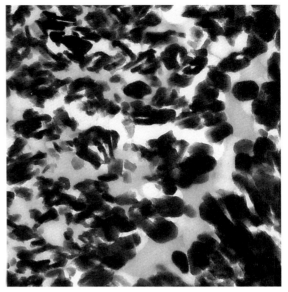

Fig. 11-12. Higher magnification of the borderland between rod and interrod enamel separated by a widened periprismatic gap. Extensive intercrystalline spaces are evident, although parts of the separation between crystals may be artificially produced during section preparation. Virtually all crystals show varying degrees of central and peripheral dissolution.

an overall reduction in the dimension of the crystals as well as the formation of "hairpins", which reflects the partial dissolution of the center of some crystals (Figs. 11-12 and 11-13). Along the diffusion pathways, i.e. the periprismatic gaps, the bordering crystals often appear larger and more irregular than those normally found in the sound enamel. Such rhomboid crystals are often referred to as "caries crystals" and are thought to represent the results of de- and remineralizing processes taking place particularly along the major diffusion pathways through the enamel.

When polarized light microscopy is used to study enamel caries lesions, the advancing front of an enamel lesion may be separated into a translucent zone and a dark zone.[47] If a translucent zone is present at the advancing front of the lesion, the dark zone is the "second zone of alteration" from normal enamel, before its transition into the body of the lesion. The translucent zone reflects a pore volume of approximately 1%, representing a significant increase when compared with sound enamel (pore volume approximately 0.1%).[52] The pores in this zone are primarily located at the already established diffusion pathways such as the rod peripheries.

Micro-dissection of ground sections through caries lesions made it possible to describe the

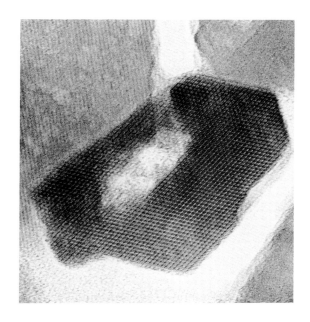

Fig. 11-13. High resolution transmission electron micrograph of a human enamel crystal from the body of the lesion of a non-cavitated caries lesion. The crystal is sectioned perpendicular to the C-axis and shows central dissolution. Notice the distinct lattice patterns indicative of hydroxyapatite. Courtesy of Dr. C Tohda, Tokyo Dental College, Japan.

chemical characteristics of the various zones.[60] It is of interest that the fluoride content of the translucent zone is greater relative to adjacent sound enamel. In addition, a loss of magnesium was also detected, and on a weight basis the translucent zone enamel has a lower carbonate content relative to sound enamel. The overall findings suggest that the caries attack at the advancing front preferentially removes magnesium and carbonate rich material (which probably originates from dissolution of the mineral phase). Microchemical analyses of the dark zone[23] showed an average reduction of 6% of mineral per unit volume when compared to sound enamel.

As was implied earlier, the chemical events taking place at the plaque-enamel interface would suggest that fluoride present in the plaque fluid would gradually become incorporated into the enamel surface zone as the lesion gradually develops, assuming a slowly developing lesion over months to years. Recently detailed microprobe analyses of the fluoride distribution within lesions have shown a highly varying – but always substantially elevated – concentration in the well-mineralized surface layer[43] (Figs. 11-14 and 11-15).

Once the enamel surface breaks down, and a true cavity starts to form (Fig. 11-16), the environmental conditions change substantially because the cavity is inaccessible to plaque removal and the diffusion of saliva deep into such lesions is questionable. Plaque pH remains low for prolonged periods of time, favoring the growth of aciduric microorganisms. This results in a more acidic environment with a lowering also of the resting plaque pH values[18] (see Fig. 11-17). Thus, a vicious circle is created, but very little is known at this stage about subsequent microchemical events and how fluoride affects the metabolic and chemical processes within carious cavities.

197

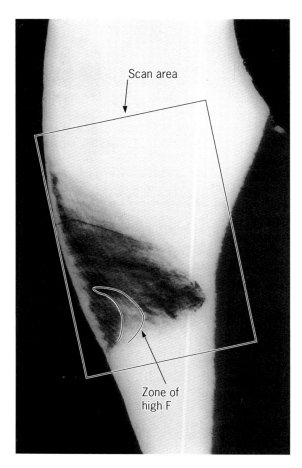

Figs. 11-14, 11-15. Microradiograph through non-cavitated enamel caries lesion extending almost to the enamel dentin junction. The framed area indicates where microanalyses of the fluoride content have been performed as shown in Fig. 11-15A and 11-15B . Both the topographical map and the surface, three-dimensional representation show very little increase in fluoride concentration in the deepest part of the lesion, but a large increase about 0.3 mm beneath the surface in the part of the lesion appearing more radiopaque in the microradiograph. Courtesy of E. Pearce and M. Joost Larsen.[43]

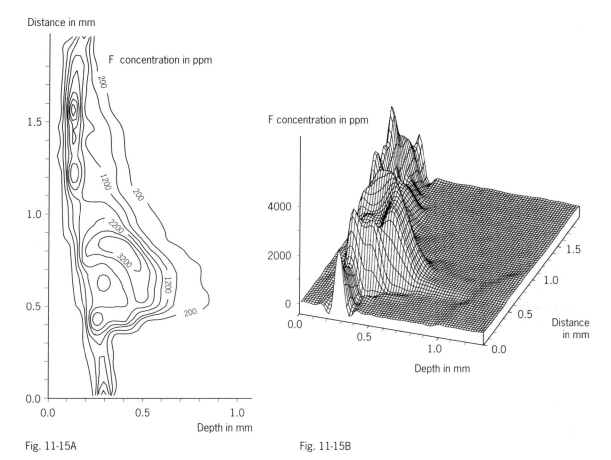

Distance in mm
F concentration in ppm
200
1200
200
2200
3200
1200
200
1.5
1.0
0.5
0.0
0.0
0.5
1.0
Depth in mm

Fig. 11-15A

F concentration in ppm
4000
2000
0
0.0
0.5
1.0
Depth in mm
1.5
1.0
0.5
0.0
Distance
in mm

Fig. 11-15B

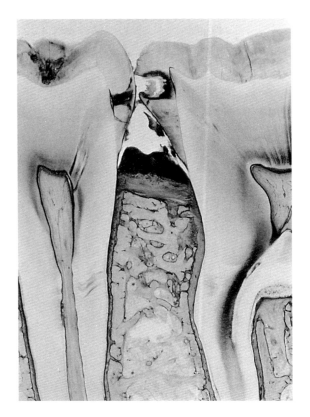

Fig. 11-16. Undemineralized section prepared in mesiodistal direction of human maxilla showing parts of a premolar and molar tooth corresponding to the approximal contact areas. The approximal caries lesions involve the pulpo-dentinal organ. In the premolar, however, the surface enamel is still intact, although the demineralization is extensive, whereas in the molar approximal surface cavitation has occurred almost to the enamel-dentin junction. Notice how such a cavity is inaccessible and therefore impossible to keep free from microbial deposits. From the Hanagawa collection with the kind permission of Professor Yanagisawa, Tokyo Dental College, Japan.

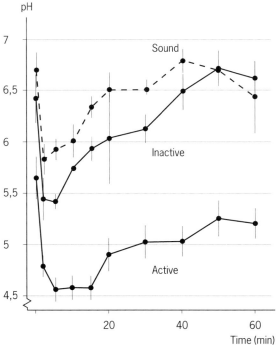

Fig. 11-17. Stephan response curves obtained from sound occlusal surfaces, inactive occlusal caries lesions and deep, active occlusal caries lesions following a controlled sucrose rinse. The bars indicate standard errors. Notice that resting pH values are substantially lower in the active caries cavities as compared to inactive and sound surfaces. Moreover, the pH drop in the caries cavity is more pronounced, and even 60 minutes after a rinse remains below pH 5.5. From Fejerskov et al. 1992.[18]

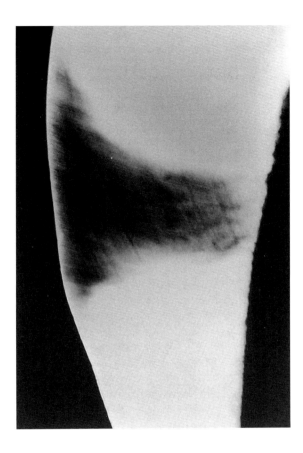

Fig. 11-18. Microradiograph of non-cavitated enamel caries lesion classified as inactive or arrested in the clinic. The subsurface demineralization extends throughout the enamel to the enamel-dentin junction. Notice that although the approximal surface area has been partly abraded away, the lesion is covered by a highly mineralized surface zone.

Arrest of caries lesion progression

At any given stage of caries lesion development the disease may be arrested by simply removing the causative agent, i.e. the microbial deposit from the diseased site. If we couple with this the knowledge that saliva is supersaturated with respect to both hydroxyapatite and fluorapatite, we would then expect the mineralized hard tissues to gradually regain mineral by deposition from the supersaturated solution. In fact, very early enamel caries lesions may regress and even disappear when the cariogenic challenge is removed. However, it must be remembered that when a lesion "disappears" on a bitewing radiograph, it may his-

tologically be found to penetrate the entire depth of the enamel even into the dentin.[49] Such a lesion will have a certain degree of porosity, and it will persist lifelong as a caries "scar". This can be white in color or, due to exogenous uptake of stain, can become yellowish or dark brown. The surface texture of the lesion may change over time, becoming hard and shiny, but a true remineralization in the sense that all of the lost mineral is redeposited seldom takes place. This is apparent from the microradiograph shown in Fig. 11-18, where a lesion with a known history of arrest for several years following removal of the neighboring tooth shows a persistent extensive subsurface demineralization with well-mineralized surface zones of highly varying thickness. This is a fascinating problem and numerous attempts have been made, and are still being made, to develop a technique to bring about remineralization throughout the entire demineralized lesion.[51] At present, fluoride plays a key role in these attempts because of its established effect on the redeposition of calcium and phosphate in demineralized areas. In the following sections, examples of past and present research into the remineralization of demineralized enamel will be presented. Before doing so, however the lesion characteristics of occlusal and root surfaces will be described.

Occlusal caries

Occlusal caries is often referred to in clinical and epidemiologic studies as "pit and fissure caries". This is because the deep fissures, grooves or pits in the occlusal surface of the tooth are natural entrapment areas where microbial deposits can accumulate and grow for prolonged periods of time. However, even without daily toothbrushing, gross microbial accumulations will be eliminated from occlusal surfaces once the teeth erupt into functional occlusion. Even so, if the surface has not been kept clean during the period of tooth eruption, it is likely that in the grooves and pits and fissures, demineralization will have reached a stage where substantial subsurface demineralization has occurred, although it may not be immediately visible on clinical inspection.

It is, however, very important to appreciate that the pits and narrow fissures in and of themselves may not necessarily comprise sites on the tooth surfaces which are particularly susceptible to dental caries. This knowledge became evident about 20 years ago, when *in vivo* experiments were conducted in an experimental fissure caries model.[19,56] Even during experiments where the fissures were allowed to

accumulate dental plaque for almost a year and were daily exposed to frequent sucrose applications, these fissures did not develop signs of lesion formation, as long as, the occlusal surfaces were in functional occlusion. Carvalho and coworkers[7-9], applying these observations, performed ordinary dental plaque control of molar occlusal surfaces during and subsequent to tooth eruption, with the result that these surfaces were kept mostly caries free.

If, however, occlusal surfaces and pits are not kept free from large amounts of microbial deposits, caries lesions develop in a manner similar to what has been described for the smooth surfaces. The spread of lesions will differ from those on smooth surfaces simply because of the structural arrangements of the enamel rods in the walls surrounding fissures and grooves.[21,58]

In deep fissures, caries lesions characteristically develop along the walls just below the entrance to the fissure.[57] Lesions then most often progress symmetrically (Fig. 11-19) and spread laterally until they reach the enamel-dentin junction. Because of the particular anatomy in the fissures and this pattern of spread, the overall appearance of the occlusal surface may appear intact until a relatively large lesion has developed (Fig. 11-20). Such lesions can be difficult to diagnose and pushing the tip of a probe into the entrance of the fissure may result in substantial damage (which clinically will be reflected as "sticking"). The specimen shown in Fig. 11-20 originated from an individual who had been exposed to numerous topical fluoride applications and it is tempting to interpret the very pronounced hypermineralized surface zone as being caused by the accumulation of fluoridated apatite in the surface. In fact, this interpretation would be in accordance with the clinical observation that in contemporary populations with improved oral hygiene and exposeure to a variety of topical fluorides, it is difficult to diagnose occlusal and approximal lesions until they have reached a stage where

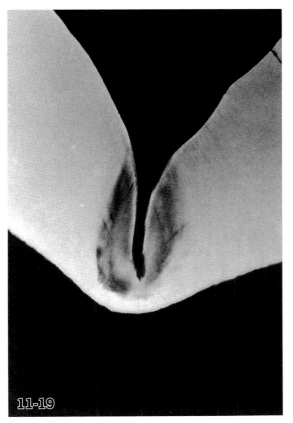 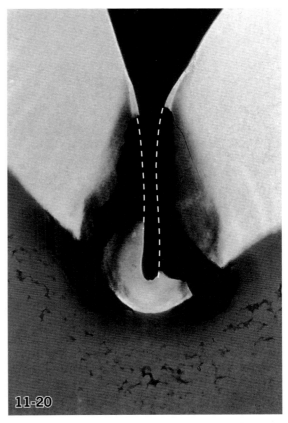

Figs. 11-19, 11-20. Microradiographs of deep occlusal fissures showing how the subsurface demineralization occurs just deep to the entrance to the fissure and spreads slong the direction of the enamel rods. As a result of the oblique course of the rods towards the enamel-dentin junction, the subsurface demineralization results in a pattern of dissolution undermining the occlusal surface. Notice how the caries demineralization can spread and involve the dentin without disruption of the surface zone at the entrance of the fissure. Most of the enamel lost in the caries lesion in Fig. 11-20 is a likely result of preparation of the ground section.

the caries has penetrated deeply into the tissue over a narrow area.

Once a distinct cavity has been formed in the occlusal surface the environmental conditions are similar to those described earlier for ap- proximal surfaces; and unless the cavity is either kept relatively plaque-free by mechanical/chemical cleaning, or the lesion excavated and a filling inserted, the caries will continue to spread until the surface is destroyed.

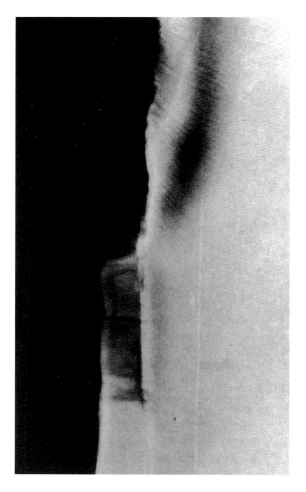

Fig. 11-21. Microradiograph of an active root surface caries lesion. In the lower part, the root cement still remains with an obvious subsurface dissolution in the cementum. In the upper half, the cementum has been lost, but notice how the mineral dissolution occurs deep to a relatively well mineralized surface layer in the root dentin.

Root surface caries

Root surface caries has recently been the focus of substantial interest,[4,17,38] and detailed descriptions of the microbiology and histopathology of root surface caries are available. Combining this knowledge with a number of clinical studies reveals that the response of root surface caries to fluoride treatments is very similar to that of coronal caries, i.e. daily exposure to various fluoride sources results in fewer lesions developing in a population (for review see[17]).

From a structural point of view, root surface caries can be regarded, in principle, as dentinal caries not surrounded by enamel. Therefore, root surface caries lesions are exposed more directly to the oral salivary environment, and this probably explains why root surface caries penetrates less deeply but has a strong tendency to spread over a large surface area, especially if the root surface has been plaque covered for a substantial period of time. The most striking structural feature of root surface caries is that of a subsurface demineralization of the tissue (Fig. 11-21). Even at the very early stages, where a root surface covered by a layer

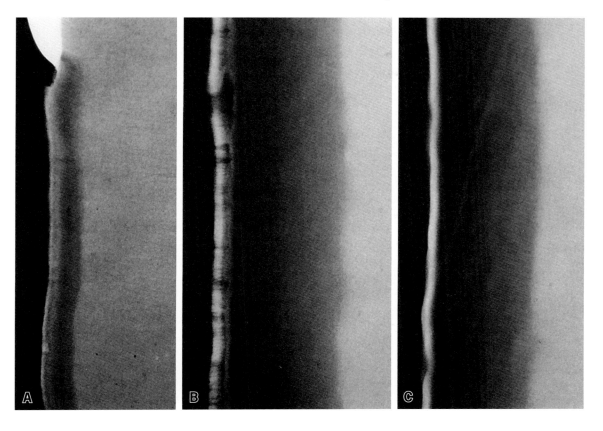

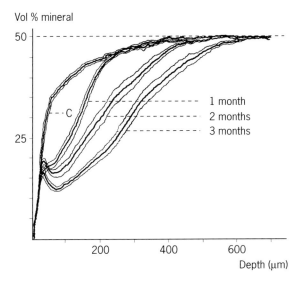

Figs. 11-22, 11-23. Microradiographs and scans of mineral content of root surface caries lesions experimentally produced in the oral cavity in human root surfaces which have been covered by dental plaque for 1 month (Fig. 11-22A), 2 months (Fig. 11-22B) and 3 months (Fig. 11-22C), respectively. Notice how a subsurface caries lesion gradually develops over time concomitant with a build up of mineral in the surface layers of cementum. With time, mineral loss increases in depth and extent. The fine lines in the scans reflect the magnitude of the standard error around the mean values. From Nyvad *et al.* 1989[42]).

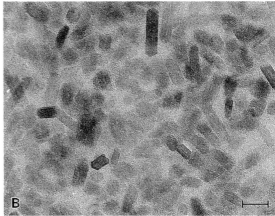

Fig. 11-24. High resolution transmission electron micrographs of sound human cementum surface (Fig. 11-24A) and a well mineralized surface zone covering a root caries lesion (Fig. 11-24B). Notice a substantial difference in size of the crystals, with much larger crystals corresponding to the surface zone of the caries lesion as compared to sound surfaces. The typical lattice pattern is clearly seen in the larger crystals which also demonstrates central dark lines. The bar indicates 100 Å. From Tohda et al. 1995.[59]

of cementum is exposed in the oral cavity, lesion formation within the cementum may occur as a loss of mineral deep to a somewhat unaffected surface layer. However, root surface caries, in contrast to enamel caries, is characterized early in its development by the invasion of microorganisms into the tissues.[40]

Recently, controlled in situ studies on patterns of both mineral loss and distribution in root surfaces during caries lesion development have been conducted.[42] Figs. 11-22 and 11-23 are microradiographs and densitometry profiles demonstrating the build-up of a relatively well-mineralized surface zone concomitant with an increased subsurface loss of mineral.

Based on such observations it was suggested some years ago that, in principle, the physico-chemical events taking place during lesion formation in enamel and root surfaces may be rather similar[39,] despite the fact that the tissues are structurally and chemically very different.

It is evident that the surface zone covering root surface caries lesions contain a higher fluoride content than that of the surrounding normal root surfaces[59] and that the crystals in carious cementum (Fig. 11-24) are substantially greater than those of normal cementum. These differences together with the increased concentration of fluoride have been interpreted as an indication of that the apatitic phase in cementum undergoes similar modifications during lesion development as those described for enamel during early stages of lesion formation.

Remineralization – demineralization

As we have now shown, in enamel the development of a caries lesion is a continuum stretching from its initiation, the loss of few calcium and phosphorus ions through its progression to a white spot (subsurface) lesion, and finally to frank cavitation.

The literature on the effects of fluoride on this continuum of caries lesion development in dental hard tissues, especially with regard to the histologic and ultrastructural characteristics of the lesions, is voluminous. Many of these *in vitro* and *in vivo* studies have been exquisitely designed, carefully executed and meticulously documented; the results, however, are not definitive. The reason for this is the complexity of the interactions which occur at the dental hard tissue and plaque interface where the caries lesions develop. The dissolving mineral is not pure but a complex mixture of hydroxyapatites containing carbonate, magnesium, fluoride, and several other ions. The tissue itself also contains water and organic material, which in enamel is 3% by weight, but in dentin and cementum is as high as 30%. The surface of the hard tissue is covered by an organic pellicle and a heterogeneous biofilm all bathed in saliva, which is of variable composition. And finally, at least three times per day the whole system is deluged by food and liquid of various composition and consistency.

These complicating events are well illustrated in an *in situ*, human study investigating the effect of a fluoridated toothpaste on enamel remineralization.[36] In this study, in Table 11-1, subject 1, sections of *in vitro* produced lesions sandwiched together showed marked remineralization on one side of the mouth but negligible remineralization on the other, when exposed to the fluoride-containing paste. When a placebo paste (without fluoride) was used, marked demineralization occurred on the side of the mouth that showed no remineralization and negligible demineralization on the side which had shown marked remineralization. Such variation was also seen in some of the other panelists, although in the group as a whole, measurable remineralization did occur in the panelists exposed to fluoride. How is it possible, therefore, to pinpoint the precise affect of one ion, like fluoride, on the structural characteristics of the caries lesion?

Table 11-1
Percent change in artificial caries lesions treated
in vivo for four weeks*

Subject	Side	Active Treatment		Placebo Treatment	
		Area	Depth	Area	Depth
1	Right	81	12	11	21
		56	0	8	0
		50	16	8	0
	Left	-14	0	-9	-19
		-5	0	-239	-38
		37	0	-186	-64
2	Right	55	0	4	0
		66	0	22	-7
		–	–	33	19
	Left	54	0	-48	0
		48	22	-20	-13
		45	0	-1	0
3	Right	22	0	26	12
		27	0	4	0
		29	0	-26	0
	Left	36	0	10	0
		16	0	25	0
		11	0	5	0
4	Right	11	0	-2	0
		-9	0	-12	-11
		-33	0	-12	0
	Left	41	0	1	0
		44	0	-5	0
		30	0	-4	5
5	Right	39	26	-6	0
		31	0	30	0
		27	11	–	–
	Left	9	0	-68	-44
		-16	0	-13	-27
		0	11	–	–
6	Right	2	0	-151	-13
		24	0	-50	-15
		–	–	-11	0
	Left	18	0	-141	-112
		16	0	-140	-78
		4	0	–	–
7	Right	4	0	-2	0
		-14	0	11	0
		-17	0	–	–
	Left	6	0	14	0
		-5	0	13	0
		-14	0	–	–

*Negative signs indicate demineralization or increase in lesion depth.

207

Much of the speculation as to the precise effects of fluoride stems from rigorously controlled *in vitro* experiments which demonstrate that fluoride affects both the demineralization and remineralization kinetics of dental hard tissues. The results of the effect of fluoride on these two processes appears to be so intimately involved that it is difficult to distinguish them. Thus, although this discussion will concern itself primarily with the structural alterations brought about by fluoride as it affects remineralization, it could be argued that tissue structural changes may be an alteration of the demineralization dynamics during the development and/or consolidation of the lesion brought about by this ion.

Logic would suggest that in the absence of an oral environment which is incapable of initiating caries, an unlikely event in anyone's mouth in this day and age, there must be a repair mechanism or, eventually, we would all exhibit high caries rates. This mechanism of repair is called remineralization, and fluoride is said to accelerate this process. From many of the simply designed, but elegantly performed, *in vitro* experiments, it has been suggested that fluoride can also affect the quality, quantity and position of reprecipitated mineral in the artificially produced carious lesion. It is also argued on the basis of these same experiments that fluoride: (i) will, at very low concentrations [sub 1 ppm (52.6 µM/L)] when in solution, initiate mineral phase transformations, for example, dicalcium phosphate dihydrate (DCPD) into fluorapatite[2,13] in the lesion, thus theoretically rendering the mineral less susceptible to further acid dissolution; (ii) may foster the production of larger crystals in certain zones of the lesion, again rendering the crystals less susceptible to acid attack;[2,6] (iii) and will,depending on the calcium and phosphorus concentrations in the remineralizing solutions (including saliva and plaque fluid) help deposit mineral preferentially in the various zones in the subsurface lesion, the zones most often

mentioned being the surface zone[13,54] and the base of the body of lesion, which could include the dark zone.[15,48,50]

However, in naturally developing lesions with mixed apatite systems containing contaminating ions and organic moieties (both internally and externally derived) how is fluoride's effectiveness as a mineral phase initiator affected? Under these same conditions how effective would fluoride be in fostering the growth of larger apatite crystals when, in fact, there are many examples of organic molecules, especially proteins, when absorbed on to crystal surfaces acting as crystal growth inhibitors[24,45]? Thus the presence of organic material, which has been demonstrated in natural white spot lesions in enamel in relative high concentrations, would argue against fluoride being able to affect such crystal growth.[5,47] This, coupled with the extreme difficulty and relative subjectivity of measuring the crystal size of apatites in enamel caries lesions, makes the reports of fluoride's ability to affect to any great extent crystal growth, equivocal. However, in numerous *in situ* studies, remineralization has been demonstrated when dealing with demineralized lesions affecting the outermost enamel surface, only (100-150 µm). As we have shown, this surface zone is certainly highly susceptible to chemical changes as a result of the intermittent pH fluctuations, and in cementum, where the organic content is so high that it allows for precise sampling and measurement of crystals, there is no doubt that fluoride accumulates in the surface zone covering caries lesions – and that this zone contains apatite crystals significantly larger than those in sound, normal tissue.[59]

When it comes to natural caries lesions, however, with subsurface demineralization located several hundreds of microns deep within the tissues, the surface zone will most probably act as a diffusion barrier.[30] Thus, the ability of fluoride to affect the disposition of calcium and phosphate deep in a lesion would seem to depend greatly on the porosity of the surface of the lesion.[14] It should be appreciated that in both *in vitro* and *in situ* experiments where subsurface deposition has been demonstrated, lesions were produced *in vitro* under "pure" conditions, that is, without the complex interactions of contaminating ions, organic molecules and pH fluctuations, and one must ask just how representative are these of the "naturally" occurring lesions. Certainly, natural lesions have been shown to be particularly resistant to remineralization even under ideal laboratory, remineralizing conditions.[53]

There is some evidence from epidemiologic data gathered during fluoridation studies, and clinical studies testing a variety of fluoridated products of the lack of progression of small caries lesions (presumably white spot lesions) in enamel, diagnosed either on x-rays or visually. In some cases, disappearance of these lesions has even been reported.[3] This would argue strongly for fluoride being able to influence the structure of natural lesions throughout its depth and, in the case of nonprogression, may be a consolidation of this surface zone. However, in the past it has been argued that the disappearance of caries lesions diagnosed via bitewing x-rays is because of an original misdiagnosis and/or the vagaries of the technical aspects of taking reproducible x-rays over time. Less credence is now placed on this later argument as more *in vivo* longitudinal data indicate that approximal caries lesions may diminish in size.

Many authors have reported *in vitro* experiments which have demonstrated the need of fluoride to be present at high concentrations in the enamel and at relatively low concentrations in the demineralizing media for the surface zone to form.[10,12,34,44] Chow[10] in a recent article make a nice point as to what these relative amounts are and what concentration the mineral based fluoride equates to in solution once the mineral is dissolved. Certainly, the 13 ppm of fluoride in apatites in which subsurface le-

Table 11-2

Effect of fluoride concentration on lesion development in human enamel when present in solutions undersaturated with respect to enamel mineral[a]

F (ppm)	C	SSL	NL	DS(FA)[b]
0.004	89	11	–	0.7
0.009	53	40	7	1.6
0.024	20	80	–	3.7
0.054	10	90	–	8.3
0.154	–	90	10	28.5
0.504	–	20	80	96.8
1.004	–	–	100	187.0

a From Margolis *et al.*[33] Degree of saturation with respect to enamel (equal to 4.4×10^{-9}) was the same in all solutions. Results obtained following exposure of enamel surfaces (n = 10 - 18) to solutions for 72 h. C, percent of teeth showing cavitation; SSL, percent of teeth showing subsurface demineralization; NL, percent of teeth showing no detectable mineral loss.
b Degree of saturation with respect to fluorapatite.

sions were produced by Anderson & Elliot[1] is very low and when the mineral is dissolved it would translate into a concentration in the media of 0.003 ppm once the Ca^{++} concentration in the solution has been reduced to 3 mM. This is far below any concentration advocated by those authors arguing for fluoride's major structural effect during lesion development being the formation of the surface zone (Table 11-2). In fact, it is so low that its affect on the kinetics of the reaction is probably nonexistent. Anderson & Elliot explain the production of the subsurface lesion and, therefore, the surface zone by a coupled diffusion theory.[1] However, recently Margolis & Moreno[34] have produced data which show the effect of low fluoride concentrations on lesion development in human enamel, when present in solutions undersaturated with respect to enamel mineral (see Table 11-2; see also Chapter 14). It is apparent that concentrations as low as 0.5-1.0 ppm fluoride in solution has a dramatic effect on lesion development. These data thus fully support the studies by Larsen *et al.* from 1976[31] where they emphasized that the predominant cariostatic effect of fluoride derives from it being present in very low concentrations in the oral environment, whereas the concentration of fluoride in the enamel within the range physiologically occurring in man (see Chapter 14) has a negligible effect on the solubility behavior of enamel.

Much of what has been discussed about enamel probably pertains to dentin and the dentin/cementum complex. However, the effect of fluorides on the structure of caries lesions in dentin and root surfaces is further complicated by the "live" reaction of the dentin to caries and the high organic content of the tissue. For example, recent work would suggest that a major component of the noncollagenous proteins, phosphoprotein, in dentin may block dentin's ability to remineralize[11] and the presence or absence of fluoride may be of little consequence until this moiety is removed.

The "natural" caries lesion development in the mouth is complex and the multifactorial effects of fluoride on this process, which are reflected in the structural changes occurring during lesion development, only complicate the issue even more. An interesting dimension has been added by meticulously reexamining the clinical caries data from what is probably the best followed up water fluoridation study so far[22] (see also Chapter 15). When lesions were recorded at non-cavitated stages ("white spot lesions") and were added to the cavitated lesions (resistance to withdrawing the probe), then there was no differences in carious prevalence between the non-fluoridated city of Culemborg and the fluoridated city of Tiel. This might be interpreted, simplistically, as the fluoride interfering with the progression of the lesion rather then its initiation. For this to happen, fluoride would have had to effect a structural metamorphosis of the lesion in which mineral phase transformations could have occurred, larger crystals could have formed, and mineral could be deposited in various zones of the lesion. Of particular importance in this process would have been the ability of fluoride to cause the consolidation and ensure the maintenance of the surface zone by catalyzing the deposition of mineral into this zone. Of all the effects of fluoride, this last effect may be the most important.

Thus, at present it is envisioned that the presence of fluoride in small but elevated concentrations in the plaque fluid during lesion development both slows down the rate of lesion development (demineralization) and at the same time enhances deposition of fluoridated apatite into the lesion surface ("remineralization").

Literature cited

1. Anderson P, Elliot JC. Microradiographic study of the formation of caries-like lesions in synthetic apatite aggregates. Caries Res 1985; 19: 403-6.

2. Arends J, Gelherd TBFM. *In vivo* remineralization of human enamel. In: Leach S, Edgar M, eds. Remineralisation and demineralisation of teeth. Oxford: IRL Press 1986: 1-16.

3. Backer Dirks O. Posteruptive changes in dental enamel. J Dent Res 1966; 45: 503-11.

4. Beck J. The epidemiology of root surface caries. J Dent Res 1990; 60: 1216-21.

5. Bibby BG. Organic enamel material and caries. Caries Res 1971; 5: 305-22.

6. Brown WE. Physicochemical mechanisms of dental caries. J Dent Res 1974; 53: 204-16.

7. Carvalho JC, Ekstrand KR, Thylstrup A. Dental plaque and caries on occlusal surfaces of first permanent molars in relation to stage of eruption. J Dent Res 1989; 68: 773-9.

8. Carvalho JC, Ekstrand KR, Thylstrup A. Results of 1 year of non-operative occlusal caries treatment of erupting permanent first molars. Community Dent Oral Epidemiol 1991; 19: 23-8.

9. Carvalho JC, Ekstrand KR, Thylstrup A. Results of 3 years of non-operative occlusal caries treatment of erupting permanent first molars. Community Dent Oral Epidemiol 1992; 20: 187-92.

10. Chow LC. Tooth-bound fluoride and dental caries. J Dent Res 1990; 69: 595-600.

11. Clarkson BH, Feagin FF, McCurdy SP, Sheetz JH, Speirs R. Effects of phosphoprotein moieties on the remineralization of human root caries. Caries Res 1991; 25: 166-73.

12. Dijk JWE van, Borggrevan JMPN, Driessens FCM. Chemical mathematical simulation of caries. Caries Res 1979; 13: 169-80.

13. Elder B, Nancollis GH. Physical and chemical aspects of the mineralization and demineralization of tooth components. In: Bowen WH, Tabek LA, eds. Cariology for the nineties. Rochester: University of Rochester Press 1993: 186-96.

14. Featherstone JDB. Diffusion phenomena and enamel caries development. In: Guggenheim B, ed. Cariology today. Basel: Karger 1984: 259-68.

15. Featherstone JDB, Glena R, Shariati M, Shields CP. Dependence of *in vitro* demineralization of apatite and remineralization of dental enamel on fluoride concentration. J Dent Res 1990; 69: 620-5.

16. Fejerskov O, Larsen MJ, Richards A, Baelum V. Dental tissue effects of fluoride. Adv Dent Res 1994; 8: 15-31.

17. Fejerskov O, Nyvad B. Root surface caries in humans: a review. In: Embery G, Rølla G, eds. Clinical and biological aspects of dentifrices. Oxford: Oxford University Press 1992: 105-30.

18. Fejerskov O, Scheie AA, Manji F. The effect of sucrose on plaque pH in the primary and permanent dentition of caries-inactive and -active Kenyan children. J Dent Res 1992; 71: 25-31.

19. Fejerskov O, Silness J, Karring T, Löe H. The occlusal fissure of unerupted third molars as an experimental caries model in man. Scand J Dent Res 1976; 85: 142-9.

20. Fejerskov O, Thylstrup A. Dental enamel. In: Mjör IA, Fejerskov O, eds. Human oral embryology and histology. Copenhagen: Munksgaard 1986: 50-89.

21. Fejerskov O, Thylstrup A. Pathology and treatment of dental caries. In: Thylstrup A, Fejerskov O, eds. Textbook of cariology. Copenhagen: Munksgaard 1986: 204-34.

22. Groeneveld A, van Eck AAMJ, Backer Dirks O. Fluoride in caries prevention: Is the effect pre- or posteruptive? J Dent Res 1990; 69: 751-5.

23. Hallsworth AS, Robinson C, Weatherell JA. Mineral and magnesium distribution within the approximal carious lesion of dental enamel. Caries Res 1972; 6: 156-68.

24. Hay DI, Moreno EC. Hydroxyapatite interactive proteins. In: Bowen WH, Tabak LA, eds. Cariology for the nineties. Rochester: University of Rochester Press 1993: 71-84.

25. Kidd EAM, Thylstrup A, Fejerskov O. The histopathology of enamel caries in fluorosed primary teeth. Caries Res 1981; 15: 346-52.

26. Kostlan J. Translucent zones in the central part of the carious lesions of enamel. Brit Dent J 1962; 113: 244-8.

27. Larsen MJ. Emaljens opløselighed caries og erosioner. Thesis. Aarhus: Royal Dental College 1975.

28. Larsen MJ, Bruun C. Enamel/saliva – inorganic chemical reactions. In: Thylstrup A, Fejerskov O, eds. Textbook of cariology. Copenhagen: Munksgaard 1986: 181-203.

29. Larsen MJ, Bruun C. Caries chemistry and fluoride - mechanisms of action. In: Thylstrup A, Fejerskov O, eds. Textbook of clinical cariology, 2nd edn. Copenhagen: Munksgaard 1994: 231-57.

30. Larsen MJ, Fejerskov O. Chemical and structural challenges in remineralization of dental enamel lesions. Scand J Dent Res 1989; 97: 285-96.

31. Larsen MJ, von der Fehr FR, Birkeland JM. Effect of fluoride on the saturation of an acetate buffer with respect to hydroxyapatite. Arch Oral Biol 1976; 21: 723-8.

32. Margolis HC. An assessment of recent advances in the study of the chemistry and biochemistry of dental plaque fluid. J Dent Res 1990; 69: 1337-42.

33. Margolis HC, Duckworth JH, Moreno EC. Composition of pooled resting plaque fluid from caries-free and caries susceptible individuals. J Dent Res 1988; 67: 1468-75.

34. Margolis HC, Moreno EC. Physiochemical perspectives on the mechanisms of systemic and topical fluorides. J Dent Res 1990; 69: 606-13.

35. McCann HG. Inorganic components of salivary secretions. In: Harris RS, ed. Art and science of dental caries research. New York: Academic Press 1968: 55-73.

36. Mellberg JR, Castrovince LA, Rotsides ID. In vivo remineralization by monofluorophosphate dentifrice as determined with a thin section sandwich method. J Dent Res 1986; 65: 1078-83.

37. Newman P, Macfayden EE, Gillespie FC, Stephen KW. An in-dwelling electrode for in vivo measurement of the pH of dental plaque in man. Arch Oral Biol 1979; 24: 501-7.

38. Nyvad B. Microbial colonization of human tooth surfaces. Thesis. APMIS 1993; 101: 1-45.

39. Nyvad B, Fejerskov O. Active and inactive root surface caries – structural entities? In: Thylstrup A, Leach SA, Qvist V, eds. Dentine and dentine reaction in the oral cavity. Oxford: IRL Press 1987: 165-79.

40. Nyvad B, Fejerskov O. An ultrastructural study of bacterial invasion and tissue breakdown in human experimental root-surface caries. J Dent Res 1990; 69: 1118-25.

41. Nyvad B, Fejerskov O. Development, structure and pH of dental plaque. In: Thylstrup A, Fejerskov O, eds. Textbook of clinical cariology, 2nd edn. Copenhagen: Munksgaard 1994: 89-110.

42. Nyvad B, ten Cate JM, Fejerskov O. Microradiography of experimental root surface caries in man. Caries Res 1989; 23: 218-24.

43. Pearce EIF, Coote GE, Larsen MJ. Distribution of fluoride in carious enamel [abstr.]. J Dent Res 1994; 73: 238.

44. Poole DFG, Silverstone LM. Remineralization of enamel. In: Hard tissue growth, repair and remineralization. Amsterdam: Elsevier 1973: 36-56.

45. Robinson C, Shore RC, Kirkham J, Stonehouse NJ. Extracellular processing of enamel proteins and control of crystal growth. J Biol Buccale 1990; 18: 355-61.

46. Scheie AA, Fejerskov O, Lingström P, Birkhed D, Manji F. Use of palladium touch microelectrodes under field conditions for in vivo assessment of dental plaque pH in children. Caries Res 1992; 26: 44-52.

47. Silverstone LM. The structure of carious enamel, including the early lesion. In: Melcher AH, Zarb GA, eds. Oral sciences reviews, No 3, Dental enamel. Copenhagen: Munksgaard 1973: 100-60.

48. Silverstone LM. Remineralization phenomena. Caries Res 1977; 11: 59-84.

49. Silverstone LM. Relationship of the macroscopic, histological and radiographic appearance of interproximal lesions in human teeth: in vivo study using artificial caries technique. Ped Dent 1982; Spec Iss 2: 414-22.

50. Silverstone LM. Remineralisation and enamel caries: Significance of fluoride and effect on crystal diameters. In: Leach SA, Edgar WM, eds. Oxford: IRL Press 1983: 185-205.

51. Silverstone LM. Fluorides and remineralization. In: Wei SHY, ed. Clinical uses of fluorides. Philadelphia: Lea & Febiger 1985: 153-75.

52. Silverstone LM. The primary translucent zone of enamel caries and of artificial caries-like lesions. Br Dent J 1986; 120: 461-71.

53. Silverstone LM, Wefel JS, Zimmerman BF, Clarkson BH, Featherstone MJ. Remineralization of natural artificial lesions in human dental enamel *in vitro*. Caries Res 1981; 15: 138-57.

54. ten Cate JM. *In vitro* studies on the effects of fluoride on de- and remineralization. J Dent Res 1990: 69: 614-9.

55. Tenovuo J, Lagerlöf F. Saliva. In: Thylstrup A, Fejerskov O. Textbook of clinical Cariology, 2nd edn. Copenhagen: Munksgaard 1994: 17-43.

56. Theilade E, Fejerskov O. Prachyabrued W, Kilian M. Microbiological study on developing plaque in human fissures. Scand J Dent Res 1974; 82: 420-7.

57. Thomsen JR, Tagesen J, Fejerskov O. Forekomst og fordeling af fissurcaries i klinisk "sunde" præmolarer (with English abstract). Dan Dent J 1988; 92: 1-6.

58. Thylstrup A, Fejerskov O. Clinical and pathological features of dental caries. In: Thylstrup A, Fejerskov O, eds. Textbook of clinical cariology. 2nd edn. Copenhagen: Munksgaard 1994: 111-58.

59. Tohda H, Fejerskov O, Yanagisawa T. Transmission electron microscopy of cementum crystals correlated with Ca and F distribution in normal and carious human root surfaces. J Dent Res 1996; In press.

60. Weatherell JA, Deutsch D, Robinson C, Hallsworth AS. Assimilation of fluoride by enamel throughout the life of the tooth. Caries Res 1977; 11: 85-115.

CHAPTER 12

FLUORIDE IN ORAL FLUIDS AND DENTAL PLAQUE

G. Rölla • J. Ekstrand

Introduction – Fluoride in saliva – Fluoride in plaque – Fluoride in the crevicular fluid
Fluoride and dental enamel – Fluoride reservoirs in or on oral soft tissue
Amount of plaque, nature of plaque bacteria and their role in the cariostatic effect
of fluoride in plaque fluid

Introduction

The marked caries reduction recorded in many countries over the last two decades is thought to be mainly the result of the widespread and frequent use of fluoride-containing toothpaste. The caries reduction has been experienced in all age groups, and can be correlated with the introduction of fluoride-containing toothpaste. There seem to be no other factors which can explain the decline in dental caries, which has occurred worldwide during the same period, in geographic regions as far apart as the Scandinavian countries and Australia/New Zealand.[3,20,21,23,43,44]

The caries-inhibiting effect of fluoride has previously been attributed to ingestion and subsequent incorporation of the ion during enamel formation, resulting in a more acid-resistant surface. This is usually referred to as the systemic cariostatic effect of fluoride. As discussed also in other chapters of this textbook, the fluoride ion has a local cariostatic effect on the teeth and components of the dental plaque.

The clinical importance of any possible systemic effect is uncertain.[9,26] The most important mode of action of topical fluoride is probably the enhancement of remineralization and inhibition of demineralization (see also Chapters 11 and 14).

The plaque fluid, the aqueous phase within the plaque, is in contact with the enamel surface, with the plaque bacteria (which produce the organic acids) and with saliva and gingival fluid. Plaque fluid transports organic acids as well as fluoride, calcium, phosphate and other ions to the enamel surface. To be biologically active these have to be in solution. The balance between these factors, of which fluoride and pH are the most important, determines whether the tooth mineral will dissolve or not. It is thus the fluoride present in plaque fluid and not the fluoride incorporated into the enamel which is decisive for re- or demineralization of enamel. The plaque fluid is the site at which fluoride influences the re- and demineralization process.[6,15]

The fluoride in the plaque fluid may origin-

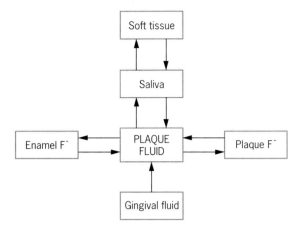

Fig. 12-1. Sources of fluoride in plaque fluid.

ate from many sources: calcium fluoride on the enamel beneath the plaque, calcium fluoride in plaque and fluoride in saliva and gingival fluid (Fig. 12-1). It is well known that dental plaque is normally richer in fluoride than the fluids to which it is exposed[15] (i.e. saliva, plaque fluid and gingival fluid). Plaque thus appears to be able to retain and concentrate fluoride (Fig. 12-2).[7,51] This is probably an important aspect of the cariostatic effect of fluoride, because an inverse relationship between a high fluoride content of plaque and a low caries activity is known to exist.[18]

In the following chapter the data concerning fluoride in saliva, in plaque and plaque fluid and in gingival fluid will be reviewed. These data will be discussed in relation to recent concepts of the mechanisms by which fluoride exerts its cariostatic effect in the oral cavity.

Fluoride in saliva

The concentration of salivary fluoride from the parotid and submandibular/sublingual glands is about two-thirds of the plasma fluoride con-

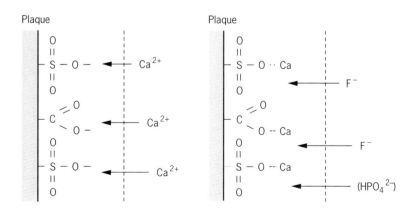

Fig. 12-2. A possible mechanism by which salivary fluoride may be concentrated and bound in plaque. The sulfate, carboxyl and sulfate groups on the left represent fixed negative charges in plaque known to be present on the bacterial surfaces and in the plaque matrix. The charges attract calcium ions. Some of these bound calcium ions have a free charge which can bind fluoride.[42]

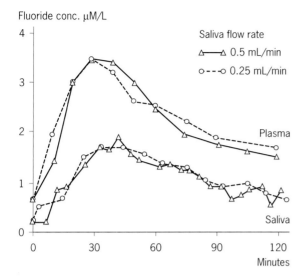

Fig. 12-3. Plasma (the two upper curves) and parotid saliva (the two lower curves) fluoride concentrations after intake of 1 mg fluoride as NaF capsules.[34]

centration,[13,32-34] and seems to be independent of flow rate in contrast to most electrolytes (Fig. 12-3). In subjects living in a low fluoride area, the saliva fluoride concentration is less than 1 μM/L.[31] The fluoride concentration in whole saliva is related not only to the fluoride excreted from the glands but also to dietary fluid intake and dental fluoride preparations.[4,5,31] In

a study in children living in low or high fluoride areas (0.1 and 1.2 ppm, respectively) the saliva levels were 0.3 and 0.9 μM/L. A diurnal fluctuation in the saliva fluoride concentration was also seen in the high fluoridated area (Fig. 12-4).[35]

This resting saliva fluoride level will be influenced not only by the fluoride concentration

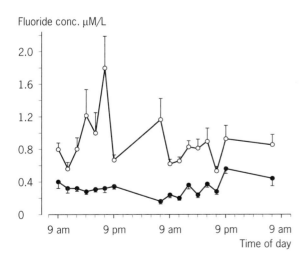

Fig. 12-4. The diurnal mean salivary fluoride concentration during 46 hours in a 0.2 ppm F area (bottom curve) and 1.2 ppm F areas. (n = 27; age 12 years). The vertical bars indicate standard error of the mean.[35]

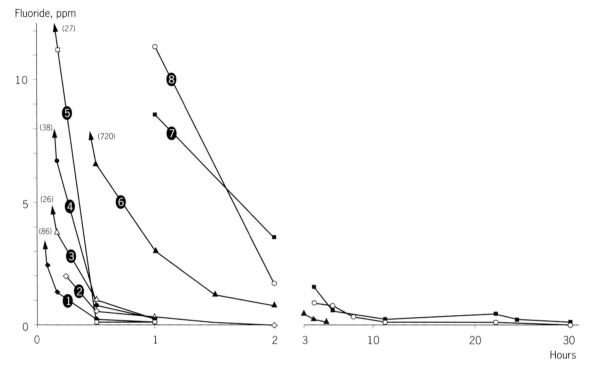

Fig. 12-5. Mean fluoride concentrations in saliva at different times after various topical fluoride treatments. Curves numbered 1-8 represent the following treatments: 1: toothbrushing with MFP dentifrice (0.50 mg F) followed by 10-second mouthrinse with water. 2: toothbrushing with NaF dentifrice (0.50 mg F) without subsequent rinsing. 3: chewing of chewable F tablets (0.42 mg F). 4: chewing of plain F tablets (0.50 mg F). 5: chewing of F-containing chewing gum (0.50 mg F). 6: mouthrinse with 0.2% NaF solution. 7: topical application of APF (1.2% F). 8: topical application of neutral 2% NaF solution. Figures on top of curves denote initial F concentrations after 2-3 minutes.[15]

in the drinking water but also by regular daily use of a fluoride dentifrice/mouthrinse. Studies have shown that the resting saliva fluoride concentration can increase to about twice the original concentration,[10] probably through equilibrium with a higher level of fluoride in plaque, or with other possible retention sites in contact with saliva.

The low concentration of fluoride and the small volume of resting saliva present in the oral cavity (about 1 mL) indicate that fluoride from the ductal saliva is not normally an im-portant source of fluoride in plaque or plaque fluid. However, following topical application of fluoride in the form of mouthrinses, toothpaste, or any other fluoride vehicles, there is a 100- or even 1000-fold increase in salivary fluoride concentration, depending on the fluoride concentration of the fluoride agent (Fig. 12-5).[4,5] This high concentration of fluoride in saliva falls rapidly. Two and sometimes three exponential phases in the decline of the saliva fluoride concentration curve are seen.[14] Depending on the concentration and type of flu-

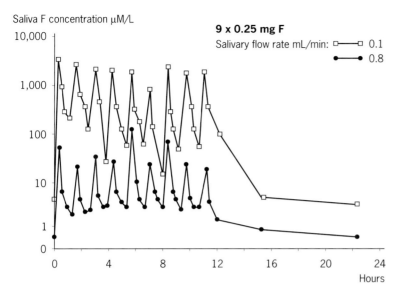

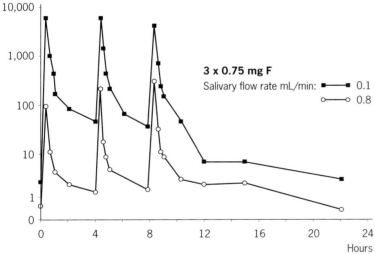

Fig. 12-6. Fluoride concentration in whole saliva in two subjects (resting salivary flow rate of 0.1 and 0.8 mL/min respectively) after repeated intake of 0.25 mg × 9 (upper graph) and 0.75 mg × 3 (lower graph) fluoride as slow-release lozenges.[15]

oride agent, the saliva fluoride concentration is reduced to a few ppm within an hour, and within the next 3-6 hours returns to the baseline level.[8,14]

The clearance of saliva fluoride varies considerably because of large individual variations in salivary flow rates (Fig. 12-6), the volume of fluoride distribution in the oral cavity and individual variation in anatomy, and the number of teeth.[16,25,36]

Saliva is in direct contact with the plaque fluid and plaque, as mentioned above. It ap-

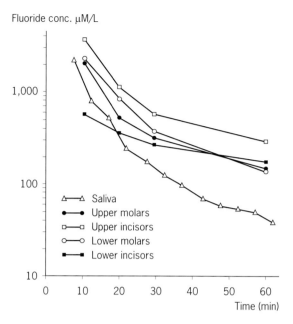

Fluoride conc. μM/L

△—△ Saliva
●—● Upper molars
□—□ Upper incisors
○—○ Lower molars
■—■ Lower incisors

Time (min)

Fig. 12-7. Plaque-fluid fluoride and salivary fluoride after a one minute 0.2% NaF rinse (10 mL). Saliva concentrations are plotted at the midpoint of the 5-minute collection interval. The left and right molar sites are combined into maxillary and mandibular sites. Data from one subject.[53]

pears that a transfer of fluoride from saliva to plaque or plaque fluid may occur during or immediately after mouthrinsing (or similar procedures): a 10-mL volume of rinsing solution is diluted in only 1-2 mL of saliva, giving a high salivary fluoride concentration.[19] This is probably conducive to fluoride transfer to plaque and plaque fluid. When the mouthrinse is spat out, both the volume of fluid in the mouth and the concentration of fluoride decrease, and saliva again becomes less important as a source of plaque fluoride.

Fluoride in plaque

Fluoride in plaque exists in ionic and bound forms: as in saliva, the concentration is determined by the frequency of fluoride exposure and the fluoride concentration of the source. Sources of plaque fluoride include the diet, saliva and crevicular fluid. Dental plaque (wet weight) contains a total of 5-10 ppm fluoride

wet weight.[51] Only a small part is present as free ions (%), the amount being dependent on exposure to fluoride.

There is a correlation between salivary fluoride level and fluoride in the plaque fluid.[8,53] Plaque fluid fluoride concentrations are much higher than salivary fluoride concentrations. This may be due to slower elimination of the ion from the plaque, due to the thickness of the salivary film, or release of fluoride from sources of fluoride in the plaque such as calcium fluoride. There seems to be a large variation between the plaque fluid fluoride concentration at various sites in the mouth (Fig. 12-7).[53] Plaque fluid collected in the region of the maxillary incisor site maintains a much higher concentration of fluoride than the other sites.[53] The pH of the plaque appears to be an important factor, low pH being associated with low fluoride concentrations.

The nature of fluoride in plaque is uncertain. It has been reported that strong mineral acid is needed to dissolve all the fluoride in

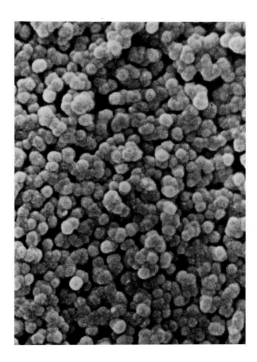

Fig. 12-8. Scanning electron microscope (SEM) observation of an enamel surface treated with 2% neutral NaF for 24 hours. The surface is covered with small, round particles. These are alkali soluble and probably consist of CaF_2. The size and number of particles formed during fluoride exposure of enamel are dependent on the concentration and pH of the fluoride solution and on the exposure time.

plaque.[12,37] It has been suggested that fluoride may be stored inside the plaque bacteria.[22,48] However, this is only a very small amount, which increases during acidic conditions because of the formation of hydrogen fluoride (HF), an undissociated weak acid with a pKa of 3.4 formed at low pH. Hydrogen fluoride penetrates the bacterial cell membrane, reducing the fluoride content of plaque fluid. This mechanism thus can not explain the observed release of fluoride from plaque at low pH (see also Chapter 13).

Another possibility is that calcium fluoride forms in the plaque during mouthrinsing or toothbrushing with fluoride (Fig. 12-8). There is some experimental evidence to support this hypothesis[24,29] (Fig. 12-9). During and after a mouthrinse (or toothbrushing), the plaque fluid is supersaturated with respect to calcium fluoride because plaque fluid contains considerable amounts of calcium. This fluoride will be mobilized when the pH falls below 6 (Figs. 12-10 and 12-11),[42] accounting not only for the fluoride in plaque, and the release of fluoride and calcium from plaque during caries challenges, but also for the need for strong mineral acid to dissolve plaque fluoride.

A third possible mechanism would be retention of fluoride associated with plaque bacteria surfaces (Fig. 12-12).[42,45] These surfaces represent a formidable total surface area, with a net negative charge and abundant phosphate and carboxyl groups.[28] In the oral environment, which is rich in calcium, the acidic groups on the surfaces of bacteria will acquire counterions, mainly calcium. Fluoride can thus be associated with calcium counterions[42,45] (Fig. 12-11). This fluoride would also be released (with calcium) when the pH approaches the pK of the acidic groups; they release F^- and Ca^{2+} at low pH. Because the total surface area is so large, this mechanism could also account quantitatively for the fluoride retained in plaque.

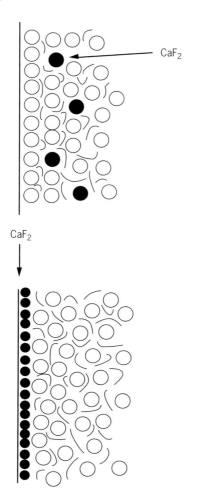

Fig. 12-9. Calcium fluoride can form in dental plaque by interaction between calcium in the plaque fluid and fluoride from a mouthrinse (top). Calcium fluoride may form on the enamel surface during toothbrushing, in particular on demineralized enamel. This is later covered by plaque (bottom). Both sources can supply the plaque-fluid with F⁻ during periods of low pH.

Fluoride in the crevicular fluid

The crevicular fluid, which enters the oral cavity via the gingival crevice, is closely related to serum. Its fluoride concentration is low[27,52] and closely related to plasma fluoride concentration. It is unlikely to be an important source of fluoride for plaque or plaque fluid.

Fluoride and dental enamel

Large amounts of fluoride may be acquired by enamel exposed to fluoride toothpaste during toothbrushing, which is subsequently covered by plaque. Calcium fluoride is the fluoride phase which forms first under such conditions. The pH cycling which occurs in the plaque covering this fluoride-rich enamel contributes to its rapid mobilization and transfer of flu-

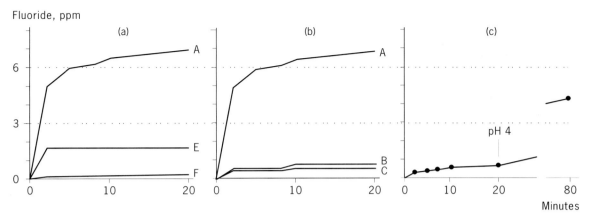

Fig. 12-10. (a) Solubility of calcium fluoride in water (A), in saliva (E) and in water after 1 hour of exposure to human saliva (F); (b) solubility of calcium fluoride in water (A), in 1 M phosphate buffer pH 7 (B) and solubility in water by CaF_2 exposed to phosphate buffer for 60 minutes (C); (c) solubility of saliva-treated calcium fluoride in distilled water. When the pH is reduced to 4 (or 5) the solubility increases, indicating that the protective layer formed during saliva treatment is acid soluble (see Fig. 12-11).

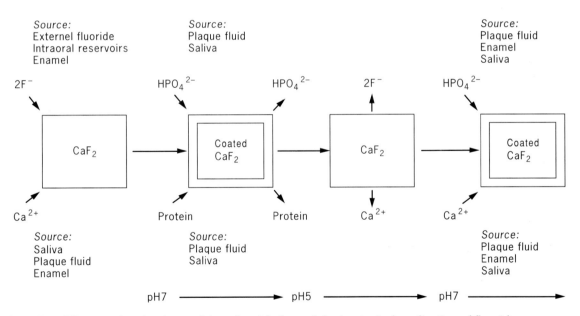

Fig. 12-11. Diagram showing how calcium fluoride formed during topical application of fluoride can serve as a fluoride reservoir which increases the release of fluoride when pH approaches 5, but otherwise conserves the fluoride available. Such reservoirs may be present in the plaque matrix and of the enamel underneath plaque, and may greatly influence both re- and demineralization processes in the enamel and the metabolism of dental plaque.

223

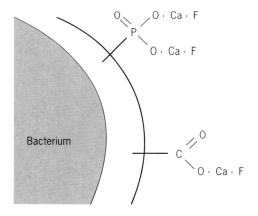

Fig. 12-12. A possible mechanism of fluoride binding by bacterial surfaces.[41]

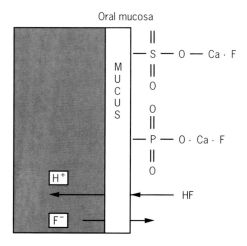

Fig. 12-13. Suggested mechanisms for fluoride retention by soft tissue.

oride to the plaque fluid (Figs. 12-10 and 12-11). Demineralized enamel takes up particularly high amounts of fluoride.

Fluoride in enamel, in the form of calcium fluoride, is abundant and available for transfer to the plaque fluid.[42] This fluoride reservoir can release fluoride and calcium during caries challenges (Fig. 12-11).

Enamel (and dentin) not covered by plaque may also take up fluoride, which is subsequently slowly released. This source is prob-ably less important than fluoride deposited beneath the plaque, as discussed above. The reaction between the fluoride in toothpaste and dental enamel is probably not mediated through saliva, because the paste is applied directly to the tooth enamel. This fluoride is replenished regularly and this reservoir is thus scarcely depleted. This probably makes toothpaste a particularly appropriate fluoride vehicle.

Fluoride reservoirs in or on the oral soft tissue

It has recently been shown that soft tissue can acquire fluoride during topical applications.[11] Some is absorbed through the tissue, and this uptake is pH dependent, because fluoride penetrates more easily when protonated (HF). This fluoride is dissociated (Fig. 12-13) after the absorption, and may not necessarily be easily released. However, some of the fluoride in soft tissues is associated with calcium; pretreatment with calcium ions increases fluoride retention, whereas treatment with EDTA decreases retention.[29] This mechanism may be interpreted in terms of the presence of acidic groups on the surface of the tissues, and retention of fluoride based on interaction with calcium counterions (Fig. 12-13). Connective tissue has sulfate- and carboxyl groups, whereas the cell membranes contain phosphate groups (in phospholipids). The mucus on the surface of the epithelium also has acidic groups. The soft tissue-retained fluoride may supply the saliva with fluoride after a mouthrinse, but is probably not a major source of fluoride.

Effect of plaque fluid fluoride and de- and remineralization of enamel lesions

Demineralization of enamel will not occur under dental plaque when the plaque fluid is saturated with respect to the minerals present in tooth enamel, viz. hydroxyapatite, carbonated hydroxyapatite, partly fluoridated hydroxyapatite and fluorapatite. The concentrations of calcium and phosphate in the plaque fluid and the pH of this fluid determine whether demineralization or remineralization will occur. Another factor crucial to the fate of the enamel surface is the concentration of fluoride in the plaque fluid.[53] Fluoride catalyzes the transformation of calcium phosphates to hydroxyapatite during remineralization periods and participates in the deposition of fluoridated hydroxyapatite and fluorapatite. Both these minerals are less soluble than hydroxyapatite, and the fluoride ions thus contribute to the integrity of dental enamel, even when the plaque fluid is undersaturated with respect to hydroxyapatite (below approximately pH 5.5).

Amount of plaque, nature of plaque bacteria and their role in the cariostatic effect of fluoride in plaque fluid

The cariostatic effect of fluoride is limited; if plaque pH falls below about 4.5 the plaque fluid becomes undersaturated with respect to fluorapatite and demineralization will occur, regardless of the presence of fluoride.[43] It has been shown in human in situ experiments that shark enamel, which consists of fluorapatite (33,000 ppm F), is demineralized when placed in the human oral cavity. This was seen within 1 month, when a 1-mm-thick layer of plaque covered the teeth. This also occurred if excess fluoride was present in the liquid phase above the enamel, because mouthrinsing with fluoride had no effect on the demineralization of shark enamel during these conditions (see Chapter 14).[55]

The oral hygiene of many patients at high risk for developing caries is often inadequate.[56] This probably causes the pH to fall to such a low level that even fluoride is unable to inhibit caries development completely. In such cases the oral hygiene has to be improved, or combinations of fluoride and antibacterial agents used. The role of the latter would be to prevent the pH from falling to a level at which fluorapatite dissolves (Fig. 12-14).

The pH of plaque fluid is obviously dependent on the nature of the bacteria in plaque; acidogenic and aciduric bacteria produce more

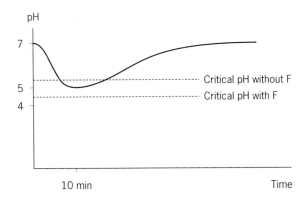

Fig. 12-14. A Stephan curve illustrating schematically how fluoride inhibits caries. A challenge which would cause demineralization in the absence of fluoride does not cause demineralization in the presence of fluoride. If pH drops below the critical pH with fluoride, caries can develop, even in the presence of fluoride. Large amounts of plaque may cause this situation (bad oral hygiene).

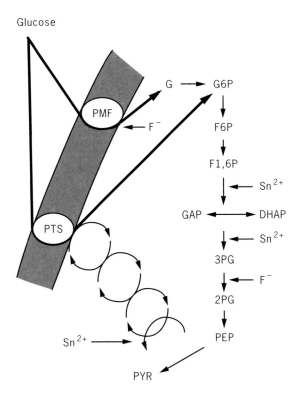

Fig. 12-15. The diagram illustrates how stannous ions inhibit bacterial fermentation of glucose. Oxidation of thiol groups is presumably the mechanism involved. Other metal ions such as Zn^{2+}, Cu^{2+} and Ag^+ have similar properties.[47]

acid than other bacteria. The number of bacteria at a specific site is also important, because more bacteria produce more acid. The thickness of plaque and the age of plaque have been related to its pathogenicity. It has also been shown that the volume of extracellular polysaccharides in plaque is important in this respect.[54] One explanation is that fermentable carbohydrates penetrate deeper in the loose, polysaccharide- containing plaque, and acid formation occurs closer to the enamel surface than in denser plaque with less polysaccharides. Here the fermentable carbohydrate is catabolized close to the plaque surface, and further from the enamel surface.

Effect on dental plaque of combinations of fluoride and metal ions

Stannous fluoride has been extensively used in preventive dentistry, in mouthrinses, for topical application and in dentifrices. It is now well established that in addition to its general fluoride effect, stannous fluoride possesses an antiplaque effect, due to the antibacterial effect of stannous ions.[17,30,49,50] Stannous ions are known to oxidize thiol groups and thus inhibit enzymes which are dependent on such groups (Fig. 12-15). The oxidation of thiol groups by Sn^{2+} ions is pH-dependent, and negligible at low pH.[39] Aqueous solutions of (freshly prepared) stannous fluoride have a pH of 3-4 due to the buffering effect of HF formation in the solution, whereas aqueous solutions of other stannous salts ($SnCl_2$) reach a much lower final pH. Such solutions have no antibacterial activity.[38,39] Zinc ions and cuprous ions can also oxidize thiol groups in the same way as stannous ions. This effect is not limited to the fluoride salts. The principle of the antibacterial mechanism of stannous fluoride is shown in Fig. 12-15. Zinc ions, cuprous ions and silver ions all work according to the same mechanism. Several studies have shown that the anticaries effect of stannous fluoride is in the same range as that of sodium fluoride.[2,30,40] The effect of the stannous ions as such thus appears to be of no clinical significance. On the other hand, it has been shown that cuprous ions give an additive effect to the cariostatic effect of fluoride in rats.[1] The main effect of metal ions may be the prevention of gingivitis.[46]

Literature cited

1. Afseth J, Amsbaugh SM, Monell-Torrens E, et al. Effect of topical application of copper in combination with fluoride in drinking water on experimental caries in rats. Caries Res. 1984; 18: 134-40.

2. Andres C, Shaeffer J, Winderer Jr A. Comparison of antibacterial properties of stannous fluoride and sodium fluoride mouthwashes. J Dent Res 1974; 53: 457-60.

3. Brunelle JA, Carlos JP. Recent trends in dental caries in U.S. children and the effect of water fluoridation. J Dent Res 1990; 69 (Spec Iss): 723-7.

4. Bruun C, Giskov H, Thylstrup A. Whole saliva fluoride after toothbrushing with NaF and MFP dentifrice with different F concentration. Caries Res 1984; 18: 282-8.

5. Bruun C, Lambrou D, Larsen MJ, Fejerskov O, Thylstrup A. Fluoride in mixed human saliva after different topical treatments and possible relation to caries inhibition. Community Dent Oral Epidemiol 1982; 10: 124-9.

6. Carey C, Tatevossian A, Vogel GL. The driving forces in human dental plaque fluid for demineralisation and remineralisation of enamel. In: Leach SA, ed. Factors relating to demineralisation and remineralization of the teeth. Oxford: IRL Press 1986; 163-73.

7. Dawes C, Jenkins N, Hardwick J, Leach S. The relation between the fluoride concentrations in the dental plaque and in drinking water. Br Dent J 1965; 119: 164-7.

8. Dawes C, Weatherell JA. Kinetics of fluoride in oral fluids. J Dent Res 1990; 69 (Spec Iss): 638-44.

9. Driessens FC. Mineral aspects of dentistry. Basel: Karger, 1982: 133-8.

10. Duckworth R, Morgan S. Oral fluoride retention after use of fluoride dentifrices. Caries Res 1991; 25: 123-9.

11. Duckworth R.M. Fluoride in plaque and saliva. Thesis, University of Amsterdam 1993: 71-86.

12. Edgar WM. Fluoride metabolism in dental plaque, bacteria and man. In: Ferguson DB, ed. The environment of the teeth, Frontiers of Oral Physiology, Vol. 3. Basel: Karger 1981: 19-37.

13. Ekstrand J, Alván G, Boréus L, Norlin A. Pharmacokinetics of fluoride in man after single and multiple oral doses. Eur J Clin Pharmacol 1977; 12: 311-7.

14. Ekstrand J, Lagerlöf F, Oliveby A. Some aspects of the kinetics of fluoride in saliva. In: Leach SA, ed. Factors relating to demineralisation and remineralization of the teeth. Oxford: IRL Press 1986: 91-8.

15. Ekstrand J, Spak CJ, Vogel G. Pharmacokinetics of fluoride in man and its clinical relevance. J Dent Res 1990; 69 (Spec Iss): 550-5.

16. Ekstrand J. Pharmacokinetic aspects of topical fluorides. J Dent Res1987; 66: 1061-5.

17. Ellingsen J, Svatun B, Rölla G. The effects of stannous and stannic ions on the formation and acidogenicity of dental plaque in vivo. Acta Odontol Scand 1980; 38: 219-22.

18. Gaugler RW, Briton WF. Fluoride concentration in dental plaque of naval recruits with and without caries. Arch Oral Biol 1982; 275: 269-72.

19. Geddes DAM, McNee SG. The effect of 0.2 % (48 mM) NaF rinses daily on human plaque acidogenicity in situ (Stephan Curve) and fluoride content. Arch Oral Biol 1982; 275: 765-9.

20. Glass RL. Fluoride dentifrices: the basis for the decline in caries prevalence. J Roy Soc Med 1986; 79: 15-7.

21. Jenkins G. Recent changes in dental caries. Br Med J 1985; 291: 1297-8.

22. Jenkins GN, Edgar WM, Ferguson DB. The distribution and metabolic effects of human plaque fluorine. Arch Oral Biol 1969; 14: 105-19.

23. Karlsbeek H, Verrips GHW. Dental caries prevalence and the use of fluorides in different European countries. J Dent Res 1990; 69 (Spec Iss): 728-32.

24. Lagerlöf F, Ekstrand J, Rølla G. Effect of fluoride addition on ionized calcium in salivary sediment and in saliva. Scand J Dent Res 1988; 96: 399-404.

25. Lagerlöf F, Oliveby A, Ekstrand J. Physiological factors influencing salivary clearance of sugar and fluoride. J Dent Res 1987; 66: 430-5.

26 Larsen MJ. Demineralization of human enamel. Scand J Dent Res 1974; 82: 491-5.

27. MacFayden EE, Hilditch TE, Stephen KW, Horton PW, Campell JR. Distribution of fluoride in gingival fluid and dental plaque of dogs. Arch Oral Biol 1979; 24: 427-31.

28. Marquis R, Burne, Parsons DT, Casiano-Colon AE. Arginine deiminase and alkali generation in plaque. In: Bowen WA, Tabac L, eds. Cariology for the nineties. Rochester: University of Rochester Press 1993; 309-17.

29. Matsuo S, Rølla G, Lagerlöf F. Effects of fluoride addition on ionized calcium in salivary sediment and in saliva containing various amounts of solid calcium fluoride. Scand J Dent Res 1990; 98: 482-5.

30. Mercer V, Muhler J. Comparison of a single application of stannous fluoride with a single application of sodium fluoride or two applications of stannous fluoride. J Dent Child 1961; 28: 84-6.

31. Oliveby A, Ekstrand J, Lagerlöf F. Effect of salivary flow rate on salivary fluoride clearance after use of a fluoride-containing chewing gum. Caries Res 1987; 21: 393-401.

32. Oliveby A, Lagerlöf F, Ekstrand J, Dawes C. Studies on fluoride concentration in human submandibular/sublingual saliva and their relation to flow rate and plasma fluoride levels. J Dent Res 1989; 8: 146-9.

33. Oliveby A, Lagerlöf F, Ekstrand J, Dawes C. Studies on fluoride excretion in human whole saliva and its relation to flow rate and plasma fluoride levels. Caries Res 1989; 23: 243-6.

34. Oliveby A, Lagerlöf F, Ekstrand J, Dawes, C. Influence of flow rate, pH and plasma fluoride concentration on fluoride concentration in human parotid saliva. Arch Oral Biol 1989; 34: 191-4.

35. Oliveby A, Twetman S, Ekstrand J. Diurnal fluoride concentration in whole saliva in children living in a high- and a low-fluoride area. Caries Res 1990; 24: 44-7.

36. Oliveby A, Weetman DA, Geddes DAM, Lager-

löf F. The effect of salivary clearance of sucrose and fluoride on human dental plaque acidogenicity. Arch Oral Biol 1990; 35: 907-11.

37. Ophaug RH, Jenkins GN, Singer L, Krebsbach PH. Acid diffusion analysis of different forms of fluoride in human dental plaque. Arch Oral Biol 1987; 32: 459-61.

38. Opperman R, Johansen J. The effect of fluoride and non-fluoride salts of copper, silver and tin on the acidogenicity of dental plaque in vivo. Scand J Dent Res 1980; 88: 476-80.

39. Opperman R, Rølla G, Johansen J, Assev S. Thiol groups and reduced acidogenicity of dental plaque in the presence of metal ions in vivo. Scand J Dent Res 1980; 88: 389-96.

40. Rølla G, Amsbaugh S, Monell-Torrens E, Ellingsen JE, Afseth J, Ciardi J, Bowen W. Effect of topical application of stannous fluoride, stannous chloride and stannous tartrate on rat caries. Scand J Dent Res 1983; 91: 351-5.

41. Rølla G, Bowen W. Concentration of fluoride in plaque – A possible mechanism. Scand J Dent Res 1977; 85: 149-51.

42. Rølla G, Saxegaard E. Critical evaluation of composition and use of topical fluorides with special emphasis on the role of calcium fluoride in caries inhibition. J Dent Res 1990; 69 (Spec Iss): 780-5.

43. Rølla G, Øgaard B, Cruz RA. Fluoride containing toothpastes, their clinical effect and mechanism of cariostatic action – A review. Int Dent J 1991; 41: 171-4.

44. Rølla G, Øgaard B. Reduction in caries incidence in Norway from 1970 to 1984 and some considerations concerning the reason for this phenomenon. In: Frank R, O'Hickey S, eds. Strategy for dental caries prevention in European countries according to their laws and regulations. Oxford: IRL Press 1987: 145-54.

45. Rølla G. Effects of fluoride on initiation of plaque formation. Caries Res. 1977; 11: 243-61.

46. Rølla G, Ellingesen JE, Gaare D. Clinical effects and possible mechanisms of action of stannous fluoride. Int Dent J 1994; 44: 99-105

47. Scheie A, Assev S, Rølla G. The effect of SnF$_2$ and NaF on glucose uptake and metabolism in S. mutans OMZ 176. In: Leach SA, ed. Factors relating to demineralization and remineralization of the teeth. Oxford: IRL Press 1986: 99-104.

48. Singer L, Jarvey BA, Venkateswarlu P, Armstrong WD. Fluoride in plaque. J Dent Res 1970; 49: 455.

49. Skjørland K, Gjermo P, Rølla G. Effect of some polyvalent cations on plaque formation in vivo. Scand J Dent Res 1978; 86: 103-7.

50. Svatun B, Gjermo P, Eriksen H, Rølla G. A comparison of the plaque inhibiting effect of stannous fluoride and chlorhexidine. Acta Odontol Scand 1977; 35: 247-50.

51. Tatevossian A. Fluoride in dental plaque. J Dent Res 1990; 69 (Spec Iss): 645-52.

52. Whitford GM, Pashley DH, Pearson DE. Fluoride in gingival crevicular fluid and a new method for evaporative water loss correction. Caries Res 1981; 15: 399-405.

53. Vogel GL, Ekstrand J. Fluoride in saliva and plaque fluid after a 0.2 % NaF rinse: Short term kinetics and distribution. J Dent Res 1992; 71: 1553-7.

54. Zero D, Van Houte J, Russo J. The intraoral effect on enamel demineralization of extracellular matrix material synthesized from sucrose by streptococcus mutans. J Dent Res 1986; 65: 918-23.

55. Øgaard B, Rølla G, Dijkman T, Ruben J, Arends J. Effect of fluoride mouthrinsing on caries lesions development in shark enamel: an in situ model study. Scand J Dent Res 1991; 99: 372-7.

56. Øgaard B, Seppa L, Rølla G. The relations between oral hygiene and approximal caries in 15 year olds. Caries Res 1994; 4: 297-300.

FLUORIDE EFFECTS ON ORAL BACTERIA

I.R. Hamilton • G.H.W. Bowden

Introduction – Fluoride in dental plaque – Fluoride uptake by oral bacteria
Metabolic effects of fluoride – Fluoride and dental plaque ecology
A model of fluoride effects on plaque ecology

Introduction

Fifty years have passed since the first demonstration of the inhibition of carbohydrate metabolism by low concentrations of fluoride with pure cultures of oral streptococci and lactobacilli (for review see Hamilton[6]). The interest shown by dental researchers in the glycolysis-inhibiting properties of fluoride was natural because of the central role played by the saccharolytic dental plaque microflora in the caries process of acid end-product formation during sugar metabolism. Since that early report, a significant literature has accumulated reporting the effects of fluoride on various biochemical processes carried out by the oral bacteria in or from dental plaque. The current evidence indicates that fluoride has a multitude of direct and indirect effects on the bacterial cell, some of which may have a significant influence on the acid-producing (acidogenic) microorganisms in dental plaque (Table 13-1).

Any discussion of the fluoride effects on oral bacteria in dental plaque must consider the concentrations of F likely to be found in the microbial environment, and the type and properties of the bacteria likely to be most influenced by the inhibitor. In this chapter, we will briefly examine the distribution of fluoride in dental plaque, the uptake of fluoride by oral bacteria, the results of *in vitro* experiments which focus on the mechanisms of fluoride interaction with individual bacteria and, finally, the *in vivo* effects of fluoride and the role of the inhibitor in the ecology of the oral microflora.

Fluoride in dental plaque

The distribution of fluoride in dental plaque has been discussed in Chapter 12; however, it may be useful to reiterate some points in relation to the oral microflora found in plaque. Bacteria in the various individual plaque ecosystems form a complex and highly dense mass (e.g. ~ 10^{11} cells per g wet weight) which receives an intermittent and variable food supply. The pH of each system is governed by the num-

Table 13-1
Some biological effects of fluoride on bacteria

Parameter	Specific effect	
	Direct	**Indirect**
Growth	Energy metabolism	
Colonization	Adherence to tooth	
Macromolecular synthesis	Lipoteichoic acid Peptidoglycan	Glycogen
Glycolysis	Enolase	Phosphotransferase sugar transport system
Transmembrane gradients	H^+/ATPase Dissipates proton gradients Efflux of K^+ and P_i	Dissipates proton gradients Acidification of cytoplasm Dissipates proton gradients
Other enzymes	Acid phosphatase Pyrophosphatase Pyrophosphorylase Peroxidase Catalase	

ber and types of bacteria, the nutrient intake, as well as the flow rate and composition of saliva. Some habitats, such as fissures and carious lesions, occasionally have pH values as low as 4.0 following active glycolysis, while smooth tooth surfaces may be exposed to pH values above 8.0 during periods of sleep when saliva flow is minimal and plaque bacteria degrade protein to alkaline end-products.

The concentration of fluoride in dental plaque is known to vary with the fluoride content of water and dietary constituents, the amount of plaque, the pH of the environment and the fluoride content of enamel. With the introduction of the fluoride electrode, the estimates of the total plaque fluoride concentration have decreased 2-5-fold compared with those from earlier colorimetric analyses. Values for total plaque fluoride obtained by hot acid extraction procedures in independent studies vary considerably, but usually range from 5-10 mg F/kg wet weight of plaque in low fluoride areas to higher values (10-20 mg/kg) in areas with fluoridated water.[43]

Earlier descriptions of the fluoride distribution in dental plaque suggested three compartments – free fluoride ion (F^-), ionizable (loosely bound) fluoride and tightly-bound fluoride, based on the extraction procedures employed.[15,25,43] More recent estimates suggest only two compartments, one consisting of free fluoride ion representing less than 5% of the total F and a second major fraction (95%) extracted by cold perchloric acid and considered to be "bound" fluoride.[43] The extreme reactivity of fluoride ensures that it will bind to a variety of biologically active molecules, such as charged matrix proteins, cytoplasmic enzymes,[25,26] cell membranes and cell wall components,[55] with the interactions likely to be electrostatic in nature and not involving covalent bonding.

As a consequence of this reactivity, fluoride can be found both inside and outside the bacterial cells in dental plaque. For example, fluoride is known to be transported into the bacterial cell, with 90% appearing in the cytoplasm, the majority in a bound state.[26] In addition to intracellular fluoride, the inhibitor has also been observed external to bacterial cells in the plaque matrix and much of this extracellular F may be calcium fluoride, particularly after the application of high concentrations of fluoride.[37] Extracellular plaque calcium fluoride is believed to be stabilized by inorganic phosphate and matrix protein, with fluoride released during periods of low pH. Clearly, F in the form of calcium fluoride would be retained in plaque and would be more substantive than free F or fluoride in other salt forms, such as NaF.

Fluoride uptake by oral bacteria

Any discussion of fluoride uptake by bacteria must take into consideration the various forms of F in solution, the composition and physiologic status of the various plaque bacteria and the immediate environment occupied by the microflora. For example, plaque pH is a major factor and, therefore, the flow rate and buffering capacity of saliva, the carbohydrate content of the diet and the caries status of the individual will have an influence on F activity. In solution, fluoride is a relatively weak acid and can be found as F ion (F^-), HF and HF_2^-, although HF_2^- is of no significance above pH 4. The dissociation of HF to H^+ and F^- has a pK_a of 3.45 and, consequently, at plaque pH levels above 5.0, more than 98% of the free fluoride will be ionized with only 1.4% present as HF. At pH 4.0, 12% of the fluoride will be in the HF form, with this increasing as the pH decreases. Thus, we can see that, although the plaque pH can vary, the vast majority of the fluoride present will be F^- and it is this form that will be involved in binding the various plaque components.

As fluoride is extremely reactive, F binding undoubtedly occurs by electrostatic interaction and this will be relatively random and nonspecific. Studies employing ^{18}F have examined binding by various oral bacteria[53] and differences have been observed between different organisms. In addition, ^{18}F has been employed to show differences in binding to cell walls and membranes of various strains of *Streptococcus mutans* and *Actinomyces viscosus*.[8] In spite of the observed differences in F binding, this information does not correlate with the inherent F resistance of oral bacteria (Table 13-2). For example, ^{18}F binding to the oral streptococci is approximately equal to that for lactobacilli[53] and yet growth and metabolism of the latter bacteria is 10-50-fold less sensitive to fluoride than the streptococci. This should not be unexpected since F will react with a host of positively charged cations and macromolecules in cells, and most of these interactions will not affect the active sites of enzymes. Thus, observed differences in the F sensitivity of the various bacteria seen in Table 13-2 must be related to the physiologic character of the individual species.

There is general agreement that fluoride interacts with the bacterial cell rapidly and in a pH-dependent fashion, a fact that has been verified many times in the past 40 years. Early work with *Streptococcus sanguis* showed that F uptake was concentrative (i.e. occurs against a concentration gradient) such that cells incubated at pH 5.5 with 1 μg F/mL (1 ppm) accumulated up to six times as much intracellular F as the external medium.[25] This and subsequent

Table 13-2
Minimum concentration of fluoride necessary to overcome the inherent fluoride resistance of some oral bacteria[a]

Organism	No. of strains	Concentration of F (µg/ml) at pH		
		7.0	6.5	5.5
Fusobacterium sp	2	115	_b	–
Streptococcus sp				
S. mitis	1	115	–	–
S. mutans	1	> 135	135	20
	50	–	20-50	5-10
S. 'mitior'	35	–	10-80	–
S. sanguis	1	230,	–	–
	3	–	10-30	–
Veillonella sp	8	200	200	–
Prevotella sp				
P. intermedia	1	230	–	–
P. melaninogenica	1	230	–	–
Actinomyces sp				
A viscosus[c]	9	60-200	–	–
A. naeslundii genosp. 1	2	930	–	–
A. odontolyticus	1	930	–	–
Lactobacillus sp				
L. casei	5	2900-6000	–	–
	3	–	–	300
L. brevis	3	–	–	120

[a] Data derived form Refs. 7-11 and unpublished observations.
[b] No data
[c] Now reclassified to Actinomyces naeslundii genospecies 2.

work by various laboratories[21,35,51,53,54] has shown that F uptake occurs in the absence of an energy source, in the presence of metabolic inhibitors, at a wide range of temperatures, under aerobic and anaerobic conditions and is stimulated by Ca^{2+}. In addition, fluoride is taken up by F-resistant as well as by F-sensitive strains of oral streptococci, indicating that the resistance does not result in the exclusion of the inhibitor from the cell.[24]

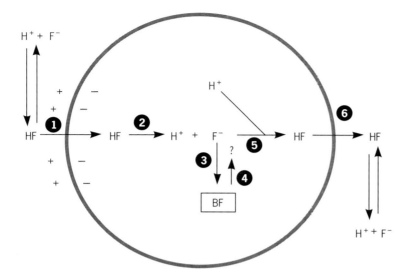

Fig. 13-1. Fluoride accumulation, distribution and efflux from bacterial cells.

Pertinent to our understanding of fluoride uptake into bacterial cells are the observations that F accumulation does not involve an energy-dependent active transport process and that uptake increases as the external pH decreases. This latter observation suggests that F uptake has characteristics typical of weak acid permeation into cells, with HF as the permeant form (Fig. 13-1, reaction 1). During carbohydrate metabolism, when the external pH is decreasing due to the formation of acid end-products, acidogenic oral bacteria, such as the streptococci, naturally attempt to maintain the intracellular pH above that in the external environment.[17] As a consequence, the difference between the intracellular pH (pH_i) and the external pH (pH_e), or the pH gradient (i.e. $\Delta pH = pH_i - pH_e$), will increase as the pH_e is decreased. Thus, more F will accumulate in the cell at low pH values when the ΔpH is large than at neutral pH when the ΔpH is small. This important relationship is the basis for the well-known pH-fluoride effect.[1] Inherently fluoride-resistant organisms, such as Lactobacillus casei,

avoid the inhibiting effects of F by maintaining a negligible ΔpH until the external pH is near 5.0, while F-sensitive bacteria, such as S. mutans, generate increasing pH gradients as the pH decreases from 7.0.[20]

The entry of HF into the more alkaline cytoplasmic compartment of the cell results in its dissociation to H^+ and F^- (Fig. 13-1, reaction 2). This uptake will continue until the HF concentrations in the external and internal compartments are equal and equilibrium is reached. At this point, $\Delta pH = 0$. The intracellular dissociation of HF has two separate and major effects on the physiology of the cell. The first is the release of F^- to interact with cellular constituents, including various F-sensitive enzymes (Table 13-1), causing inhibition of enzyme activity. One assumes that the F responsible for enzyme inhibition is part of the bound-F pool (Fig. 13-1, reaction 3), which constitutes the vast majority (> 95%) of the cellular fluoride.

The second major effect of HF dissociation in the cell is the release of protons (H^+), resulting in the acidification of the cytoplasmic compartment. Normally, protons are pumped from the cell by the membrane, proton-extruding AT-Pase (H^+/ATPase) and via acid end-product efflux; however, as we will see later, fluoride interferes with these processes. Consequently, the decrease in the cellular pH resulting from HF influx will make the cytoplasm a less favorable environment for the activity of many of the essential enzymes required for growth. Acidification of the cytoplasmic compartment is now recognized as a significant factor in the fluoride inhibition of growth and metabolism.

Another consequence of cytoplasmic acidification will be the efflux of fluoride from the cell as HF once the intracellular pH has reached a point where internal HF concentration exceeds the external level (Fig. 13-1, reaction 5). In addition to the internal pH, this will also depend on the availability of free F^- in the cell. Since F efflux from the cell has been observed experimentally to occur very rapidly, one assumes that the intracellular pH is an important factor in the generation of F^- from the bound cellular form.[32,50,51]

Many of the studies showing the direct relationship between fluoride uptake and the magnitude of transmembrane pH gradients have been carried out with *S. mutans* and it has been possible to demonstrate intracellular F concentrations 5-12-fold higher than that of the external medium depending on the experimental conditions.[24,50,51] With *S. mutans* in acidic environments (i.e. below pH 5.8), fluoride is transported in and out of the cell rapidly. Since the ΔpH in acidic environments is large, significant amounts of HF are transported into the cell, leading to rapid acidification of the cytoplasmic compartment and this is normally followed by the slow efflux of F from the cell. This process may only happen in cells in buffer and not in growing cells since there is evidence that cells grown with fluoride take it up and retain it more readily than cells grown without fluoride and subsequently exposed to it.[15] This may be related to the fact that F is sequestered in the bound fraction in the cell. However, this fraction is normally saturated at low levels of external fluoride and it is conceivable that only the ionizable F fraction is involved in the efflux of fluoride ion.

Experimental evidence has been obtained for the fluoride-associated dissipation of the pH gradient in oral streptococci.[23,50] These studies have also shown that fluoride-resistant cells take up more fluoride than fluoride-sensitive cells and are able to maintain a high ΔpH and intracellular fluoride levels with relatively minor inhibition of glycolysis.

The concept of HF as the permeable form of fluoride has been disputed by some workers. It has been suggested that a significant uptake of fluoride is not necessary for inhibition since cells incubated in buffer at pH 5.0 in the presence of 10 μg F/mL and readjusted to pH 7.0 were as active as control cells not exposed to fluoride at low pH.[15] Cited as further evidence for this view were results of experiments with *S. sanguis*, which showed that the fluoride content of resting cells at pH 5.5 was only slightly higher than that in pH 7.0 cells, while cells of the organism made permeable by freezing-thawing were no more sensitive to fluoride at neutral pH than undamaged cells.

There are plausible reasons for suggesting that fluoride may interact with external elements of cells to inhibit cellular metabolism. However, the above findings do not necessarily exclude HF uptake because of the nature of pH gradients in oral bacteria. Oral streptococci do not maintain large ΔpH values near neutrality and the preparation of resting cells by washing with buffer dissipates established pH gradients.[17] Consequently, since fluoride uptake requires a pH gradient, the adjustment of the pH of cell suspensions from 5.0 to 7.0 will result in a loss of ΔpH with the resultant extrusion of fluoride from the cells as HF. Permeabilization of cells would also destroy the pH gradient, effectively reducing fluoride uptake, while resting cells incubated at pH 5.5 would be expected

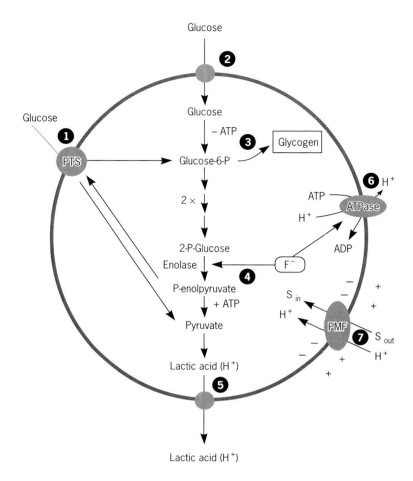

Fig. 13-2. Essential reactions involved in carbohydrate metabolism by acidogenic oral bacteria: (1) sugar transport via the P-enolpyruvate (PEP) phosphotransferase system (PTS), (2) an ATP-dependent sugar transport system, (3) glycogen-synthesizing pathway, (4) enolase, (5) lactic acid (H$^+$) efflux, (6) proton-extruding ATPase, and (7) solute transport in symport with protons driven by proton motive force (PMF).

to have a low ΔpH value unless high concentrations of K$^+$ ions and an energy source were present.

Thus, a summary of the evidence would suggest that under conditions of active carbohydrate metabolism, where pH values will routinely range from pH 7.0 to below 5.0, fluoride will be taken up by dental plaque as HF and, upon entry into the more alkaline cytoplasmic compartment, will dissociate into F$^-$ and H$^+$. The protons will acidify the cytoplasm, reducing the ΔpH, while fluoride would be available for interaction with cellular cations and macromolecules to inhibit cellular processes.

Metabolic effects of fluoride

Glycolytic pathway

The major and long-established target for fluoride in the bacterial cell is the metalloenzyme, enolase, which converts 2-P-glycerate (2PGA) to P-enolpyruvate (PEP) in the glycolytic pathway (Fig. 13-2, reaction 4). Enolase requires Mg^{2+} ions for activity and fluoride: Mg^{2+} complexed, probably in association with phosphate, removes Mg^{2+} ion from the catalytic site, thereby inhibiting enzyme activity. While much of the early historic work on enolase was

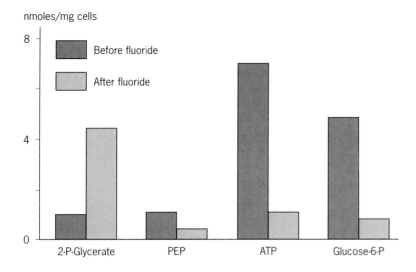

nmoles/mg cells

Fig. 13-3. Effect of the addition of NaF (2.4 mmol/L) on the intracellular concentration of 2-P-glycerate, P-enolpyruvate (PEP), ATP and glucose-6-P in intact cells of *Streptococcus salivarius* metabolizing glucose.[5,22]

carried out with cell-free enzyme preparations, direct evidence for the inhibitory action of F on the enzyme has been demonstrated *in vivo* with intact oral streptococci.[5,7] Washed cells of *S. salivarius* and *S. mutans* metabolizing glucose at pH 7.2 were exposed to 2.4 mM fluoride and then extracted with perchloric acid before and after the addition of the inhibitor. Analysis of various glycolytic intermediates revealed that the addition of F resulted in the rapid increase in the intracellular concentration of 2PGA and a reduction in the level of PEP (Fig. 13-3). Such effects were observed to a lesser degree at F concentrations as low as 60 µM fluoride.[22] The immediate accumulation of the substrate of the enolase reaction, 2PGA, upon the addition of fluoride and a decrease in the product, PEP, provides unequivocal evidence for the F sensitivity of the enzyme in acidogenic oral bacteria. In addition, Fig. 13-3 clearly demonstrates that cellular ATP was also reduced significantly by the addition of fluoride, reflecting, in part, the reduced flow of PEP to pyruvate by pyruvate kinase. Thus, F influences not only the formation of PEP, but also the generation of the key metabolite, ATP, which is central to cell maintenance and growth.

The same effects on 2-PGA, PEP were seen with cells metabolizing glucose at a lower pH value (i.e. 5.8) except that the same inhibition could be observed at lower F concentrations. More recent studies reveal that cells of *S. mutans* metabolizing glucose at pH 5.5 will require 10-12-fold less F to achieve complete inhibition than cells incubated at pH 7.0. For example, glucose metabolism by chemostat-grown cells incubated in a pH stat at pH 7.0 were completely inhibited by 10 mM NaF, while the same cells incubated at pH 5.5 required only 0.8 mM NaF for the same results.[19] Inhibition of growth exhibits similar F/pH effects. Thus, acidogenic oral bacteria metabolizing sugar in the presence of fluoride will become progressively more inhibited as the pH declines in what can be viewed as a "self-regulating process".

Sugar transport

The study with *S. salivarius* and *S. mutans* depicted in Fig. 13-3 revealed that the formation of the first intermediate of the glycolytic pathway, glucose-6-P, was immediately and rapidly inhibited by fluoride indicating an effect on glucose transport.[5] Oral streptococci and other acidogenic oral bacteria transport glucose via the P-enolpyruvate phosphotransferase system (PTS), resulting in the formation of intracellular glucose-6-P (equation 1).

Glucose + PEP -----> Glucose-6-P + Pyruvate (1)

This transport process, also responsible for the uptake of other "PTS sugars", is actually a phosphoryl-cascade system transferring phosphate from PEP to the incoming sugar (Fig. 13-2, reaction 1) via two nonspecific, cytoplasmic proteins, Enzyme I and HPr, and a sugar-specific, membrane component, Enzyme II, often associated with a sugar-specific Enzyme III.

As shown in Fig. 13-3, the addition of fluoride to cells of *S. salivarius* metabolizing glucose resulted in a severe reduction in the formation of glucose-6-P. The glucose-PTS was itself unaffected by fluoride since the PEP-dependent phosphorylation of glucose by permeabilized cells was not inhibited by the inhibitor. Clearly, the inhibition of glucose-6-P formation was due to a reduction in the availability of the phosphoryl donor, PEP, the product of the fluoride-inhibited enolase reaction.

Proton-extruding ATPases
An important physiological parameter for acidogenic oral bacteria is the maintenance of intracellular pH homeostasis during metabolism that generates extracellular acids. Cellular enzymes usually function within a narrow pH range and acidification of the cytoplasm would severely reduce the metabolic activity necessary for maintenance and growth. With oral streptococci, the cytoplasmic pH is maintained above the external medium by pumping protons out of the cell by two mechanisms: via a membrane-associated, proton-extruding ATPase (H$^+$/ATPase), energized by ATP hydrolysis (Fig. 13-2, reaction 6), and by acid end-product efflux (Fig. 13-2, reaction 5). The efflux of protons by this latter mechanism would be de-

pendent on the internal/external ratio of the acid end-product, however, considerable cellular energy would be conserved by this process. This system appears to function only for the efflux of lactic acid in the streptococci and not for the other major acid end-products derived from sugar metabolism, such as acetic, formic, propionic and succinic acids.

Proton extrusion by either of these processes immediately creates a pH difference (ΔpH) between the cytoplasm and the external medium, as well as an electrical difference or $\Delta\Psi$. The potential energy in these gradients, known as the transmembrane proton electrochemical gradient, or proton motive force (PMF), can be utilized to do biologic work, such as ATP synthesis, flagellar motion and solute transport. The driving force for such work is the movement of protons (H+) down the concentration gradient from the high external compartment to the lower internal compartment. This re-entry of H$^+$ into the cell completes the proton circuit and this will rapidly result in equilibrium (i.e. Δp = 0) unless protons are continually pumped out of the cell.

Relatively little is known about the H$^+$/ATPase in oral bacteria, however, research has shown that this enzyme is important in the maintenance of acid tolerance by oral bacteria, allowing aciduric bacteria, such as *S. mutans*, to metabolize carbohydrate at low pH values on the tooth surface.[18] The H$^+$/ATPase in oral bacteria is inhibited by fluoride[42] and, as a consequence, the maintenance of cellular pH homeostasis will be compromised, particularly at low pH. This disruption of intracellular pH regulation is a significant factor in the antimicrobial effect of fluoride and illustrates its multiple effects on cell physiology. The H$^+$ released on entry of HF in the cell will acidify the cytoplasm because of the reduced capacity to extrude protons via the H$^+$/ATPase due to fluoride inhibition. Furthermore, the F inhibition of the glycolytic pathway results in less ATP for the H$^+$/ATPase reaction (Table 13-2), as well as fewer acid end-products that can participate in proton efflux.

The H^+/ATPase in isolated membranes of *S. mutans* was originally shown to be more sensitive to fluoride than that of *L. casei*, with 3 mM fluoride being required to inhibit the initial rate of ATP hydrolysis by 50% compared with 25 mM for the latter organism.[42] Inhibition was reversible at low F levels, but non-reversible at high fluoride concentrations with the F interacting directly with the membrane-associated F_1F_0 holoenzyme. More recent results[41] have indicated that F inhibition is dependent on aluminum through A1:F complexes, the previously observed differences in sensitivity between the two organisms being due to differences in the levels of aluminum.

One factor that will ameliorate the F effect at low pH is the ability of oral bacteria to adapt to acidurance. Oral streptococci grown in a low pH (< pH 6.0) environment for prolonged periods exhibit altered cellular physiology, such that the pH optimum for sugar transport and glycolysis is reduced and the cells are also less permeable to protons.[18] Notably, the glycolytic rate increases in such environments, thereby increasing ATP formation and carbon flow to metabolic end-products. This is also associated with an increase in the specific activity of H^+/ATPase as the pH decreases. Thus, adapted cells have an increased capacity for proton pumping which tends to compensate for the inhibiting properties of fluoride at low pH.

Proton motive force

A variety of metabolic processes in bacteria are driven by the potential energy in transmembrane proton electrochemical gradients. One important function of the pH and electrical gradients that make up PMF is to drive solute transport, particularly sugar and amino acid uptake. Oral streptococci are known to generate proton motive force during growth and metabolism, although the maximum energy derived is normally less than in other bacteria, rarely exceeding 150 mV.[23] This is due in large measure to the small ΔpH values generated by these bacteria with gradients of less than one pH unit (59 mV) even during metabolism at pH values as low as 5.5. As predicted from our previous discussion, fluoride dissipates pH gradients in cells at most pH values and will also reduce $\Delta\Psi$ in cells exposed to low pH. Thus, the addition of fluoride to bacteria will dissipate proton motive force and disrupt those processes depending on this energy.

Early studies with *S. mutans* indicated that, in addition to the PEP phosphotransferase sugar transport system, glucose could be transported by a secondary non-PTS process under conditions of low pH, high glucose concentrations and high growth rates.[6] Cells grown under these conditions were sensitive to proton ionophores, suggesting that the non-PTS system was coupled to proton motive force probably via a symport process coupling glucose uptake with proton movement into the cell. However, subsequent results with *S. mutans* have shown that 6-deoxyglucose, a non-PTS glucose analog, was not taken up in response to artificially generated pH and electric gradients, indicating that secondary transport is not linked to the proton motive force. More recent information suggests that the non-PTS transport system in *S. mutans* is ATP dependent and would be inhibited by fluoride through the reduction in the supply of ATP via the glycolytic pathway (Fig. 13-2, reaction 2).

Although limited information is available on other solute processes in oral bacteria, amino acids are known to be transported by PMF-linked transport mechanisms (Fig. 13-2, reaction 7). Recent studies[14] with *S. mutans* Ingbritt have suggested that the branched-chain amino acids, leucine, valine and isoleucine, are transported via a PMF driven, carrier-mediated process with a proton:substrate stoichiometry of 1. Such processes are undoubtedly widespread among oral bacteria and these transport systems would be sensitive to fluoride because the proton gradients that drive transport would be dissipated.

Macromolecular synthesis

Surprisingly little is known about the specific effects of fluoride on the biosynthesis of macromolecules in bacterial cells, particularly those related to protein synthesis and cell division. Generally, high concentrations of fluoride are required to inhibit growth, with values approximating 200 mg F/kg cells being required for 50% inhibition of growth.[52] It is difficult to separate the known inhibitory effects of fluoride on energy metabolism from the reactions involved in biosynthesis. Fluoride at concentrations as low as 1-2 mM is known to inhibit exogenous glycerol uptake into lipoteichoic acid by *S. mutans* BHT, whereas amino acid incorporation into cellular protein per mg of cells was not affected by 10 mM NaF, despite significant decreases in cell yield (43%). Lipoteichoic acid is believed to play a role in membrane stability, in the regulation of the flow of cations across the membrane and in the colonization of *S. mutans* on hydroxyapatite. Fluoride has also been shown to increase peptidoglycan turnover in strains of *Streptococcus, Bacillus* and *Neisseria,* which results in a reduced level of this macromolecule in the cells. In cells with highly active autolytic systems, such as *Neisseria* and *Bacillus*, this reduction can result in cell lysis. *S. mutans* and *S. sanguis* show only sporadic or partial lysis in fluoride-containing media.

Probably the most studied effect of fluoride on synthesis is in relation to the intra- and extracellular carbohydrate polymers synthesized by the oral streptococci. The intracellular polysaccharide of the oral streptococci has a glycogen-like structure and is synthesized to varying degrees by most species. Oral bacteria synthesize glycogen to act as an energy source during periods when the exogenous energy source is depleted (i.e. between meals). The slow degradation of glycogen results in the formation of low concentrations of lactate, acetate, formate and ethanol for prolonged periods, creating an acidic environment in dental plaque long after any exogenous dietary sugar source has disappeared. Theoretically, this could contribute to the demineralization of enamel should the plaque pH be in the "critical region".

Early experiments with *S. salivarius* demonstrated that glycogen synthesis was completely inhibited immediately following the addition of relatively low levels of fluoride.[5] On the other hand, the degradation of glycogen by the same cells in the absence of exogenous glucose occurred at an appreciable rate at concentrations of fluoride 15 times that capable of inhibiting synthesis completely. Since the enzymes involved in glycogen synthesis are fluoride insensitive,[22] it is apparent that the F effect on glycogen formation was due to the unavailability of glucose-6-P (Fig. 13-2, reaction 3) since ATP synthesis in the glycolytic pathway has priority over glycogen formation.

The synthesis of extracellular polysaccharides (EPS) of the glucan and fructan types by the oral streptococci, and in particular, by *S. mutans* and *S. sanguis*, has received a considerable amount of attention over the past 15 years. These polymers, synthesized during sucrose metabolism, are important in stabilization of oral bacteria in plaque ecosystems. Most of the attention has been directed at glucan (dextran) synthesis by *S. mutans,* which involves a group of membrane-bound glucosyl transferases. Two groups of glucans have been recognized, water-soluble glucans with a predominantly α 1-6 backbone and an insoluble glucan (mutan) with a high concentration of α 1-3 linkages. The latter polymer has high affinity for protein and hydroxyapatite and is particularly resistant to microbial degradation. The extracellular fructan (levan) polymer synthesized by fructosyltransferase from sucrose is readily degraded by plaque bacteria.

A variety of studies have been undertaken to determine whether fluoride has an influence on glycosyltranferase activity and synthesis. Currently, there seems to be a general agreement that EPS formation by the oral streptococci is not fluoride sensitive. In fact, few enzymes involved in direct sucrose metabolism appear to be fluoride sensitive. Of these enzymes, both fructosyl- and glucosyltransferase appear to be particularly fluoride resistant, although studies with *S. mutans* have shown increases in the fructan to glucan ratio in the EPS formed in the presence of fluoride. Partially purified glucosyltransferase from *S. mutans* 6715 was unaffected by 500 μg/M NaF.[38] Furthermore, studies with plaque samples showed that NaF did not block sucrose-mediated extracellular polysaccharide formation at concentrations as high as 300 μg/mL NaF, indicating that all of the plaque enzymes involved in EPS formation were fluoride insensitive. High concentrations of NaF (500 μg/mL) were also shown to have no influence on the sucrose-dependent adherence of *S. mutans* to glass, nor could this level of fluoride promote desorption of bacteria from such surfaces. Consequently, fluoride would appear to have a negligible effect on sucrose-dependent EPS formation and associated enzyme activity.

Other fluoride effects

Fluoride is known to inhibit metalloenzymes, such as phosphatases, pyrophosphatases and phosphorylases, many of which require magnesium for activity. As a general rule, Mg^{2+}-requiring enzymes are fluoride sensitive, although other cations, as well as pH, will affect the inhibition patterns. For example, alkaline phosphatases are relatively insensitive to fluoride, while acid phosphatases are particularly sensitive. This has some relevance to oral bacteria and it has been suggested that membrane-bound acid phosphatases in *S. mutans* are activated at acid pH to hydrolyze enamel matrix phosphate during demineralization.[31] This re-

sults in the uptake of enamel phosphate by those bacteria colonizing the enamel surface. The addition of fluoride would inhibit phosphatase activity and result in phosphate efflux from the cells where it would be incorporated into enamel during remineralization.

Fluoride and plaque metabolism

The previous discussion has highlighted the multiple inhibitory effects of fluoride on carbohydrate metabolism by pure cultures of oral bacteria from *in vitro* experiments. The key question naturally arises as to whether the bound intracellular and extracellular fluoride that is present in dental plaque can be released and whether the released F is available at a concentration high enough to inhibit bacterial function. Considerable controversy surrounds this topic with various researchers on both sides of the question. It is perhaps useful to quote the summary[16] of a recent International Conference on Fluorides on the role of F in dental plaque: "The role fluoride plays in cariostasis by affecting plaque metabolism has been overshadowed in recent years by studies of its influence on remineralization and demineralization; nevertheless, the plausibility that the anticaries effect of fluoride is biological is clear".

A review of the data by Tatevossian[43] has suggested that plaque would contain 5-10 mg total F/kg wet cells in areas with low fluoride concentrations in the drinking water and somewhat higher values from individuals receiving water containing 1 μg F/mL (1 ppm). Comparing these values with the concentrations producing certain physiological effects in oral streptococci, it is clear that complete inhibition of carbohydrate metabolism will not occur *in vivo*. For example, complete inhibition of metabolism by *S. salivarius* at pH 7.2 occurs at 2.4 mM NaF with 10 mg dry weight of cells per mL, or an equivalent of 680 mg F/kg wet weight.[5] Even calculations invoking the increased effectiveness of F at pH 5.5 (i.e. 10-

12-fold less F required for the same effect) would reduce the value to only 56-68 mg/kg. However, partial inhibition of metabolism has been observed at NaF concentrations at low as 0.06 mM with washed cells of *S. salivarius* incubated at pH 7.2. This is the equivalent of 17 mg F/kg wet weight of cells, which is at the upper level of those plaque samples from individuals exposed to 1 µg F/mL. However, extrapolation of the F effect to pH 5.5 would suggest that the same degree of inhibition would occur at 1.4-1.7 mg F/kg wet weight of cells, well within the suggested range for plaque fluoride. This suggests that as the plaque pH falls during metabolism, there would be sufficient fluoride to bring about an inhibition in the rate of acid formation. The fluoride effect would be small, but perhaps sufficient to have an anti-caries effect.

Fluoride and dental plaque ecology

The previous sections have clearly defined the variety of fluoride effects on oral bacteria. It is apparent that the significant question in relation to fluoride, bacteria, and caries is whether the effects seen *in vitro* occur *in vivo* and contribute to the anticaries activity of fluoride. Examination of the microbial ecology of dental plaque has provided useful insights into its development and the etiology of dental caries.[3] Fluoride is one of many environmental factors that will influence plaque ecology and the following sections will examine the potential of this aspect of fluoride.

Dental plaque is a bacterial biofilm community comprising a wide variety of genera, species and varieties of organisms.[4] As a biofilm it follows a series of stages during its development to a point where its composition is relatively stable and in balance with the local environment. The major phases of development are:

- Adsorption and adherence of bacterial cells to the tooth pellicle
- Growth of the adherent cells and competition among different bacterial populations, and
- Stability of the biofilm community.[29]

Throughout its development, dental plaque is subjected to a variety of factors governing its composition, including nutrients, immune mechanisms, environmental pH and ecosystem-generated antibacterial compounds. The changes in plaque that result from the influences of such factors may be very subtle and difficult to detect.

Fluoride, which is accepted as one of the most effective prophylactic agents against caries, is commonly present in the environment of plaque. As mentioned previously, attempts have been made to explain the anticaries activity of fluoride from numerous *in vitro* studies, including models of cell adherence and biofilm formation in addition to the metabolic effects already discussed. Very often these *in vitro* findings have been the basis of hypotheses of an anti-plaque activity by fluoride *in vivo*. However, it has proved difficult to correlate *in vitro* findings with the predicted activity *in vivo*.

Effects on biofilms

Cell adsorption and adherence
Few studies have dealt with the effect of fluoride on the earliest (1-2 hours) adherence of bacterial cells to tooth enamel. Generally, *in vitro* and *in vivo* data are available for the numbers and types of bacteria accumulating in the presence of fluoride after several hours (5-48 hours), which includes time for cell growth.[29] Some *in vitro* studies have shown that fluoride can affect the adhesion of bacterial cells in buffer to glass,[40] while others suggest that fluoride

Table 13-3

Numbers of cells of *Streptococcus mutans* accumulating on epon-hydroxyapatite (HA) and epon-fluorapatite (FHA) surface in a chemostat model[a]

Nutrient limitation and culture pH	Time of biofilm accumulation in hours							
	1.0		2.0		3.0		4.0	
	HA	FHA	HA	FHA	HA	FHA	HA	FHA
Glucose limitation								
pH 7.0	0.88[b]	0.88	1.02	1.06	1.19	1.22	1.64	1.55
pH 5.5	0.80	0.78	0.93	0.89	1.05	0.99	1.37	1.26
Nitrogen limitation[c]								
pH 7.0	1.21	1.09	2.34	2.31	3.24	3.61	4.02	3.94
pH 5.5	1.05	1.01	1.69	1.33	2.45	1.76	3.14	1.98

a Data from ref.[30]

b Cell numbers/area = $1 \times 10^6/cm^2$.

c Culture is in excess with respect to glucose.

does not affect adhesion.[38] It is also possible that fluoride may affect early adhesion *in vivo* by modifying the selective deposition of salivary macromolecules on enamel.[36] More recently, a biofilm model[29] has been used to measure the effects of fluoride liberated from the substratum on the development of associated biofilms of single species of oral bacteria.[30] The numbers of cells of *S. mutans* BM 71 accumulating on epon-hydroxyapatite (HA) and fluoride-treated, epon-fluorapatite rods (FHA) during the early stages of biofilm formation are shown in Table 13-3. It can be seen that after 1 hour, which is during the stage of adherence, there was no significant difference between cell accumulation on HA or FHA at an environmental pH of 7.0 or 5.5, although the acid environment reduced adherence at 2 hours. Taken overall, it seems most likely that fluoride *per se* does not influence the initial (0-2 hour) adherence of cells to teeth in any appreciable way

that can be demonstrated through *in vitro* models.

Growth and accumulation

After adherence, cells on the surface begin to divide and extend the biofilm. There is little doubt that cell division accounts for a major increase in biofilms *in vitro*[29] and plaque in humans.[12] However, it is difficult to determine the rate of cell division in the plaque community in humans, although some studies have been done in experimental animals. Hence, studies in humans, which differentiate between an effect of fluoride on the rate of cell division and effects on other aspects of accumulation, such as continuous adherence and coaggregation, have not been done. Therefore, most of the data from studies of plaque development *in vivo* and *in vitro* may record overall accumulation of plaque rather than biofilm cell growth.

In an *in vitro* model of plaque accumulation

on teeth,[40] a reduction occurred in the accumulation of S. mutans on enamel surfaces treated with a 1% fluoride gel and when the environment contained high concentrations (250 µg/mL) of fluoride compared to F-free controls. However, the fluoride effect was not sustained over time and after 5 days there was an equivalent accumulation of S. mutans on test and control teeth.

A statistically significant difference has been found between the growth of biofilm cells of S. mutans on HA or FHA surfaces at pH 5.5 in a medium with excess glucose.[29] Fewer cells were observed on FHA surfaces after 4 hours during the growing phase of cells in the biofilm (Table 13-3). Calculation of the time taken for the number of cells to double on HA surfaces was 1.4 hours compared with 2.5 hours for cells growing on FHA surfaces. As this reduction occurred during the growing stage of the biofilm, these values were close to the mean generation times. In this model system, fluoride did not affect accumulation on the two surfaces in environments at pH 7.0, or when the cultures were in medium with low or limiting glucose (Table 13-3), emphasizing the importance of the carbohydrate concentration and the environmental pH on the fluoride activity.

Models of plaque development with single species have been useful in studying the mechanisms of biofilm formation; however, they do not assess the role of inter-bacterial competition. In plaque in vivo and in mixed-culture model systems,[11] competition between bacterial populations is important in determining the final composition of the bacterial community. Therefore, the direct and indirect influences of fluoride on the outcome of competition between bacterial populations in plaque could play a significant role in its anti-caries activity.

When considering fluoride effects on plaque in vivo, it is important to differentiate between the amount of environmental fluoride that can occur naturally and higher levels that might be applied as a prophylactic measure. Studies by Kilian et al.[27] clearly showed that fluoride treatment of test enamel surfaces with 150 µg/mL fluoride in acetate buffer (pH 4.0), or in vivo rinsing with a 0.2% solution of NaF, did not influence the early development (5 hours) of dental plaque in humans. In addition, no significant differences were detected in the bacterial composition of plaque samples from persons living in areas with high (3-21 µg/mL) or low (0.3 µg/mL) levels of naturally occurring fluoride in the water supply.[28] This suggested that naturally available environmental fluoride, even in relatively high concentrations, was unlikely to affect the bacterial composition of plaque. The application of SnF$_2$ in vivo, however, significantly reduced plaque accumulation. More recently, the bactericidal effects of SnF$_2$ were studied in vivo and it was demonstrated that this compound reduced the numbers of S. mutans in plaque.[39] These results draw attention to the potential significance of the counterion associated with fluoride in control of plaque accumulation in vivo.[33]

Sufficiently high concentrations of NaF (e.g. 250 µg/mL in drinking water or a 1% fluoride gel) will affect the numbers of organisms in plaque in humans and animals.[2] Beighton & McDougall[8] have shown a significant effect of relatively high levels of fluoride (NaF) on the composition of rat plaque. The application of 250 µg/mL fluoride in the drinking water reduced the numbers of S. mutans in rat plaque and increased the numbers of Actinobacillus. Moreover, mixed, batch-culture models supported the suggestion that fluoride in the environment placed S. mutans at a growth disadvantage relative to Actinobacillus, resulting in enriched cultures of the latter organism. The results from the studies above identify the possibility that, rather than causing complete elimination of bacterial populations from plaque, fluoride has the potential to affect the proportions of different bacteria in plaque ecosystems.

Environmental pH and fluoride

It is apparent from the foregoing that the environment associated with dental plaque can influence its bacterial composition and, in turn, plaque composition is related to the metabolic activities of the biofilm community. Thus, there is some degree of homeostasis in plaque, as the community adjusts to changes in the environment with these adjustments involving compositional changes in the proportions of organisms and/or metabolic changes. Clearly, from our previous discussion with respect to the physiology of oral bacteria and their role in the various oral ecosystems, plaque pH is a significant environmental parameter with respect to caries and fluoride.

There is convincing evidence that fluoride reduces acid production by plaque *in vivo*[2] although the duration of the effect varies, depending on the nature of the fluoride application.[45] One significant aspect of control of acid production by fluoride is the potential effect on demineralization of enamel. Studies *in vitro* using pure cultures of *S. mutans* have shown that fluoride can reduce the amount of demineralization by up to 75%.[47] A second important effect of the reduction of plaque acid production is a higher environmental pH, which can influence competition between bacteria in plaque.

Fluoride, pH and bacterial competition

It is possible to relate some compositional changes in bacterial populations in dental plaque to its cariogenicity.[3] If a potentially pathogenic organism like *S. mutans* is so favored by a low environmental pH such that it is able to outgrow and dominate other bacteria in the community, then the area of tooth surface associated with this increase in cells is at risk of demineralization. Studies on the effects of environmental pressure on the proportions of bacterial species in communities *in vitro* have shown that a low environmental pH enhances the competitiveness of aciduric organisms,

such as *S. mutans* and *L. casei*. In particular, an *in vitro* model was used to test the effect of added fluoride on the proportions of bacteria in a defined oral microbial community growing in a chemostat and subjected to acid environments.[11] Fluoride had a significant effect on the composition of the model community through control of the environmental pH, even in the presence of glucose pulses. For example, in the absence of fluoride and pH control, the addition of glucose caused a drop in pH of the culture and *S. mutans*, *L. casei* and *Veillonella dispar* predominated in the chemostat community. However, when fluoride was added to the communities, although the proportions of *L. casei* and *V. dispar* in the community remained high and were unaffected by fluoride, the proportion of *S. mutans* did not increase.

There could be at least two reasons that are not mutually exclusive for this effect of fluoride on *S. mutans*. Firstly, *S. mutans* may have been more sensitive to fluoride than others in the community and unable to take advantage of the glucose available because of metabolic inhibition. The other related possibility is that carbohydrate metabolism was reduced by fluoride and, as a consequence, less acid was produced resulting in a higher final environmental pH. Consequently, the ecologic advantage given to *S. mutans* by its ability to metabolize carbohydrate at low pH was eliminated. It is likely that both reasons contributed to the stabilizing effect of fluoride on the populations of *S. mutans* in the community as the environmental pH decreased. In this instance, changes in the diversity of the community were not seen, as all of the species were present before and after the addition of fluoride. These results are in keeping with the anticaries effects of fluoride and the *in vivo* observations by Kilian *et al.*[27,28] that naturally occurring fluoride does not significantly influence the bacterial composition of plaque. Thus, fluoride in the plaque appears to act by reducing the metabolic activity of acidogenic and aciduric bacteria exposed to carbohydrate, thereby preventing severe decreases in the environmental pH. Maintenance of the plaque pH at higher levels reduces the risks of enamel demineralization and prevents the emergence of aciduric odontopathic bacteria.

Survival of plaque populations

Several reasons can be advanced for the relative stability of plaque composition *in vivo* in the presence of fluoride. The simplest is that the levels of fluoride present or applied to plaque are not sufficiently high for an appropriate period of time to exceed the inherent resistance or bactericidal levels for the organisms. This is so with *Lactobacillus* and *Veillonella* species, which are resistant to high levels of fluoride.[2] Even bacteria which are completely inhibited by low levels of fluoride may persist in the plaque biofilm and grow again once conditions are favorable. An example of this survival was seen in a study of the competition between *S. mutans* and *L. casei* growing together at pH 7.0 in the presence of fluoride in continuous culture.[9] *S. mutans* dominated the culture in the absence of fluoride; however, the addition of 20 mM NaF to the culture resulted in the inhibition of growth and the elimination of *S. mutans* from the fluid phase of the culture. *L. casei* became dominant and this situation continued for 5 days when F-free medium was applied again. Within 2 days, *S. mutans* resumed its dominant role in the culture. The most likely reason for the survival of *S. mutans* in the culture was that cells of this organism survived on the surfaces of the culture vessel as a biofilm.

Another significant survival mechanism available to plaque bacteria is adaptation to normally harmful levels of fluoride. Phenotypic adaptation by oral bacteria to fluoride *in vitro* has been demonstrated on many occasions.[2] Phenotypic adaptation differs from a stable mutation to resistance by microorganisms in that it is not permanent. Bacteria acquiring phenotypic resistance to an agent like fluoride only retain the resistance while the active agent is in the environment. Therefore, organisms which develop phenotypic resistance to fluoride either *in vitro* or *in vivo* lose the characteristic when they are grown in fluoride-free environments. This phenomenon was demonstrated in plaque from xerostomic patients treated with fluoride gels.[13] Strains of *S. mutans* which had developed phenotypic resistance to fluoride lost their resistance after laboratory culture on fluoride-free medium.

One important outcome of phenotypic adaptation to fluoride *in vivo* could be that plaque bacteria resistant to fluoride effects retain or regain their pathogenicity or cariogenicity. There is little evidence that phenotypic adaptation occurs *in vivo* in humans receiving normal levels of fluoride,[10] but plaque from patients on high fluoride concentration regimens for long periods of time may contain strains resistant to relatively high levels of fluoride.[13,40] Thus, although it may be a rare event, high levels of fluoride *in vivo* may trigger phenotypic adaptation to fluoride resistance.

Adaptation to fluoride by *S. mutans* was observed *in vivo* with rats fed fluoride in their diets (20 mg/kg) and drinking water (20 mg/L).[44] In this experiment, the amount of acid in resting plaque and that produced following a 10% sucrose rinse was significantly lower in rats receiving a F-containing diet and drinking water than in F-free control rats. However, acid production by the latter control plaque was severely inhibited when 4 mM fluoride was added to the sucrose rinse, while acid formation by the fluoride-adapted plaque was not inhibited. In spite of these results, it is not clear that the adapted strain would have any ecologic advantage over the non-adapted strain since no difference was observed in the amount of plaque that accumulated on the teeth in the control and F-fed rats.

In another rat study, van Loveren and his coworkers[48] have provided useful data relating to the significance of adaptation to fluoride and the anticaries activity of fluoride. These workers tested the ability of an *in vitro* fluoride-adapted strain of *S. mutans* and its fluoride-sensitive parent to cause caries in rats. The results showed that fluoride in the drinking water did not influence the numbers of either strain of *S. mutans* in the plaque of the animals. In the absence of fluoride, the adapted strain caused less severe fissure caries lesions than did the parent strain, which supports observations by others that strains adapted to fluoride may be less cariogenic. Analysis of the effect of fluoride on the amount of caries in test and control animals showed no differences. Taken together, the results suggest that adaptation to fluoride by organisms in plaque may reduce its cariogenicity, but that adaptation does not modify the anticaries effects of fluoride *in vivo*.

An *in vitro* plaque model, employing oral streptococci, has been used to study the relationship of adaptation to fluoride resistance and enamel demineralization.[49] The *S. mutans* strains in this study were adapted laboratory strains and recent isolates that were relatively resistant or sensitive to fluoride and included *S. sobrinus* 6715 and fluoride-resistant variants. The results showed that strains resistant to fluoride did not all have the same characteristics in terms of acid production or demineralization. The fluoride-resistant variants of *S. sobrinus* produced less acid than the parent even in the presence of fluoride. In contrast, the *S. mutans* strains resistant to fluoride, including the recent isolates, produced more acid and caused more demineralization than the fluoride-sensitive strains in the presence or absence of fluoride. Thus, it is not possible to make generalizations on the degree of acidogenicity or the potential effects of fluoride on strains adapted to fluoride.

In their most recent study, van Loveren *et al.*[46] examined the ability of a fluoride lacquer to protect enamel against demineralization. Isolates of *S. mutans* and *S. sobrinus* adapted to fluoride and the parental strains were used in the model. The results of this study again showed that strains varied in their characteristics. Although fluoride treatment protected the enamel in all cases, the protection was reduced for fluoride-resistant strains of *S. sobrinus*. In contrast, the protection afforded by fluoride against enamel demineralization was the same for fluoride-resistant strains of *S. mutans* or the parental isolates.

Another possibility for the survival of bacteria in the presence of fluoride is the selection of stable, fluoride-resistant mutants. Relatively stable fluoride-resistant mutants have been generated *in vitro*[2] and Brown *et al.*[13] reported the isolation of only a single stable mutant from humans treated with high levels of fluoride. Thus, the data available suggest that the selection of stable mutants resistant to fluoride *in vivo* is a rare event.

In summary, there is little evidence that exposure of humans to normal prophylactic levels of fluoride (e.g. 1 µg/mL F) in fluoridated-drinking water results in the adaptation of plaque bacteria to fluoride resistance. On the other hand, there is evidence that exposure of plaque bacteria to high levels of fluoride (10 µg/mL NaF gel daily) for prolonged periods does result in a degree of fluoride resistance.[13] Apparently, adaptation to fluoride resistance does not negate any protective effect that fluoride may have against caries and the pressures exerted by fluoride on plaque bacteria *in vivo* very rarely select out or promote stable mutants resistant to fluoride.

A model of fluoride effects on plaque ecology

A possible model for the action of fluoride on plaque ecology is shown in Fig. 13-4. The consumption of high concentrations of refined carbohydrate results in an acidic plaque environment (Fig. 13-4, pathway 2) If this state persists,

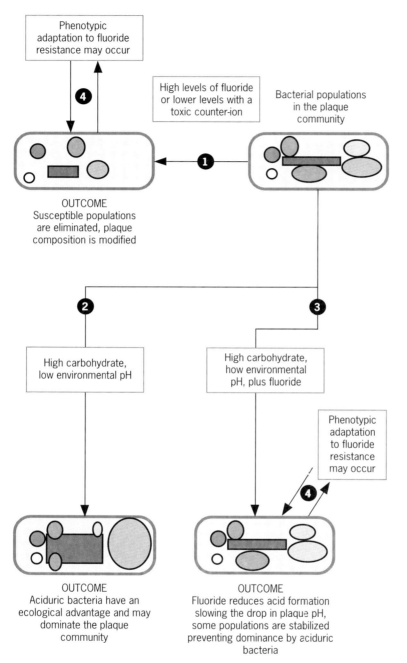

Fig. 13-4. Model for the effects of fluoride on plaque ecology.

the plaque community will be dominated by acidogenic and aciduric bacteria, such as *S. mutans* and lactobacilli, which can result in the demineralization of tooth enamel. Fluoride given in relatively high levels on a continuous basis and fluoride at lower concentrations with a toxic counterion can reduce the numbers of bacteria in plaque (Fig. 13-4, pathway 1).

The application of normal prophylactic levels of fluoride, such as a 0.2% NaF rinse (Fig. 13-4, pathway 3), probably will not modify the early adherence or colonization of tooth pellicle by oral bacteria. However, such concentrations of fluoride can cause demonstrable effects on metabolism and cell division, reducing the growth rate of susceptible cells in biofilms. This latter effect is only apparent in low pH environments, when cells have ample carbohydrate available. A very significant action of fluoride on cell metabolism is the reduction of acid formation by plaque bacteria, which in turn regulates the pH of plaque. Regulation of plaque

pH by subminimal inhibitory concentrations of fluoride is directly related to preventing changes in the proportions of organisms in the bacterial community. Collectively, the effects on cell growth and acid production maintain plaque homeostasis in the presence of carbohydrate, denying an ecologic advantage to acidogenic and aciduric bacteria.

Fluoride does not encourage the selection of stable resistant mutants *in vivo* and, although phenotypic adaptation can occur (Fig. 13-4, pathway 4), it is uncommon under normal conditions. Acquisition of such resistance does not place the adapted cells at an advantage over fluoride-sensitive strains and, by definition, phenotypic resistance is lost in the absence of fluoride in the environment. Bacteria, such as *Lactobacillus*, are naturally resistant to fluoride but do not became dominant in its presence and are apparently controlled by other unknown factors in the environment.

Literature cited

1. Borei H. Inhibition of cellular oxidation by fluoride. Ark Kemi Miner Geol 1945; 20A: 1-215.

2. Bowden GHW. Effects of fluoride on the ecology of dental plaque. J Dent Res 1990; 69 (Spec Iss): 653-9.

3. Bowden GHW. Which bacteria are cariogenic in humans? In: Johnson N, ed. Dental caries markers of high and low risk groups and individuals. Vol 1. Cambridge: Cambridge University Press 1991: 266-86.

4. Bowden GHW, Ellwood DC, Hamilton IR. Microbial ecology of the oral cavity, In: Alexander M, ed. Advances in microbial ecology, Vol 3. New York: Plenum 1979: 135-77.

5. Hamilton IR. Effects of fluoride on enzymatic regulation of bacterial carbohydrate metabolism. Caries Res 1977; 11 (Suppl. 1): 262-91.

6. Hamilton IR. Effects of changing environment on sugar transport and metabolism by oral bacteria. In: Reizer J, Peterkofsky A, eds. Sugar transport and metabolism in Gram-positive bacteria. Chichester: Ellis Horwood 1987: 94-131.

7. Hamilton IR. Biochemical effects of fluoride on oral bacteria. J Dent Res 1990; 69 (Spec Iss): 660-7.

8. Beighton D, McDougall WA. The effects of fluoride on the percentage bacterial composition of dental plaque, on caries incidence and on the *in vitro* growth of *Streptococcus mutans*, *Actinomyces viscosus and Actinobacillus sp*. J Dent Res 1977; 56: 1185-91.

9. Bowden GHW, Hamilton IR. Competition between *Streptococcus mutans* and *Lactobacillus casei* in mixed continuous culture. Oral Microbiol Immun 1989; 4: 57-4.

10. Bowden GHW, Odlum O, Nolette N, Hamilton IR. Microbial populations growing in the presence of fluoride at low pH isolated from dental plaque of children living in an area with fluoridated water. Infect Immun 1982; 36: 247-54.

11. Bradshaw DJ, McKee AS, Marsh PD. Prevention of population shifts in oral microbial communities *in vitro* by low fluoride concentrations. J Dent Res 1990; 69: 436-41.

12. Brecx M, Theilade J, Attstrom R. An ultra-structural quantitative study of the significance of microbial multiplication during early plaque growth. J Periodont Res 1983; 18: 177-86.

13. Brown IR, White JO, Horton IM, Driezen S, Streckfuss JL. Effect of continuous fluoride gel use on plaque fluoride pretention and microbial activity. J Dent Res 1983; 62: 746-51.

14. Dashper SG, Reynolds EC. Branched-chain amino acid transport in *Streptococcus mutans* Ingbritt. Oral Microbiol Immunol 1993; 8: 167-71.

15. Edgar WM, Fluoride metabolism in dental plaque, bacteria and man, In: Ferguson DB, ed. The environment of the teeth. Basel: Karger, 1981; 19-37.

16. Geddes DAM, Bowen WH. Summary of Session III: Fluoride in saliva and dental plaque. J Dent Res 1990; 69 (Spec Iss): 637.

17. Hamilton IR. Growth, metabolism and acid production by *Streptococcus mutans*. In: Hamada S, Michalek SM, Kiyono H, Menaker L, McGhee JR. eds Molecular microbiology and immunobiology of *Streptococcus mutans*. Amsterdam: Elsevier Science Publishers 1986; 145-55.

18. Hamilton IR, Buckley ND. Adaptation of *Streptococcus mutans* to acid tolerance. Oral Microbiol Immunol 1991; 6: 65-71.

19. Hamilton IR, Ellwood DC. Effects of fluoride on carbohydrate metabolism by washed cells of *Streptococcus mutans* grown at various pH values in a chemostat. Infect Immun 1978; 19: 434-42.

20. Hamilton IR, Boyar RM, Bowden GH. Influence of pH and fluoride on the properties of an oral strain of *Lactobacillus casei* grown in continuous culture. Infect Immun 1985; 48: 664-70.

21. Harper DS, Loesche WJ. Inhibition of acid production from oral bacteria by fluorapatite-derived fluoride. J Dent Res 1986; 65: 30-3.

22. Kanapka JA, Khandelwal RL, Hamilton IR. Fluoride inhibition of glucose-6-P formation in *Streptococcus salivarius*: Relation to glyocgen syntheisis and degradation. Arch Biochem Biophys 1971; 144: 596-602.

23. Kashket S, Kashket ER. Dissipation of proton motive force in oral streptococi by fluoride. Infect Immun 1985; 48: 19-22.

24. Kashket S, Preman RJ. Fluoride uptake and fluoride resistance of oral streptococci. J Dent Res 1985; 1290-2.

25. Kashket S, Rodriguez VM. Fluoride accumulation by a strain of human oral *Streptococcus sanguis*. Arch Oral Biol 1976; 21: 459-64.

26. Katayama T, Edgar WM, Jenkins GN, Johnson B. Preliminary fractionation of fluoride-binding constituents of human oral *Streptococcus sanguis*. Arch Oral Biol 1981; 26: 341-42.

27. Kilian M, Larsen MJ, Fejerskov O, Thylstrup A. Effects of fluoride on the initial colonization of teeth *in vivo*. Caries Res 1979; 13: 319-29.

28. Kilian M, Thylstrup A, Fejerskov O. Predominant plaque flora of Tanzanian children exposed to high and low water fluoride concentrations. Caries Res 1979; 13: 330-43.

29. Li YH, Bowden GHW. The accumulation of selected oral gram positive bacteria on mucin conditioned glass surfaces. Oral Microbiol Immunol 1994; 9: 1-11.

30. Li YH, Bowden GHW. The effect of surface fluoride on the accumulation of biofilms of oral bacteria. J Dent Res 1994; 73: 1615-26.

31. Luoma H. Phosphorus translocation between enamel and *Streptococcus mutans* in the presence of sucrose and fluoride with observations on the acid phosphatase of S. mutans. Caries Res 1980; 14: 248-57.

32. Luoma H, Tuompo H. The relationship between sugar metabolism and potassium translocation by caries-inducing streptococci and the inhibitory role of fluoride. Arch Oral Biol 1975; 20: 749-59.

33. Maltz M, Emilson CG. Susceptibility of oral bacteria to various fluoride salts. J Dent Res 1982; 61: 786-90.

34. Mandell RL. Sodium fluoride susceptibilities of suspected periodontopathic bacteria. J Dent Res 1982; 62: 706-8.

35. Mante S, Yotis WW. Fluoride accumulation by

Streptococcus mutans from a low ionic medium. Caries Res 1982; 16: 138-46.

36. Rolla G. Effects of fluoride on initiation of plaque formation. Caries Res 1977; 11 (Suppl 1): 243-61.

37. Rolla G, Saxegaard E. Critical evaluation of the composition and use of topical fluorides, with emphasis on the role of calcium fluoride in caries inhibition. J Dent Res 1990; 69: (Spec Iss): 780-5.

38. Schachtele CF. Effects of fluoride on enzymatic regulation of bacterial carbohydrate metabolism. Discussion. Caries Res 1977; 11 (Suppl 1): 278-87.

39. Schaeken MJM, De Long MH, Franken HCM, Van der Hoeven JS. Effects of highly concentrated stannous fluoride and chlorhexidine regimes on human dental plaque flora. J Dent Res 1986; 65: 57-61.

40. Streckfuss JL, Perkins D, Horton IM, Brown LR, Driezen S, Graves L. Fluoride resistance and adherence of selected strains of *Streptococcus mutans* to smooth surfaces after exposure to fluoride. J Dent Res 1980; 59: 151-8.

41. Sturr MG, Marquis RE. Inhibition of proton-translocating ATPases of *Streptococcus mutans* and *Lactobacillus casei* by fluoride and aluminum. Arch Microbiol 1990; 155: 22-7.

42. Sutton SVW, Bender GR, Marquis RE. Fluoride inhibition of proton-translocating ATPases of oral bacteria. Infect Immun 1986; 55: 2597-603.

43. Tatevossian A. Fluoride in dental plaque and its effects. J Dent Res 1990; 69: (Spec Iss): 645-52.

44. van der Hoeven JS, Franken HC. Effect of fluoride on growth and acid production by *Streptococcus mutans* in dental plaque. Infect Immun 1984; 45: 356-9.

45. van Loveren C. The antimicrobial action of fluoride and its role in caries inhibition. J Dent Res 1990; 69 (Spec Iss): 676-81.

46. van Loveren C, Buijs JF, ten Cate JM. Protective effect of topically applied fluoride in relation to fluoride sensitivity of mutans streptococci. J Dent Res 1993; 72: 1184-90.

47. van Loveren C, Fielmich AM, ten Brink B. Comparison of the effects of fluoride and the ionophore nigericin on acid production by *Streptococcus mutans* and the resulting *in vitro* enamel demineralization. J Dent Res 1987; 66: 1658-62.

48. van Loveren C, Lammens AJ, ten Cate JM. *In vitro* induced fluoride resistance of *Streptococcus mutans* and dental caries in rats. Caries Res 1989; 23: 358-64.

49. van Loveren C, Spitz LM, Buijs JF, ten Cate JM, Eisenberg AD. *In vitro* demineralization of enamel by F-sensitive and F-resistant mutans streptococci in the presence of 0, 0.05 or 0.5 mM/L NaF. J Dent Res 1991; 70: 1491-6.

50. Vicaretti J, Thibodeau E, Bender G, Marquis RE. Reversible uptake and release by *Streptococcus mutans* GS-5 and FA-1. Curr Microbiol 1984; 10: 317-22.

51. Whitford GM, Schuster GS, Pashley HD, Venkateswarlu P. Fluoride uptake by *Streptococcus mutans* 6715. Infect Immun 1977; 18: 680-7.

52. Yoon NA, Berry CW. The antimicrobial effect of fluorides (acidulated phosphate, sodium and stannous) on Actinomyces viscous. J Dent Res 1979; 58: 1824-9.

53. Yost KG, vanDemark PJ. Growth inhibition of *Streptococcus mutans* and *Leuconostoc mesenteroides* by sodium fluoride and ionic tin. Appl Environ Microbiol 1978; 35: 920-4.

54. Yotis WW, Brennan PC. Binding of fluoride by oral bacteria. Caries Res 1983; 17: 444-54.

55. Yotis WW, Mante S, Brennan PC, Kirchner FR, Glendenin LE. Binding of fluorine-18 by the oral bacterium, *Streptococcus mutans*. Arch Oral Biol 1979; 24: 853-60.

56. Yotis WW, Zeb M, McNulty, Kirchner FR, Reilly C, Glendenin LE. Binding of 18F by cell membranes and cell walls of *Streptococcus mutans*. Infect Immun 1983; 41: 375-82.

CHAPTER 14

PHYSICOCHEMICAL ASPECTS OF FLUORIDE-ENAMEL INTERACTIONS

J.M. ten Cate • J.D.B. Featherstone

Introduction – Enamel as a substrate for fluoride – Localization of fluoride in the enamel
Availability of fluoride in the tooth environment: transport and diffusion phenomena
The active role of fluorides in the caries process
Sources, forms and reactions of different types of fluoride – Conclusions

Introduction

This chapter describes the current understanding of the physicochemical mechanisms by which fluoride interacts with enamel during the caries process and during the reversal of the caries process. There have been many schools of thought over the years as to the relative importance of the different ways in which fluoride acts to reduce dental caries. It is now well accepted that two major aspects of fluoride action, and in some opinions the primary mode of action, are the inhibition of demineralization and the enhancement of remineralization. The process of dental decay is very simple in concept but very complicated in detail.

Briefly, the plaque bacteria metabolize fermentable carbohydrates, producing organic acids such as lactic, acetic and propionic acids. These acids can diffuse through the plaque into the enamel and dissolve mineral (calcium, phosphate and fluoride) wherever there is a susceptible site (Fig. 14-1). If this mineral diffuses out of the tooth and into the oral environment, then demineralization occurs. If this process is reversed, the mineral is reabsorbed into the tooth and the damaged crystals are rebuilt, and we then have remineralization. Fluoride acts by inhibiting mineral loss at the crystal surfaces and by enhancing this rebuilding or remineralization of calcium and phosphate in a form more resistant to subsequent acid attack. This overall process is covered in more detail in the following pages.

For many years it was thought that the incorporation of fluoride into the apatite-like enamel crystals during their development was the most important mode of action and that this incorporation of fluoride made the crystal highly resistant to subsequent acid attack during caries after the tooth had erupted. This mode of action is now known to have little importance in comparison with the two processes described above.

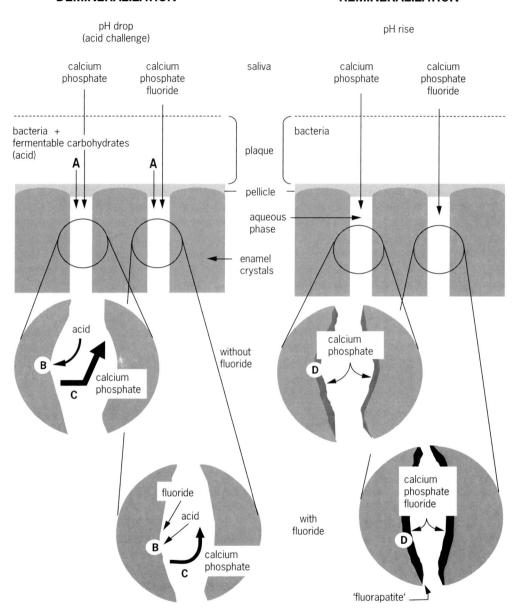

Fig. 14-1. Schematic diagram illustrating demineralization and remineralization of enamel during periods of acid challenge (left) and subsequent pH-rise (right). Steps in the caries process are designated by: A. diffusion into the tooth; B. demineralization at the crystal surface; C. diffusion of mineral components outwards; and D. remineralization at the crystal surface. Saliva serves as a source for calcium and phosphates. The two sets of inserts represent events with and without fluoride.

Table 14-1
Principal inorganic components, including major trace
elements in dental enamel[12]

Component	Range	
Ca	33.6-39.4%	w/w (on dry weight basis)
P	16.1-18.0%	w/w
CO_3	2.7- 5.0%	w/w
Na	4,500-23,600	µg/g (ppm)
Cl	2,500-15,500	µg/g
Mg	1,300- 5,700	µg/g
K	60- 1,000	µg/g
Zn	9- 1,500	µg/g
Si	20- 1,200	µg/g
Sr	10- 1,400	µg/g

Enamel as a substrate for fluoride

The nature of enamel apatite
The various ways in which fluoride interferes with the development of carious defects can all be described in terms of chemical reactions between fluoride and the inorganic component of the mineralized tissues which make up the dentition.

In order to understand those reactions, it is necessary to understand the chemical, histologic and morphologic structure of the mineralized tissues. Such information is available in standard textbooks on oral histology.

Since the majority of studies to date have concentrated on chemical reactions with fluoride and dental enamel, we will restrict ourselves to this tissue. The same principles, however, apply to apatite reactions with fluoride in cementum and dentin. In the following, a description of the sound tissue will be given, and the changes occurring during a caries attack will be discussed. This will include a brief outline of the chemical reactions taking place. Information on the histologic appearance of a demineralization defect - necessary for an understanding of the processes of de- and remineralization, is given in Chapter 11.

Dental enamel has the highest mineral content of all the mineralized tissues in the body. It comprises 96 weight % of a crystalline calcium phosphate mineral close in composition to hydroxyapatite. Pure hydroxyapatite has a unit cell (building block) formula of $Ca_{10}(PO_4)_6(OH)_2$. It is one of the intrinsic properties of minerals of this type, however, that the crystal lattice can contain large amounts of foreign ions as impurities. Likewise, dental enamel contains many chemical elements in 'trace' or small amounts. These impurities may be present either in the crystal lattice or in an adsorbed state at the crystal surface. A compilation is given in Table 14-1. It should be specifically noted that enamel contains 2-5% carbonate incorporated in the crystal lattice and that this plays a major role in enamel reactivity (see below). Enamel crystals must

Table 14-2

Enamel, related minerals and their solubilities

Abbreviation	Name	Formula	-log (sol. prod.)	Ref.
	Enamel		104-144	51
HAP	hydroxyapatite	$Ca_{10}(PO_4)_6(OH)_2$	117.2	16
FAP	fluorapatite	$Ca_{10}(PO_4)_6 F_2$	121.2	16
DCPD	brushite	$CaHPO_4.2H_2O$	6.73	36
CaF_2	calcium fluoride	CaF_2	10.44	36
OCP	octacalcium phosphate	$Ca_8(HPO_4)_2(PO_4)_4. 5H_2O$	46.9	43
FHAP	fluoridated hydroxyapatite	$Ca_{10}(PO_4)_6(OH)_xF_y$ (with x+y = 2)		

therefore be considered as carbonated apatite wich incorporates with many other trace elements, including fluoride. Several of these elements affect enamel reactivity.[13]

The composition of dental enamel is not homogeneous. All constituents are present in different concentrations at the anatomic surface and at the dentinoenamel-junction (DEJ). The density and the content of organic material and water also vary. Such variations are found not only in transverse sections, but also between different areas of teeth: for instance cervical enamel has a lower mineral density than occlusal enamel.[52]

As a result of precipitation and exchange reactions from the external fluids the composition of enamel changes both during the pre-eruptive formation phase and after eruption. One result of this is that pre- and posteruptive maturation both yield a fluoride gradient in the enamel with typical values of 3000 ppm F at the anatomic surface and 100 ppm F at the DEJ (see Chapter 5). The fluoride content of the outer enamel surface depends on different parameters such as preeruptive fluoride administration, posteruptive fluoride regimens, presence of plaque, abrasion and attrition.[59]

Histologic examination shows that enamel is arranged in so-called prisms or rods. These are cylinder-like structures 4-6 µm in diameter, extending from the DEJ to the anatomic surface, where they reach the surface at an angle of 90°-120°. Although the prisms can, at a first approximation, be described as cylinder-like, in cross-section their appearance is described as "key-hole-shaped". These prisms are made up of clusters of small crystals (or crystallites) approximately hexagonal in cross-section, with a diameter of about 40 nm (about 1000th of a hair's breadth), which extend from the DEJ to the anatomic surface.[50]

Although the mineral phase is about 96% weight this is only 85% by volume. The remaining 15% volume consists of water, protein and lipid (fatty material). This protein and lipid (present in approximately equal amounts),[46] together with a large proportion of the water constitute the diffusion channels between crystals and prisms for acid, minerals and fluoride to pass in or out of the enamel during de- or remineralization.

Solubility of enamel apatite-like mineral

The variability in composition and the presence of impurities, particularly carbonate, in the crystal lattice are responsible for the greater solubility of dental enamel apatite than hydroxyapatite and also that the variation in this solubility throughout the enamel.

In Table 14-2 the reported apparent solubility products for dental enamel and hydroxyapatite are given, the former being calculated using the formula below for the solubility product of hydroxyapatite

$$K_{sp} = a_{Ca}^{10} \; a_{PO_4}^{6} \; a_{OH}^{2}$$

in which a_{Ca} = calcium ion activity in solution, a_{PO_4} = phosphate ion activity in solution, a_{OH} = hydroxyl ion activity in solution.

The mineral hydroxyapatite contains constituents which, when solubilized, are transformed when the pH changes.

$$Ca_{10}(PO_4)_6(OH)_2 \rightleftarrows 10 \; Ca^{2+} + 6 \; PO_4^{3-} + 2 \; OH^-$$

$$PO_4^{3-} + 3H^+ \rightleftarrows HPO_4^{2-} + 2H^+$$
$$\rightleftarrows H_2PO_4^- + H^+ \rightleftarrows H_3PO_4$$

$$OH^- + H^+ \rightleftarrows H_2O$$

acid pH

$$\rightleftarrows$$

alkaline pH

This simple series of chemical reactions is the rationale for caries: at low pH the equilibrium concentrations of calcium and phosphate are greater than at high pH. Somewhere in the pH range between 5 and 6, the equilibrium concentrations equal the values for the oral fluids. Above that value, precipitation of mineral may occur from a supersaturated solution; below that value, dissolution of mineral occurs in an undersaturated solution.

The same principles apply to dissolution of the substituted apatite that occurs in enamel. As indicated above (Table 14-1) enamel apatite is similar to hydroxyapatite but contains numerous metal ion substitutions and, most importantly, 2-5% carbonate by weight replacing phosphate groups. The enamel mineral is much more reactive than pure hydroxyapatite (Table 14-2) as a result of these impurities. Hydroxyapatite-like mineral is not the only crystalline form of calcium phosphate that can be found in the body. Calcium phosphate may precipitate in various crystalline forms, all differing in solubility and with characteristic Ca/P ratios (Table 14-2).

Some of these minerals form as a result of the interaction between the oral fluids and the mineralized tissues and can be found in calculus, in a white spot lesion or as a precursor in mineral precipitation reactions. Fluoride plays a major role in the transformations between minerals. The fluoride ion speeds up these reactions dramatically. Two such transformations can be described schematically:

$$DCPD + F^- \rightarrow FAP$$

$$HAP + F^- \rightarrow FHAP \text{ or } FAP$$

FHAP indicates fluoridated hydroxyapatite where some of the OH groups, not necessarily 50%, are replaced by F.

Although nature appears to have a choice between different calcium phosphates, the type of mineral formed depends on strict chemical thermodynamic and kinetic laws. In the absence of fluoride, hydroxyapatite is thermodynamically the most stable phase. An extremely important observation is that in the presence of traces of fluoride, fluorapatite (or fluorhydroxyapatite) is thermodynamically favored. FAP and HAP have equal solubilities at about 10^{-6} ppm F and are much less soluble than carbonated apatite, which enamel crystals are made up of (Table 14-2).

The formation of hydroxyapatite from other $Ca-PO_4^-$ salts at the temperature conditions in the oral cavity will not occur through a 'solid state' reaction, since such reactions only proceed at measurable rates at high temperatures (1000°C). Similarly, the formation of FAP from HAP, or dental enamel crystals, by a solid state transformation is very slow. Alternatively, minerals may be transformed by a dissolution-precipitation mechanism. For this to happen the reaction has to proceed through an intermediate aqueous phase. In the oral environment this implies that one mineral (for instance HAP-like enamel) dissolves, or at least the surface dissolves, and that the constituents reprecipitate in a different chemical form (pure HAP or FHAP), preferably excluding impurities such as carbonate. Such dissolution and precipitation reactions in the oral cavity slowly render the exposed mineralized tissue less soluble. Acid-soluble mineral is first washed out and is usually displaced by an improved mineral. This applies particularly if ions are present during the precipitation phase in concentrations differing from the conditions during amelogenesis or preeruptive maturation. When, during this cycle of acid attack and subsequent mineral replacement, fluoride is present in the oral environment at sufficiently elevated concentrations, it will be incorporated to a greater extent than during the enamel formation. During the so-called posteruptive maturation of the enamel a gradual change in composition takes place, which results in a shift in solubility towards that of FAP.

Localization of fluoride in the enamel

In Chapter 5 and in the above, the distribution of fluoride in enamel and the fluoride gradient from the surface of enamel into the underlying regions have been described. The high concentration of fluoride in the outer few µm of enamel (3000-6000 ppm) is consistent with the presence of a fluoridated hydroxyapatite (as described above), most likely with crystal surfaces which appear as fluorapatite to the surrounding fluid. Fluoride occurs in various forms throughout the enamel and can be incorporated into or onto the crystal as part of the apatite crystalline lattice structure, strongly adsorbed to the crystal surface, weakly adsorbed to the crystal surface, or not form part of the crystal structure, or in some other phase as a secondary crystal growth of, for example, calcium fluoride (CaF_2) on the enamel apatite crystal surface. Each of these possibilities will be addressed in turn.

Fluoride in the crystal

Fluoride is incorporated into the crystal structure as part of the apatite during enamel development and the concentration of the fluoride is dependent upon the fluoride intake during enamel development and on the fluoride environment post-eruptively as described above. It was once thought that the incorporation during enamel development causes a major difference in caries resistance. Recent studies have clearly shown that fluoride incorporation into the crystal does not inherently affect the reactivity of the enamel crystals. Studies with synthetic apatites incorporating fluoride at concentrations up to 1000 ppm in carbonated apatite showed that their dissolution rates in acid were no different from non-fluoride-containing carbonated apatite, and that the carbonate was the principal driving force for the reactivity to acid.[45,21] These experiments were conducted so that the volume of acid was large and any fluoride dissolving out of the crystal did not have an observable effect at the surface.

Similar studies carried out with dental enamel of different origin have yielded contradictory conclusions. A correlation between flu-

oride content and demineralization susceptibility has been found, while other studies failed
to do so (for review see Mellberg & Ripa[41]).
Although this inconsistency might be explained by differences in the chosen experimental conditions, of which acid challenge
seems to be a very important one, the conclusion can be drawn that firmly incorporated fluoride is of much lesser importance than fluoride present in the fluid surrounding the crystals during de- and remineralization. This is
described in detail later in this chapter.

Fluoride can be weakly or strongly adsorbed
at the crystal surface. If it is incorporated into
the concentrated layer of ions in the immediate
fluid surrounding the crystal, the fluoride is
strongly held by the underlying calcium ions
during an acid challenge. Hence, fluoride at the
crystal surface is important, whereas the composition of underlying apatite will be relatively
unimportant. It is also possible for the fluoride
to replace hydroxyl ions in the crystal surface
and be strongly chemisorbed. In this case, it is
extremely difficult for hydrogen ions to subsequently dissolve that area of the crystal.[3] By
taking this argument one step further, and this
has been done experimentally,[54] it is possible to
show that as an enamel crystal dissolves, particularly if fluoride is incorporated in it or on it,
this will release fluoride into the external fluid
environment. The fluoride in solution will subsequently slow down an acid attack. In this
way, structurally incorporated fluoride can affect the caries process, providing the acid challenge is sufficient to dissolve some apatite with
fluoride, but not so strong that only dissolution
occurs.

Fluoride in the intercrystalline fluid

It is obvious from the above argument that it is
important that when acid penetrates between
the crystals during the caries process, fluoride
is present to slow down or inhibit the acid attack. Preferably, the fluoride should come from
the external environment or from readily so-

luble materials at the crystal surface. This will
occur if fluoride is applied frequently to the
tooth surface at concentrations low enough to
diffuse into the enamel and also if there is a
reasonably soluble fluoride form present either
at the surface or in the subsurface of the enamel.

Subsequent to an acid challenge, as the pH
rises externally and within the tooth structure,
if fluoride is present at low concentrations in
the intercrystalline fluid it will enhance either
the precipitation of new mineral incorporating
calcium, phosphate and fluoride or crystal
growth on existing, partly dissolved, enamel
crystals. Whichever happens, the fluoride present in the intercrystalline fluid will enhance
this process dramatically. The crystalline surface so formed will then be more resistant to
subsequent acid attack.

Availability of fluoride in the tooth environment: transport and diffusion phenomena

Fluoride in plaque fluid and saliva as it relates to de- and remineralization

The fluoride composition and ranges of plaque
and saliva have been described in Chapter 12
and these will be brought into perspective here
in terms of the caries mechanism. Fluoride is
present in whole saliva in concentrations ranging from undetectable to perhaps as high as 10
or even 20 ppm. What is important to the caries
process is the fluoride concentration in the
whole saliva (here taken to mean oral fluid) in
the mouth rather than the saliva in the ducts
prior to, or just after, the fluid enters the oral
cavity. Fluoride in whole saliva can be contributed to systemically as well as by fluoride
sources in the mouth. If, for example, a subject
has been given a fluoride topical gel, the concentration of fluoride in saliva could be ex-

tremely high for minutes or even hours afterwards.[6] Normal levels of fluoride in whole saliva vary between approximately 0.01 and 0.05 ppm, mostly toward the lower range. Some studies have indicated that levels as low as 0.1 ppm fluoride may be sufficient to enhance crystal growth.[5,1] Crystal growth is an important process during both de- and remineralization. Therefore, elevated levels of fluoride in saliva throughout the day will alter the balance between dissolution and crystal growth.

However, in the oral environment, the saliva is not in direct contact with the teeth and the fluoride must first pass through the plaque to the tooth surface. It has been shown (as reviewed in Chapter 12) that fluoride can be concentrated in the plaque and, hence, the plaque fluid. Plaque will therefore provide a fluoride source at the time of the acid challenge resulting from plaque metabolism. As the plaque ferments the carbohydrates (upon which we and the bacteria feed) acid is produced, the pH falls, and some of the fluoride is complexed into the form of HF, which will, together with the acids, rapidly diffuse into the tooth. Diffusion of fluoride through plaque is relatively fast, about 100-10,000 fold faster than the effective diffusion in enamel.[14,20] Hence, from a preventive point of view, it is desirable to have a source of fluoride in the plaque and plaque fluid and to have this continually replenished from the saliva. In simple terms, then, the plaque and the saliva act as a fluoride source.

Diffusion of fluoride through enamel

Enamel is a porous solid consisting of crystals in a protein/lipid/water matrix. On average, enamel is 85% by volume mineral, 3% protein/lipid in equal quantities, and the remainder water. The interprismatic spaces in the enamel are large and are filled with this organic/water matrix (compare Chapter 5). Even the intercrystalline spaces are large enough for small molecules of acid, fluoride, calcium, phosphate, etc., to diffuse through at a measurable rate. Again, these spaces are filled with water/organic material. So enamel essentially is a porous solid and everything which diffuses into and out of it must pass through this organic diffusion matrix. Recent experiments have shown that the organic material plays a large part in controlling the rate of diffusion of species into and out of the enamel. Fluoride can diffuse as F^- or as HF, but studies now indicate that the most rapid diffusion will occur as HF.[20,22,23] The importance of this from a caries perspective is that if fluoride is present in the plaque, or in the saliva adjacent to the plaque, at the time of an acid challenge to the tooth due to bacterial metabolism, then the fluoride can combine with hydrogen ions and be rapidly transported into the enamel at the same time as the acids (Fig. 14-1). Then the fluoride is available to inhibit acid attack at the crystal surface and promote remineralization as the pH again rises when the saliva buffers the acid and the carbohydrate source is exhausted.

In summary, fluoride can come from the crystal as it dissolves, it can come from the intercrystalline fluid, from the plaque, and from the saliva. If it is present at the site of acid attack or at the site of crystal growth at sufficient, but low, concentrations, it can have a major effect on caries progression or reversal (detailed description given below).

It is obvious from the above understanding of the mechanisms of fluoride action with the enamel that the predominant caries inhibitory effects are by fluoride from topical sources. The posteruptive effect at the crystal surface and in the immediate subsurface during de- and remineralization, as outlined above, clearly indicates revised rationale for the use of fluoride supplements, fluoride topicals applied in the dental office, and fluoride applied at home by water supply, toothbrushing or mouthrinsing. Experiments from several laboratories, both *in vitro* and *in vivo*, have now clearly shown that this approach is correct. Some of this evidence is summarized below.

The active role of fluoride in the caries process

It is only recently that the above mechanistic understanding of fluoride action was unveiled. For many years the effect of incorporated fluoride on the solubility of enamel was considered the only, or at least primary, cariostatic mechanism of fluoride. The hypothesis that an increased fluoride content in the enamel resulted in a lower caries susceptibility also predetermined the direction of fluoride research. Practically, it had a great impact on the type of fluoride treatments chosen in caries-preventive programs. The rationale for semiannual APF (acidulated phosphate fluoride) treatment, for instance, rested on two basic premises:

- The necessity to increase the fluoride content of the enamel to as high values as possible in a short time;

- The desire to prevent the formation of CaF_2 and other fluoride-containing precipitates that are more soluble than FAP.

In recent years research in the field has shifted to the study of the active role of fluoride from the oral fluids during de- and remineralization of caries defects.

Fluoride as an inhibitor of demineralization

When fluoride is added to acidified buffer solutions used to make artificial caries-like enamel lesions, two interesting phenomena can be observed. Firstly, the rate of lesion formation is slowed down, and secondly, fluoride has an effect on the histologic appearance of the lesion that develops.

Effect of fluoride on kinetics of lesion formation

In the laboratory it is possible to make artificial white spot lesions by immersing enamel in undersaturated, acidified buffers of pH 4-6. Commonly, acetic acid or lactic acid is used as the organic acid. The rate of lesion formation is monitored by measuring the increase in calcium or phosphate concentration in solution or by analyzing subsequent sections taken from the enamel specimen using one or more of the techniques of scanning electron microscopy, microradiography, microhardness, or polarized light microscopy. Several investigations have contributed to our knowledge of the caries mechanism in this way.

In such experiments the rate of lesion formation was found to be dependent on the degree of undersaturation of the solution to the mineral ('HAP') in enamel. Thus for lower calcium, phosphate or hydroxyl ion concentrations (that is, lower pH) a higher dissolution rate was observed.[15,42] The addition of fluoride to the solution complicated this relatively simple model. Decreasing the pH of the solution (that is, increasing the challenge) produced lesions more rapidly but was compensated for by increasing the concentration of soluble fluoride. Fig. 14-2 shows the amount of mineral dissolved during an acid challenge at various pH and F-concentrations.[7] The data given pertain to a given calcium and phosphate concentration in solution and the specific concentration values at which demineralization inhibition occurred therefore have no absolute physiologic meaning. When lower initial Ca and PO_4 ion concentrations were used, the same degree of inhibition was found for higher fluoride concentrations in solution. In principle, a similar graph could be drawn including mineral ion concentrations and ionic strength as parameters in saliva or plaque fluid and this would predict at which fluoride concentrations demineralization inhibition would occur. This, however, is not possible except in general terms (Fig. 14-3).

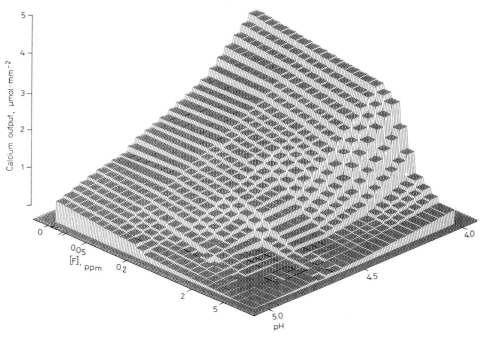

Fig. 14-2. Calcium output during enamel demineralization as a function of the initial fluoride concentration and pH of the demineralizing solutions. The demineralizing solutions initially contained 50 mM acetate buffer at pH 4.5 and 2.2 mM Ca and 2.2 mM PO$_4$ (reproduced with the permission of the publisher Karger, Basel).[7]

Effect of fluoride on lesion histology

When fluoride-deficient enamel, such as subsurface enamel, is subjected to an *in vitro* caries attack, the defect formed does not show the characteristic pattern of a subsurface lesion. Instead, a demineralization defect without a surface layer is formed.

However, when fluoride is added to the demineralizing solution, the attack results in a lesion with a completely different histologic appearance: a well formed surface layer can be discerned with a mineral content considerably higher than that of the underlying lesion body. The mineral content of the surface layer and the thickness of the surface layer are correlated with the fluoride concentration in solution.[8] For example, Fig. 14-3 shows microradiograms of lesions formed in undersaturated calcium phosphate solutions at pH 4.5 and different fluoride concentrations. As illustrated, an increase in fluoride ion concentration results not only in a thicker surface layer but also in a shallower lesion with a decreased amount of mineral removed from the lesion body.

It is important to note that the surface layer in white spot lesions does not only develop by this mechanism. When fluoride-rich (surface) enamel is subjected to caries-creating solutions, a surface layer is formed due to the lower local acid solubility as well as the favorable precipitation conditions. In this approach, less mineral is removed in this region and in addition, mineral removed from deeper regions may precipitate in the surface zone instead of diffusing out to the external solution.

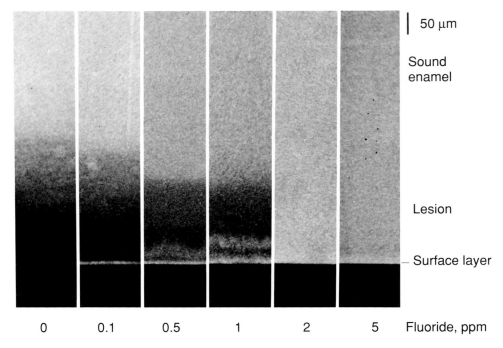

Fig. 14-3. Microradiograms of representative specimens showing the effect of fluoride concentration in solution on the formation of enamel lesions. Demineralizing solutions were made up as given in Fig. 14-2 (reproduced with the permission of the publisher Karger, Basel)[8].

Rationale for the effect of fluoride during demineralization

The active role of fluoride in the demineralization medium on the kinetics of demineralization and the histology of the lesions formed has been reported in numerous publications.

As early as 1959[40] it was reported that fluoride addition to acetic acid buffers delayed the demineralization of enamel. At a concentration of 1 ppm F in solution the rate of demineralization was slower than of fluoride-pretreated enamel in a fluoride-free buffer. A striking observation was that the fluoride acquired by the enamel from fluoride-containing solutions was only a fraction of the fluoride content of preincubated enamel. The authors concluded that precipitation of a fluoride-rich mineral at those enamel sites where demineralization is most pronounced was a possible explanation for their observations. Other investigators[57,58] also attributed the decreased acid solubility of the enamel in fluoride-containing buffers to the formation of fluoride-rich mineral covering the surface of the enamel (or apatite) crystallites.

Recent observations provide further insight into the action of fluoride on apatite dissolution. By using carbonated apatite as a model for enamel apatite the inhibitory effect of fluoride on crystal dissolution was directly demonstrated.[19,45] Dissolution of carbonated-apatite was measured in acetate buffers incorporating fluoride at 0-50 ppm in the solution. Fluoride at 1 ppm in the buffer reduced the dissolution rate of the carbonated apatite to that of hydroxy-

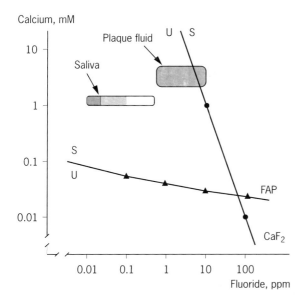

Fig. 14-4. Solubility isotherms (calcium concentrations at saturation as a function of fluoride concentration in solution) for FAP and CaF_2 at pH 7.0 and Ca/P 1.66. Regions applicable to plaque fluid and saliva are as indicated. U and S mark the areas of undersaturation and supersaturation with respect to FAP and CaF_2 on the two sides of the saturation lines.

apatite, and higher concentrations further inhibited its dissolution. The inhibitory effect was related to the logarithm of the fluoride concentration, indicating that surface-adsorbed fluoride protected dissolution sites at the crystal surfaces against acid attack.

It has also been reported that fluoride in solution affected the acid solubility of enamel and also that demineralization by EDTA was not inhibited.[29] This finding was explained by the limited number of vacant hydroxyl groups created in the EDTA-mediated demineralization. The effect of fluoride was, in the authors' view, determined by the rate of transformation of the crystallite surface to FAP. Other investigators[7] concluded that bulk solution thermodynamic considerations may not be relevant to explain the observed inhibitory effect of fluoride on enamel demineralization. Moreover, under conditions where fluorapatite became supersaturated in solution, no sudden change in demineralization rate was found. A rapid decrease in demineralization rate was, however, observed at the saturation line of CaF_2, suggesting that precipitation of this mineral may be a more effective inhibitor. As a possible explanation the authors suggested that, due to the different morphology, a calcium fluoride deposit may be more effective in blocking diffusion pathways than FAP precipitating onto the existing crystallites.

The effect of fluoride in solution on lesion formation has also been reported in a series of investigations.[37,38] The histologic appearance of the lesions was studied using microradiography and polarized light microscopy. The authors concluded that, with conditions undersaturated to both FAP and HAP, erosion takes place, while supersaturation to FAP causes a surface layer to form.

The role of fluoride during remineralization

In the preceding section the role of fluoride during the process of lesion formation was examined. From the information in the literature it has become clear that fluoride-containing minerals, precipitating under acidic conditions, inhibit enamel demineralization.

Likewise, at neutral pH, fluoride-containing calcium-phosphates may precipitate from the oral fluids.

In the first section of this chapter it was shown how saliva and plaque fluid are supersaturated with respect to HAP at above "critical pH-values". In Fig. 14-4 the solubility, expressed as mM Ca in solution, of FAP and CaF_2 are given as a function of the fluoride concentration in solution. It is obvious that plaque fluid and saliva are supersaturated with respect to FAP, but not necessarily to CaF_2.

Precipitation of mineral does not happen readily from supersaturated solutions *per se*; a substrate is needed upon which the deposit can form. In the oral environment many surfaces may act as sites for precipitation or, when such occurs in a crystalline form, crystallization. Precipitation upon a protein matrix in plaque may result in calculus formation. Mineral deposition in enamel defects may result in replacement, or partial replacement, of the lost mineral and is, therefore, called remineralization.

White spot, or carious lesion, remineralization is a widely documented phenomenon in epidemiologic, *in vivo*, as well as *in vitro* research.

In an epidemiologic survey it was shown that about 50% of the white spots diagnosed in 9-year-old children disappeared during the following 5 years as a result of the remineralizing potential of saliva.[4] At the same time, it was demonstrated that saliva and artificial mineralizing fluid produced an increase of hardness in demineralized enamel.[34,35] Since those observations many investigators have been concerned with the mechanism of this phenomenon. Remineralization of enamel lesions was found to occur by a deposition of crystalline hydroxyapatite, which *in vitro* can give rise to a complete repair of the defect. However, *in vivo*, the process proceeds considerably more slowly and a full recovery is seldom attained. Moreover, although remineralization *in vivo* takes place in a crystalline form, the crystallites never acquire as large dimensions as observed *in vitro*.[2,9,55]

The role of fluoride in the remineralization process was found to be a rather complex one. Theoretically, the matter is relatively simple: in the presence of fluoride, apatite may precipitate as FAP or FHAP (Table 14-2). Morphologically, there is no restriction to precipitation of fluoridated apatites onto a HAP crystallite matrix, as the minerals in this group all have closely related crystalline structures. As a result of the lower solubility of FAP or FHAP the thermodynamic driving force for their precipitation is greater (compared to HAP). From the foregoing the general conclusion can be drawn that fluoride stimulates apatite precipitation. Many *in vitro* experiments agree with this. Precipitation of FAP (or FHAP) on an apatite matrix is accelerated by fluoride.[1] After a few molecular layers have been deposited the substrate material reacts like a bulk FAP or FHAP mineral, e.g. when it is subjected to a dissolution experiment. In *in vitro* experiments the initial remineralization of white spot lesions or softened enamel is increased by the addition of fluoride to the remineralizing medium, and this results in an increase of the hardness of the surface of the demineralized region.[34]

When the impact of fluoride on lesion remineralization is studied a distinction should be made between the effects of high doses of fluoride of short duration and the effect of a continuous low concentration of fluoride present in the remineralizing fluid. The former case pertains to topical application or even fluoride dentifrices, while the latter situation is likely to occur in the case of drinking water fluoridation or during the periods in between toothbrushing or fluoride mouthrinsing. During and after a short-term fluoride treatment, large amounts of fluoride are adsorbed in the lesion. Chemical analysis of white spots[26,53] has revealed that these contain considerably higher amounts of fluoride than the surrounding sound enamel (cf Chapter 5), an important finding showing

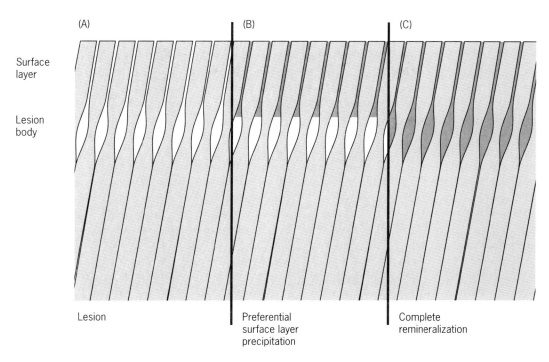

Fig. 14-5. Schematic diagram illustrating a lesion in cross-section (A). As a result of remineralization in solutions with high mineral content, surface layer precipitation will occur preferentially (B). With low mineral concentrations, remineralization may occur throughout the lesion (C).

the great affinity of demineralized regions for fluoride. As a result of this higher fluoride content, mineral precipitation will be accelerated in the outermost region of the lesion; this process draws away many of the free mineral ions from the inner pores of the lesion and, thus, effectively slows down diffusion towards the lesion interior. The result is that mineralization in the lesion body is delayed, compared to the non-fluoride control. Additionally, the excess deposition may cause the lesion pores to be blocked with mineral, resulting in an even more pronounced diffusion inhibition.

A mechanism as described above was confirmed in experiments using radioactively labeled solutions and "topical F"-treated lesions.[10] A similar mechanistic conclusion can be drawn from the results of experiments in which lesions were remineralized in solutions with different mineral ion concentrations.[56] At low supersaturation 1 mM Ca, 0.6 mM PO_4 at pH 7, remineralization took place throughout the lesion, while when using the threefold concentrations, the repair was limited to the surface layer (cf. Chapter 11). Apparently both topical fluoride concentrations and solutions with high mineral concentrations yield a preferential surface layer precipitation. This is shown schematically in Fig. 14-5.

The situation is different when fluoride is present continuously at low concentrations. Fluoride is now available simultaneously with calcium and phosphate, and it can diffuse into the lesion and precipitate as FAP or FHAP. In vitro investigations have shown that low fluoride concentrations do indeed accelerate the initial mineral deposition in lesions or softened enamel. At a constant 1 ppm F in the remineralizing solution a 2-3-fold increase in the rate of precipitation was found.[9] When fluoride was added to remineralizing solutions or saliva and teeth with caries-like lesions were immersed in these solutions, an increase in hardness was observed both *in vitro* and *in vivo*.[24, 33, 34] In these experiments, hardness was measured on the enamel surface exposed to the solution, which could mean that the actual hardness increase, reflecting mineralization, was restricted to the outermost lesion layers.

Relevant additional information concerning this can also be obtained from epidemiologic research. Early in this section, data were quoted[4] showing a considerable remineralization of natural white spots *in vivo* in a non-fluoride area. A significant difference was observed between individuals living in areas with and without drinking water fluoridation. While remineralization of lesions occurred in 50% of the individuals in the non-fluoride group, the corresponding value for the fluoride group was 22%. These findings can be interpreted by looking at the group of lesions more closely.[25] For the fluoride group, most lesions showed a glossy or shiny appearance indicative of arrested lesions, while in the non-fluoride group, a large portion had a chalky appearance. The latter type would be typical of active lesions. This leads to the conclusion that under conditions prevailing as a result of drinking water fluoridation, preferential surface layer deposition occurs after prolonged exposure periods. Based on *in vitro*, *in vivo* and epidemiologic evidence it must be concluded that preferential surface layer deposition occurs even at low fluoride concentrations, causing lesion arrestment.

In summary, fluoride, particularly when present continually, actively enhances lesion remineralization and/or arrestment.

Effect of fluoride during pH-cycling

In the oral environment there is a continual cycling of pH resulting from acid challenge and subsequent neutralization by saliva and other factors. Therefore, de- and remineralization will only occur for relatively short periods and are intimately connected. Alternating de- and remineralization of enamel *in vitro* (called pH-cycling) is a useful way to study the effect of both processes on each other.[11] Preventive regimens incorporating fluoride can be tested using this experimental approach. Recent studies along these lines have confirmed the mechanism of fluoride action outlined above.[19] Further, a single parameter can be examined with such models by keeping other variables constant. Aspects of fluoride mechanism can be examined which cannot be isolated in intraoral models. For example, low levels of fluoride in the range 0.01-0.1 ppm in the mineralizing solution in a pH-cycling model have been shown to enhance remineralization. The effect was related to the logarithm of the fluoride concentration.[18] The implications of this study are that relatively low levels of fluoride in saliva will also enhance remineralization in the mouth. Levels of 0.04-0.1 ppm F can be achieved by the regular use of fluoride products, as has been demonstrated in a recent epidemiologic study of caries risk factors.[39]

Sources, forms and reactions of different types of fluoride

The role of calcium fluoride in the caries process

Traditionally, fluoride applications were aimed at increasing the content of firmly bound fluoride in the enamel and preventing the formation of calcium fluoride. Calcium fluoride was considered to be rapidly removed because of its relatively high solubility. Experiments in which calcium fluoride deposits on enamel were leached in tap water indeed showed a rapid removal of any loosely bound fluoride.[32] It was recently demonstrated that a different situation exists in the oral fluid. *In vivo* calcium fluoride was retained for much longer periods, which was attributed to the high calcium and fluoride content of the saliva compared to tap water and, more importantly, to the formation of a phosphate- and protein-rich protective layer on the calcium fluoride globules.[47] After a single fluoride mouthrinse a considerable portion of fluoride was found to be present as calcium fluoride, even after 7 days *in vivo* leaching.[48] Additionally, under conditions of cariogenic challenge CaF_2 was found to be converted to FAP.[49] This revised understanding of the role of calcium fluoride is utilized below to help describe the action of several commercially available fluoride products.

Sources of fluoride and their effect on the physicochemical interactions of fluoride and enamel

Fluoride is available from numerous sources. Firstly, it is available naturally in all drinking water supplies at various concentrations (see Chapter 1). Fluoridation of public water supplies has been shown to be a successful method for delivering low concentrations of fluoride to whole populations every day. The primary mode of action appears to be the effect on de- and remineralization fluoride exerts from being present routinely throughout the day and night. Salivary fluoride levels are generally higher in fluoridated areas than in non-fluoridated areas, although they are still in the order of 0.02 ppm compared with 0.01 ppm respectively, unless other fluoride-containing products are utilized routinely. The diversity of fluoride agents which are available to the public is large. The three main categories can be summarized as

- Inorganic agents including NaF, SnF_2, NH_4F, etc.; in these cases the salts are readily soluble, providing free fluoride;

- Monofluorophosphate-containing agents such as Na_2FPO_3; in this case the fluoride is covalently bound in the FPO_3^{2-} ion and apparently requires hydrolysis to free the F^-;

- Organic fluorides such as amine fluoride, and silene fluorides, and many others.

Products available to the general public normally are toothpastes or mouthrinses with fluoride concentrations ranging from 1500 (or 1000) ppm fluoride as any one of the above agents in toothpaste, through mouthrinses containing 0.05% NaF to lower concentrations (approximately 250 ppm F or lower). Products which are utilized by the dental practitioner normally have a high fluoride concentration, are utilized 6-monthly or less frequently and may have any one of the above agents or related agents in the form of gels, liquids, pastes, varnishes, etc. In terms of the above physicochemical description, the use of these products can be interpreted in the following way. Daily use of fluoride toothpaste or fluoride mouthrinse in the home will provide relatively low concentrations of fluoride on a routine basis and (1) will elevate the fluoride in the saliva for periods of minutes or hours, (2) will elevate the fluoride in the plaque, and (3) will provide fluoride at the time of acid challenge and at the time of subsequent remineralization.

Frequent applications (once or twice a day) of these relatively low-level fluoride products are extremely effective in combating dental caries in the majority of the population and are probably responsible for the major reduction in dental caries in the last 10-15 years.[27] Epidemiologic studies in two towns in the Netherlands after discontinuation of water fluoridation[31] showed that between 1967 and 1980 the differences attributable to water fluoridation disappeared, and that in both towns the decay prevalence in 1980 was dramatically lower than in 1967 in either town. Although dietary habits and oral hygiene may have improved, the most important change during this period was the common usage of fluoride toothpaste.

Sodium fluoride-containing pastes
Sodium fluoride in toothpaste or other products immediately provides free F^- ion to interact with the stage of the caries process as described above.

Monofluorophosphate pastes
The MFP-containing products provide the MPF ion together with some free F^- ion, both of which can diffuse through the plaque and into the enamel, providing a source of F^- ion subsequent to hydrolysis to again interact in the way described above. Monofluorophosphate can be hydrolyzed in plaque and is also hydrolyzed under acidic conditions at the surface of apatite crystals, providing phosphate and fluoride ions.[6,17,28]

A recently carried out meta-analysis of clinical studies of efficacy of fluoride dentifrices revealed a small, but significant, difference (6%) favoring sodium fluoride dentifrices over monofluorophosphate dentifrices.[30] More important is the bioavailability of the fluoride in the toothpastes, which determines the caries-preventive effects.

Stannous fluoride
This provides fluoride ions and stannous ions, which act as an antimicrobial agent (see Chapter 3). Additionally, stannous fluoride can produce stannous phosphate fluoride precipitates which should slow down the caries process, but have staining as a side effect.[60]

Amine fluoride
This is essentially an ionic fluoride compound and readily provides free fluoride ions. Its enhanced reactivity has been attributed to the greater affinity of the hydrophilic counterions to the enamel.[44]

Topical agents
Those with high concentrations of fluoride (e.g. 1% neutral NaF gel) will promote the precipitation of calcium fluoride, CaF_2. This will provide free fluoride ions as it dissolves and may act as a long-term storehouse for fluoride during de- and remineralization. Fluoride from these topical agents will also be readily taken up into the enamel porosities (including early lesions), actively inducing lesion arrest.

Acidulated phosphate fluoride
This readily etches the enamel surface, providing calcium ions that can interact with the fluoride and precipitate large amounts of calcium fluoride, which again act in the same way. Further, the hydrogen ions present will complex with the fluoride, producing HF, which will readily diffuse deep into the enamel. There is therefore a chemical rationale for the observed clinical effectiveness of these topical agents. Other agents, such as amine fluoride and silene fluoride, again provide a complexed store of fluoride ion and may enhance diffusion through carious enamel releasing fluoride at appropriate times and appropriate sites.

Fluoride products should be used by the dentist and by the general public bearing in mind the physicochemical rationale laid out above. Frequent application of low-level fluorides will effectively inhibit demineralization and enhance remineralization by providing satisfactory levels of fluoride at the time of every acid challenge and at the time of every remineralization cycle. High-concentration fluoride topicals will provide a store of fluoride which is subsequently released over an expanded time period, providing fluoride again at the time of acid challenge and at the time of remineralization.

Conclusions

Based on the concepts developed in this chapter, the following statements are important:

- Enamel is a highly porous material consisting of apatite-like mineral crystals surrounded by water and organic components. These crystals contain carbonate and other impurities that make them more reactive to acid than pure hydroxyapatite (HAP) or fluorapatite (FAP).

- Dental caries progresses by a cycling process of acid challenge (acid from plaque bacterial metabolism) to the tooth mineral, alternating with pH increase due to saliva and other factors neutralizing the acid.

- Fluoride is present in the saliva, plaque and intercrystalline fluid, and is incorporated in the mineral crystals.

- Fluoride has a pronounced cariostatic effect primarily through its actions in the aqueous (water) phase on the tooth, and among the crystals in the tooth.

- Fluoride incorporated into the enamel mineral during tooth development has relatively little effect on the caries process. It is the fluoride incorporated posteruptively and in the aqueous phase during the caries challenge that is of primary importance.

- Demineralization (loss of mineral resulting from partial dissolution of enamel crystals) during the acid attack stage of caries is markedly inhibited if fluoride is present in solution at the time of the acid challenge. Fluoride diffuses with the acid from plaque into the enamel pores and acts at the crystal surface to reduce mineral loss. Fluoride present on crystal surfaces, for example as FAP deposited during a previous cycle, will be highly resistant to subsequent acid attack.

- Fluoride present in solution at the crystal surface during a pH rise following demineralization can combine with dissolved calcium and phosphate ions to precipitate or grow fluorapatite-like crystalline material within the tooth. Fluoride enhances this mineral gain (remineralization) and provides a material which is more resistant to subsequent acid attack. In the case of high fluoride concentrations, calcium fluoride (CaF_2) can be precipitated and this slowly redissolves providing a source of F^- ions to inhibit demineralization or promote remineralization.

- The two important factors of fluoride action in preventing or reversing caries, are therefore (1) inhibition of demineralization, and (2) enhancement of remineralization.

- Fluoride regimens employed for the prevention of dental decay should be designed and used on the basis of the above principles. High concentration 'topical preparations used at intervals of months or years by the dentist work initially not only on both de- and remineralization, but also by providing fluoride as CaF_2 or adsorbed in early lesions which is subsequently available over prolonged periods.

The most effective caries-preventive fluoride regimen, both from a theoretical perspective and as proved clinically, is the frequent (daily) low concentration application of fluoride toothpaste and/or mouthrinses.

Literature cited

1. Amjad Z, Nancollas GH. Effect of fluoride on the growth of hydroxyapatite and human dental enamel. Caries Res 1979; 13: 250-8.

2. Arends J, Jongebloed WL. Crystallite dimensions of enamel. J Biol Buccale 1979; 6: 161-71.

3. Arends J, Nelson DGA, Dijkman AG, Jongebloed WL. Effect of various fluorides on enamel structure and chemistry. In: Guggenheim B, ed. Cariology today. Basel: Karger 1984; 245-58.

4. Backer Dirks O. Posteruptive changes in dental enamel. J Dent Res 1966; 45: 503-11.

5. Brown WE. Physicochemical mechanisms of dental caries. J. Dent Res 1974; 53: 204-16.

6. Bruun C, Lambrou D, Larsen MJ, Fejerskov O, Thylstrup A. Fluoride in mixed human saliva after different topical fluoride treatment and possible relation to caries inhibition. Community Dent Oral Epidemiol 1982; 10: 124-9.

7. Cate JM ten, Duijsters PPE. Influence of fluoride in solution on tooth demineralization. I. Chemical data. Caries Res 1983; 17: 193-9.

8. Cate JM ten, Duijsters PPE. Influence of fluoride in solution on tooth demineralization. II. Microradiographic data. Caries Res 1983; 17: 513-9.

9. Cate JM ten, Arends J. Remineralization of artificial enamel lesions in vitro. Caries Res 1977; 11: 277-86.

10. Cate JM ten, Jongebloed WL, Arends J. Remineralization of artificial enamel lesions in vitro. IV. Caries Res 1981; 15: 60-9.

11. Cate JM ten, Duijsters PPE. Alternating demineralization and remineralization of artificial enamel lesions. Caries Res 1982; 16: 201-10.

12. Compiled from Curzon MEJ, Featherstone JDB. Chemical composition of enamel. In: Lazzari EP, ed. CRC handbook of experimental aspects of oral biochemistry. Boca Raton, FL: CRC Press 1983: 124, 126, 127.

13. Curzon MEJ, Cutress TW. Trace elements and dental disease. Bristol: J Wright 1983.

14. Dibdin GH. A brief survey of recent in vitro work on diffusion of small ions and molecules in dental plaque. In: Guggenheim B, ed. Cariology today. Basel: Karger 1984: 191-9.

15. Dijk JWE van, Borggreven JMPM, Driessens FCM. Chemical and mathematical simulation of caries. Caries Res 1979; 13: 169-80.

16. Driessens FCM. Mineral aspects of dentistry. Basel: Karger 1982; 14: 117.

17. Ericsson Y. The mechanism of monofluorophosphate action on hydroxyapatite and dental enamel. Acta Odont Scand 1963; 21: 341-58.

18. Featherstone JDB, Zero DT. Laboratory and human studies to elucidate the mechanism of action of fluoride-containing dentifrices. In: Embery G, Rölla G, eds. Clinical and biological aspects of dentifrices. Oxford: Medical Publications 1992: 41-50.

19. Featherstone JDB, Glena R, Shariati M, Shields CP. Dependence of in vitro demineralization of apatite and remineralization of dental enamel on fluoride concentration. J Dent Res 1990; 69(Spec Iss): 620-5.

20. Featherstone JDB. Diffusion phenomena and enamel caries development. In: Guggenheim B, ed. Cariology today. Basel: Karger 1984: 259-68.

21. Featherstone JDB, Shields CP, Khademazad B, Oldershaw MD. Acid reactivity of carbonated apatite with strontium and fluoride substitutions. J Dent Res 1983; 62: 1049-53.

22. Featherstone JDB, Cowles E. Fluoride diffusion through artificial lipid/protein/apatite membranes. Caries Res 1985; 19: 154 Abstract 3.

23. Friberger P. The effect of pH upon fluoride uptake in intact enamel. Scand J Dent Res 1975; 83: 339-44.

24. Gelhard TBFM, Arends J. In vivo remineralization of artificial subsurface lesions in human enamel I. J Biol Buccale 1984; 12: 49-57.

25. Groeneveld A. Over het werkingsmechanisme van fluoride in carieus glazuur. Ned Tandartsenbl 1976; 31: 299-304.

26. Hallsworth AS, Robinson C, Weatherell JA. Chemical pattern of carious attack. J Dent Res 1971; 50: 664.

27. Hargreaves JA, Thompson GW, Wagg BJ. Changes in caries prevalence of Isle of Lewis Children between 1971 and 1981. Caries Res 1983; 17: 554-9.

28. Ingram GS. Some factors affecting the interaction of hydroxyapatite with sodium monofluorophosphate. Caries Res 1973; 7: 315-23.

29. Jeansonne BG, Feagin FF. Fluoride action on acid resistance of unaltered human surface enamel. J Oral Path 1979; 8: 207-12.

30. Johnson MF. Comparative efficacy of NaF and SMFP dentifrices in caries prevention: a meta-analytic overview. Caries Res 1993; 27: 328-36.

31. Kalsbeek H. Evidence of decrease in prevalence of dental caries in The Netherlands. J Dent Res 1982; 61 (Spec Iss): 1321-6.

32. Kalter PGE, Flissebaalje TD, Groeneveld A. FLuoride retention in human enamel after a single phosphoric acid and mixed phosphoric acid/SnF_2 application in vitro. Arch Oral Biol 1980; 25: 15-8.

33. Koulourides T, Phantumvanit P, Munksgaard ED, Housch T. An intra-oral model used for studies of fluoride-incorporation in enamel. J Oral Pathol 1974; 3: 185-95.

34. Koulourides T, Cueto H, Pigman W. Rahardening of softened enamel surfaces on human teeth by solutions of calcium phosphate. Nature 1961; 189: 226.

35. Koulourides T, Feaging F, Pigman W. Remineralization of dental enamel by saliva in vitro. Ann N Y Acad Sci 1965; 131: 751-7.

36. Koutsoukos PG, Nancollas GH. Crystal growth of calcium phosphates – epitaxial considerations. J Crystal Growth 1981; 53: 10-9.

37. Larsen MJ. Dissolution of enamel. Scand J Dent Res 1973; 81: 518-22.

38. Larsen MJ, Fejerskov O. Surface etching and subsurface demineralization of dental enamel induced by a strong acid. Scand J Dent Res 1977; 85: 320-6.

39. Leverett DH, Proskin HM, Featherstone JDB et al. Caries risk assessment in a longitudinal discrimination study. J Dent Res 1993; 72: 538-43.

40. Manly RS, Harrington DP. Solution rate of tooth enamel in an acetate buffer. J Dent Res 1959; 38: 910-9.

41. Mellberg JR, Ripa LW. Fluorides in preventive dentistry. Chicago: Quintessence 1983: 44.

42. Moreno EC, Zahradnik RT. Chemistry of enamel subsurface demineralization in vitro. J Dent Res 1974; 53: 226-35.

43. Moreno EC, Brown WE, Osborn G. Stability of dicalcium phosphate dihydrate in aqueous solutions and solubility of octacalcium phosphate. Soil Sci 1960; 24: 99-102.

44. Mühlemann HR, Schmid H, König KG. Enamel solubility reduction with inorganic and organic fluorides. Helv Odontol Acta 1957; 1: 23-33.

45. Nelson DGA, Featherstone JDB, Dunvan JF, Cutress TW. Effect of carbonate and fluoride on the dissolution behavior of synthetic apatites. Caries Res 1983; 17: 200-11.

46. Odutuga AA, Prout RES. Lipid analysis of human enamel and dentine. Arch Oral Biol 1974; 19: 729-31.

47. Øgaard B, Cruz R, Rölla G. Fluoride dentifrices: a possible cariostatic mechanism. In: Embery G, Rölla G, eds. Clinical and biological aspects of dentifrices. Oxford: Medical Publications 1992: 305-12.

48. Øgaard B, Rölla G, Helgeland K. Uptake and retention of alkali-soluble and alkali-insoluble fluoride in sound enamel in vivo after mouthrinses with 0.05% or 0.2% NaF. Caries Res 1983; 17: 520-4.

49. Øgaard B, Rölla G, Helgeland K. Alkali-soluble and alkali-insoluble fluoride retention in demineralized enamel in vivo. Scand J Dent Res 1983; 91: 200-4.

50. Orams HJ, Zybert JJ, Phakey PP, Rachinger WA. Ultrastructural study of human dental enamel using selected area argon ion-beam thinning. Arch Oral Biol 1976; 21: 659-61.

51. Patel PR, Brown WE. Thermodynamic solubility product of human tooth enamel. J Dent Res 1975; 54: 728-36.

52. Poole DFG, Newman HN, Dibdin GH. Structure and porosity of human cervical enamel studied by polarizing microscopy and transmission electron microscopy. Arch Oral Biol 1981; 26: 977-82.

53. Sakkab NY, Cilley WA, Haberman JP. Fluoride in deciduous teeth from an anti-caries clinical study. J Dent Res 1984; 63: 1201-5.

54. Shariati M, Featherstone JDB, Shields CP, Holmen L, Thylstrup A. Inhibitory effect of fluoride and MHDP on enamel demineralization. J Dent Res 1985; 64: 364.

55. Silverstone LM. Remineralization and enamel caries: significance of fluoride and effect on crys-

tal diameters. In: Leach SA, Edgar WM, eds. Demineralization and remineralization of teeth. Oxford: IRL Press 1983: 185-205.

56. Silverstone LM, Wefel JS, Zimmerman BF, Clarkson BH, Featherstone MJ. Remineralization of natural and artificial lesions in human dental enamel in vitro. Caries Res 1981; 15: 138-57.

57. Speirs RL, Spinelli M, Brudevold F. Solution rate of hydroxyapatite in acetate buffer containing low concentrations of foreign ions. J Dent Res 1963; 42: 811-20.

58. Spinelli MA, Brudevold F, Moreno EC. Mechanism of fluoride uptake by hydroxyapatite. Arch Oral Biol 1971; 16: 187-203.

59. Weatherell JA, Deutsch D, Robinson C, Hallsworth AS. Assimilation of fluoride by enamel throughout the life of the tooth. Caries Res 1977; 11: 85-115.

60. Wei SHY, Forbes WC. Electron microprobe investigation of stannous fluoride reactions with enamel surfaces. J Dent Res 1974; 53: 51-6.

Section IV

CLINICAL USE OF FLUORIDES

CHAPTER 15

WATER FLUORIDATION

B.A. Burt • O. Fejerskov

Introduction – Discovery of fluoridated water's effects – Commentary on the 21 cities study
Pioneer fluoridation studies – World status of fluoridation – Caries prevention from water fluoridation
Partial exposure to fluoridated water – Economics of fluoridation
Water fluoridation as social policy – Summary

Introduction

Fluoridation is the controlled addition of a fluoride compound to a public water supply in order to raise the fluoride concentration to a predetermined level for the purpose of preventing dental caries. A related public health measure is defluoridation, the process of removing excess naturally-occurring fluoride from drinking water in order to reduce the prevalence and severity of dental fluorosis (or more severe skeletal disabilities when the fluoride concentration is very high).

Fluoridation reaches everyone in a community, a feature which is its greatest strength as a public health measure and its greatest limitation as social policy. Fluoridation is not a targeted approach to caries control, and support for it, or misgivings about it, are often a matter of social philosophy rather than science. Rational opposition to fluoridation today is usually on the grounds of lack of consumer choice, potential environmental issues, and concerns about the dental fluorosis that comes with fluoridation. Support for fluoridation is based on its demonstrated safety after some 50

years of use, the view that full community coverage is an advantage, and that the minor nature of the resulting dental fluorosis is of little consequence relative to the benefits of improved oral health for all. It is worth remembering that when fluoridation was first implemented some 50 years ago, a time of high prevalence and severity of caries, it was generally welcomed as a godsend.

This chapter considers the benefits and limitations of water fluoridation as a public health measure and social policy to control dental caries. The best place to begin is with a historical look at where fluoridation came from.

Discovery of fluoridated water's effects

In the early 1900s, Frederick McKay was a young dentist in Colorado Springs, USA. An observant man, he noticed that many of his patients had a form of enamel opacity that differed from the more commonly seen varieties. Locally it was known as "Colorado Brown

Stain," and was taken for granted by the residents. It seemed harmless enough, though it was disfiguring in some cases. Over the next few years, McKay's curiosity led him to investigate the condition further. He found Colorado Brown Stain highly prevalent in the district, but only among people who had been born in the area or who had moved there as babies. Since the stain was intrinsic, McKay reasoned that it must be caused by an environmental agent that was active during the period of enamel formation. McKay enlisted the collaboration of G.V. Black, a major figure in dental history, in writing the first description of what then came to be called mottled enamel.[13]

By the 1920s, McKay had reached the conclusion that the etiologic agent had to be an unidentified constituent of the water supply in some communities. In Oakley, Idaho, where the mottling was severe, McKay found that children living on the outskirts of the town, who drank water from a private spring, were free of mottling. Acting on his conclusion that the cause lay in the drinking water, he advised Oakley to abandon its existing water supply and tap this spring for a new source, which the community did in 1925. Children born in Oakley subsequently were free of mottled enamel.[61] In 1928, McKay published another of his observations, namely that caries experience was reduced by the same water that produced mottled enamel.[60] Ainsworth, in England, published a similar, but quite independent, observation soon afterwards.[1]

By 1931, new methods of spectrographic analysis led to the identification of fluoride in the drinking water from areas with endemic fluorosis, a discovery made independently in three different places at about the same time.[27,77,82] The immediate reaction was concern, because fluoride in high concentrations was known to be a protoplasmic poison. The discovery led to the appointment by the United States Public Health Service of a dentist, H. Trendley Dean, as a one-person unit to investigate the problem (this unit subsequently became the National Institute of Dental Research in 1948).

One of Dean's early steps was to develop a seven-point, ordinal-scale index of fluorosis,[29] based on the clinical appearance of the condition. The name "fluorosis" was in use by the mid-1930s.[34] Dean devised a weighted community index of fluorosis from his original seven grades of severity,[33] and later in the 1930s he condensed his original seven-point index to a six-point scale by combining the moderately severe and severe categories.[36] By 1942, Dean had mapped out the prevalence of fluorosis for most of the United States.[30]

Studies through the mid-1930s made extensive analyses of drinking waters for minerals and other chemical constituents, but none apart from fluoride could be related to fluorosis.[34,35] Dean had noted as early as the mid-1930s that mild or very mild fluorosis was found in some 12% of populations whose drinking water contained approximately 1.0 mg F/L.[35]

Dean is said to have noted quite early in his work that the milder forms of fluorosis were accompanied by lower-than-expected caries experience, and after the mid-1930s his research became more focused on the fluoride-caries relationship. He demonstrated that caries experience in 12-14-year-old children in Galesburg and Monmouth, Illinois, which received water with 1.8 mg F/L, was less than half of that seen in nearby Quincy and Monmouth, whose drinking waters containing 0.2 mg F/L.[38] He also noted that the low caries experience in Galesburg and Monmouth was accompanied by an unacceptably high level of dental fluorosis, and so he set out to define the water fluoride levels which represented the best compromise between low caries experience and a level of fluorosis which could be considered acceptable. This was done through a series of investigations which have become known collectively as the "21 Cities" study. The first part consisted of clinical data from children 12-14 years old with lifetime residence in eight suburban Chicago communities with various but stable mean water fluoride levels.[37] The project later added 13 additional communities in four other American states.[31]

The 21 Cities study was landmark epidemiology, and it led to the adoption of 1.0-1.2 mg F/L as the appropriate concentration of fluoride in drinking water for temperate climates in the United States. The results were strong presumptive evidence of cause-and-effect, though because the data were cross-sectional they could not by themselves establish cause-and-effect between fluoridated water and reduced caries experience. They did, however, set the stage for a prospective test of the fluoride-caries hypothesis, first suggested in 1943.[4] In January 1945, Grand Rapids, Michigan, became the first community to add fluoride to its municipal water supply.

Commentary on the 21 cities study

Since the results of Dean's 21 Cities study were the primary basis for the choice of 1.0 mg F/L as the optimum concentration for fluoridation, aspects of this study are worth examining in some detail. Fig. 15-1 shows the relationship between caries experience and dental fluorosis that Dean found in 12-14-year-old children in nine of the 21 cities whose water fluoride levels ranged from 0.2 to 1.3 mg/L. It can be seen that caries experience drops sharply toward 1.0-1.2 mg F/L and then tends to level out. (Dean presented his caries data as the number of teeth affected per 100 children; the DMF index had not yet been described. The mean DMFT values in Figs. 15-1 and 15-2 are derived by dividing Dean's original data by 100).

The dental fluorosis data in Fig. 15-1 is the prevalence of those with fluorosis of very mild or higher grades as Dean recorded it, but without those scored in his "Questionable" category. From these data, 1.0 mg F/L leads to substantial caries prevention, accompanied by some 12% prevalence of fluorosis, all of it in the mild to very mild categories. In this report, Dean stated that the fluorosis seen was "almost exclusively" on the later-erupting teeth, second molars and second premolars, and that "mottled enamel as an esthetic problem was not encountered."[37] Dean also said that because his index is based on the two most affected teeth in the mouth, the prevalence data overestimated the number of teeth affected. He gave as an example the 15% prevalence in Aurora, which affected only 5.1% of all erupted teeth.[37]

When the "Questionables" that Dean scored in these communities are added in, however, the picture changes to that shown in Fig. 15-2. In this Figure, caries experience has not changed, but if all fluorosis was to be minimized, regardless of severity, the trade-off between caries experience and fluorosis might be set at around 0.4 mg F/L. Adding to the interpretive difficulties of these data are the unexplained inconsistencies in the fluorosis data in both Figs. 15-1 and 15-2; Dean did not discuss why fluorosis prevalence in East Moline and Maywood, for example, was twice that seen in Aurora, despite similar water fluoride levels.

What is "Questionable" fluorosis? In the description of his original fluorosis index, Dean said that its diagnosis is "often a baffling problem,"[29] and gave a lengthy and rather discursive set of diagnostic criteria. In his subsequent, revised six-point index used in the 21 Cities study, the criteria for "Questionable" had been reduced to this description:

'The enamel discloses slight aberrations from the translucency of normal enamel, ranging from a few white flecks to occasional white spots. This classification is utilized in those instances where a definite diagnosis of the mildest form of fluorosis is not warranted and a classification of "normal" not justified.'[30]

An undertone of uncertainty can still be detected in these criteria, and one suspects that it stayed with Dean throughout his research. The

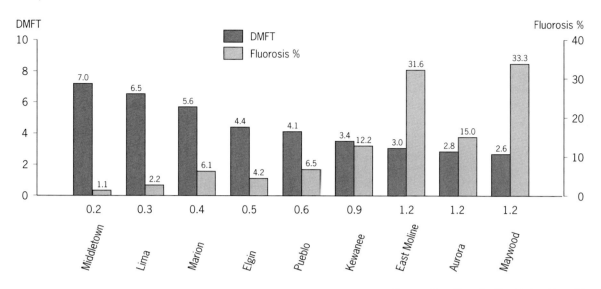

Fig. 15-1. Relation between mean dental caries experience and the prevalence of dental fluorosis among children aged 12-14 in nine of the 21 cities with water fluoride concentrations from 0.2 mg/L to 1.3 mg/L. Dean's "Questionable" diagnoses are excluded.[31,37]

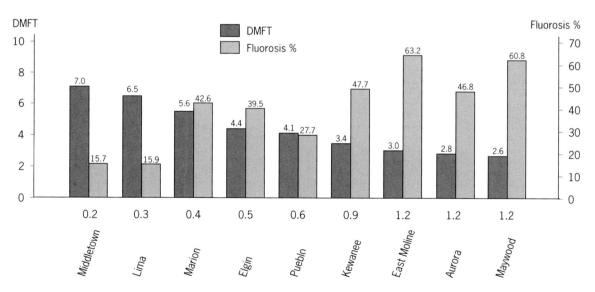

Fig. 15-2. Relation between mean dental caries experience and the prevalence of dental fluorosis among children aged 12-14 in nine of the 21 cities with water fluoride concentrations from 0.2 mg/L to 1.3 mg/L. Dean's "Questionable" diagnoses are included.[31,37]

"Questionables" were quite a large group in some of the 21 cities. In Kewanee, for example, with water containing 0.9 mg F/L, the fluorosis prevalence was listed by Dean as being 12.2% (10.6% very mild, 1.6% mild), but "Questionables" were 35%. In Marion, the prevalence of fluorosis was 6.1% (5.3% very mild, 0.8% mild), but the "Questionables" were 36.5%.[31] Dean seemed to accept that his questionable category was the earliest stages of fluorosis, for as early as 1934 he stated:

'Should an unusually large number of cases be classified as "Questionable" when, at the same time, a smaller percentage is likewise showing the milder forms of mottling of enamel, we are justified in assuming that we are dealing with what is probably a "borderline" area, an area where the causative factor in the mottling is present in the water supply quantitatively somewhere between the maximum harmless amount and the minimum amount capable of producing the very mild and the mild type of mottled enamel in from 40 to 50 percent of the children who have used the water in question exclusively from birth.'[29]

Dean's early speculations have been borne out by research since that time; Myers' 1983 review[69] showed that the prevalence of the questionable category was correlated with the fluoride concentration of the water supply. This dose-response relationship indicates that Dean's questionable category should be considered fluorosis, albeit of the very mildest manifestation.

Dean usually separated out the "Questionables" in his data tables, but with the passage of time it became common to quote only his prevalence data with very mild fluorosis as the lower boundary. By the time fluoridation was becoming social policy in the United States, the questionable category had largely come to be disregarded, because this level of fluorosis, only discernible under dental examination conditions and frequently unnoticed by affected individuals, was seen to be of little consequence when compared to severe dental caries. From our perspective of the 1990s it is hard to judge whether that approach was appropriate or not.

Some 50 years after the 21 cities study, we can now see that the choice of 1.0 mg F/L as the "optimum" concentration for fluoridated water was based on the view (implicitly rather than explicitly) that the dental caries of the day was a far greater problem than the milder levels of fluorosis. With the passage of time, the nature of the trade-off between caries and fluorosis that is inherent in the decision to fluoridate drinking water became lost, and 1.0 mg F/L often came to be seen as an absolute requirement for fluoridation. In the 1990s, however, the fact that the fluoridation decision involves this trade-off has come to be far better understood.

Pioneer fluoridation studies

Controlled fluoridation field trials began in 1945 in the United States and Canada. By that time research among people living in naturally fluoridated areas in the United States had established these facts:

- Any potential health hazards from long-term accumulation of fluoride, in areas where the fluoride level in drinking waters were low, were minimized by the healthy body's renal excretory mechanism.

- Ingested fluoride was partly deposited in bone and partly excreted.

- Although skeletal fluoride concentrations increased with age, skeletal damage could not be demonstrated in persons who ingested naturally fluoridated waters.

- Apart from dental fluorosis, no impairment to general health could be found among people who had drunk waters containing up to 8 mg F/L for long periods of time.

Table 15-1
Mean DMF teeth per child after 13-15 years of fluoridation in the four original North American fluoridation trials.
All trials began in 1945-46.

Community	Age-groups (years)	Year of study	Mean DMFT	Percent difference
Grand Rapids	12-14	1944-45	9.58	
	12-14	1959	4.26	55.5
Evanston	12-14	1946	9.03	
	12-14	1959	4.66	48.4
Brantford	12-14	1959	3.23	56.7
Sarnia (control)	12-14	1959	7.46	
Newburgh	13-14	1960	3.73	70.1
Kingston (control)	13-14	1960	12.46	

- People who drank water which contained fluoride at around 1.0 mg/L exhibited substantially less caries experience than did those who drank water with negligible concentrations of fluoride.

After the 21 Cities study, further work with fluoridation was held up by World War II. Four independent studies in controlled fluoridation were then begun in 1945 and 1946, in which the fluoride concentrations in the water supplies of the test communities were brought up from negligible to 1.0-1.2 mg/L. The purpose of these field trials was to test the hypothesis that addition of fluoride to low-concentration drinking waters would reduce caries experience. These original four studies were:

- Grand Rapids, Michigan, began in January 1945 with nearby Muskegon as the control city. This study was directed by Dean and his colleagues.[32]

- Newburgh, New York, began fluoridation in May 1945 with Kingston as the control city.[6]

- Evanston, Illinois, with Oak Park as control, began in 1946.[15]

- In Canada, the town of Brantford, Ontario, began in 1946 with Sarnia as the control. Naturally-fluoridated Stratford was also included in this study.[50]

At the end of terms ranging up to 15 years, caries experience was shown to be sharply reduced among children in each of the study populations, despite some differences in study design and examination criteria.[3,7,14,51] Results of these four pioneering studies are shown in Table 15-1. These studies also found that dental fluorosis occurred to about the same extent[8,75] as Dean had described earlier in areas of natural fluoridation,[30] namely, that some 12% of the children who grew up with water fluoridated at around 1.0 mg/L were found to have very mild to mild fluorosis.

If present-day standards of field trials are applied, all of these four studies appear rather crude. None were longitudinal, all used a sequential cross-sectional design. Sampling methods and dental examiners tended to vary from one year to the next,[2] thereby risking bias and unnecessary random error. Statistical analysis, by today's standards, was primitive, with potential confounders such as socioeconomic differences between test and control communities not factored in. Data from the control communities were not used in Grand Rapids and Evanston to compute the extent of caries reductions, with conclusions based on the weaker before-after analysis. But despite these departures from ideal design, the results were so striking and so consistent that they outweighed these design limitations, and can be taken collectively as evidence for fluoridation's effectiveness.

Among the early studies, the only true longitudinal study of fluoridation's effects was the Tiel-Culemborg study in the Netherlands.[11,12] Tiel was fluoridated in 1953, and successive cohorts of children were examined longitudinally every 2 years from the ages of 7 through 18 years until 1971. This study was rigorously controlled, more so than the original four North American studies. Even though the study was finished in 1971, subsequent data from it were analyzed a number of times down the years. The Tiel-Culemborg study has proved to be a valuable resource in the study of the effects of fluoride in general, and fluoridated water in particular.[48] It is interesting to note that in 1988, 15 years after fluoridation ceased in Tiel, Culemborg's caries experience was lower than Tiel's, even though DMF scores in Tiel that year were lower than they were when fluoridation was still operating in 1968.[54]

World status of fluoridation

There is no central agency which stores global information on water fluoridation projects. According to the most recent data from national dental associations and compiled by the Fédération Dentaire Internationale, in 1984 there were 34 countries reporting fluoridation projects reaching some 246 million people, not including naturally occurring fluoride in drinking waters.[46] While fluoridated water is used by over half of the populations of the United States, Canada, Ireland, Australia, and New Zealand, and by virtually everyone in the city-states of Singapore and Hong Kong, some of the 34 nations have only one community fluoridating, with little prospect of more. Ireland is the only nation to have a mandatory fluoridation law.

Fluoridation is not technically feasible for much of Asia and Africa because of the relative absence of municipal water systems there, and only sporadic fluoridation is found in Latin America. While fluoridation is technically feasible in Europe it is little used there outside Britain. There is no fluoridation at all in Germany, Austria, France, Belgium, Italy, Denmark, Sweden and Norway. The city of Basel, in Switzerland, has been fluoridated since 1962, but it has little company in central Europe. In Finland, Kuopio had been fluoridated for many years, but fluoridation ended there in 1992. In the Netherlands, the previously described Tiel-Culemborg fluoridation study is rightly considered a landmark, but despite that, all fluoridation in the Netherlands ceased in 1976.

Sweden had one successful experimental project in Norrkoping in the 1950s,[28] but in 1973 the Swedish parliament repealed the legislation allowing communities to fluoridate.[23] The matter was revived in 1981 when a commission appointed by the Swedish Ministry of Health and Social Affairs concluded that fluoridation was safe and effective, but it recommended no change in the law.[80]

Caries prevention from water fluoridation

There is an extensive literature on the effectiveness of water fluoridation, with studies carried out in many parts of the world. Most have been devoted to effects in children, but longer-term

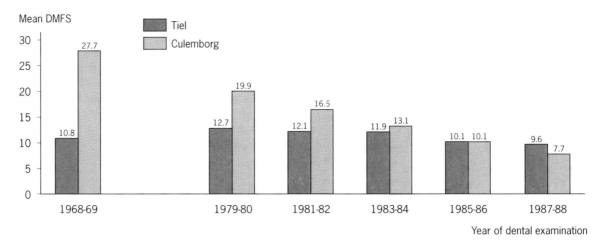

Fig. 15-3. Mean DMFS scores among 15-year-old children in Tiel and Culemborg, the Netherlands, in 1968-69 and subsequent years. Tiel ceased fluoridating in 1973.[54]

evidence is also available. Perhaps the most striking feature of these studies, which vary in the quality of their design and operation, has been the general uniformity of their results. A review of fluoridation studies among children prior to 1980, about the time that the caries decline first became fully appreciated, reported that 55 of 72 published studies found caries reductions in children's permanent teeth ranging from 40% to 70%.[68] In Britain, where fluoridated waters reach some 15% of the population, differences between fluoridated and non-fluoridated communities of around 50% are still found in both dentitions.[17,18,25,26,42,47,53,63,73] Children in fluoridated Dublin, Ireland, have DMF scores that are 45% lower than among children of the same age in non-fluoridated Glasgow, Scotland.[16]

In those countries where fluoridation is widespread, i.e. reaching more than half the population, differences in caries experience between children in fluoridated and non-fluoridated communities are now more commonly in the range of 18-35%.[19,52,70] This is clearly less

than the approximately 50% difference that was reported from the early studies, an apparent reduction that is likely to be due to the influence of fluoride coming from other sources. The use of fluoride toothpaste is almost universal in the industrialized countries, and in the highly-fluoridated countries there is also considerable indirect exposure to fluoride from food and beverages processed in fluoridated areas.[20] These latter forms of exposure are seen in all areas, whether fluoridated or not. Cariostatic effectiveness of fluoridated water also is shown in those communities where fluoridation started and stopped some years later. The outcomes have been described from three such communities in Scotland, one in Germany, and one in the USA.[10,39,57,58,79] In each instance a decline in caries was seen in young children after fluoridation began, but this decline was not continued after fluoridation stopped. Drinking water was the only substantial exposure to fluoride at the time of the studies. Perhaps the most striking example of what happens when fluoridation ceases comes from the

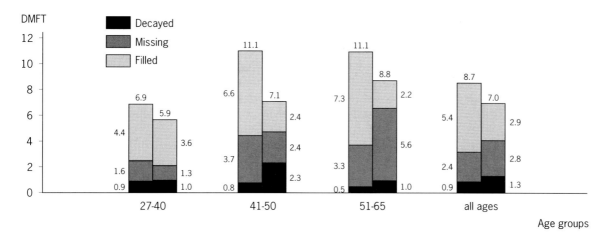

Fig. 15-4. Decayed, missing, and filled teeth in adults aged 27-65 in Deming (left-hand columns; 0.7 ppm F in drinking water) and Lordsburg (right-hand columns; 3.5 ppm F in drinking water), New Mexico, USA.[43]

Tiel-Culemborg study in the Netherlands, mentioned earlier as the site of a major longitudinal study during which Tiel was fluoridated at 1.0 mg F/L from 1953 to 1973. Fig. 15-3 shows the major difference between caries experience of 15-year-olds in the two communities that existed in 1968-69, after 15 years of fluoridation in Tiel, and then shows how these differences disappeared over subsequent years. The caries decline is evident in both communities, though far more pronounced in Culemborg.

Regarding the effect of fluoridation among adults, constant exposure to fluoridated water produces the positive effects that would be expected in light of current knowledge of how fluoride acts in the oral cavity (Chapter 10). Years ago, that close observer McKay noted that oral health was better in 45-year-old adults who drank fluoridated water than in those who did not.[62] Adults born and raised in naturally fluoridated Colorado Springs were found to have 60% lower mean DMF scores than their counterparts in low-fluoride Boulder.[76] Residents of Colorado Springs also had far fewer

teeth missing, and lower caries experience in all tooth-types was evident.[74,76] A similar profile was seen in adults from Aurora, Illinois, where the drinking water had naturally occurring fluoride at 1.2 mg/L in its drinking water,[44] and in a British study[64,65] of adults in Hartlepool (1.5-2.0 mg F/L at the time) and York (0.2 mg F/L). Both the Colorado Springs and the Aurora studies confined their results to permanent residents in order to assess lifetime effects of fluoridated water. In light of today's knowledge about fluoride's posteruptive cariostatic effects, it is a pity that purely posteruptive effects of fluoridated water were excluded from these studies.

Conclusions would also have been stronger in these three studies had they used multivariate analysis, or had they at least stratified the data to include the effects of potentially different socioeconomic status between the communities into the analyses. (In fairness, however, it has to be said that multivariate statistical techniques are far better developed today than they were in the early 1970s). However, a later study which did employ multivariate regression analysis with data from Lordsburg (3.5 mg F/L) and Deming (0.7 mg F/L), New Mexico, found tooth retention and caries experience to be better in Lordsburg, a lower socioeconomic status community. After controlling for other important variables, Deming adults had two more restored teeth per person than did those in Lordsburg, although fluorosis was naturally more severe in Lordsburg.[43] The DMFT data for these two communities are shown in Fig. 15-4.

Root caries prevalence is inversely proportional to the fluoride concentration of the drinking water.[22,78] Because virtually all industrialized countries have aging populations that keep more teeth than they used to, root caries is likely to become a greater treatment issue with the passage of years. Over a lifetime, fluoridation has been estimated to reduce coronal and root caries by about 20-40%,[70] though with today's multiple fluoride exposure, it is very difficult to attribute a degree of caries reduction to any particular form of fluoride provision.

Partial exposure to fluoridated water

In countries with extensive fluoridation, many people spend part of their lives in a fluoridated area and part in a non-fluoridated area. The evidence shows that partial exposure to fluoridation reduces caries experience proportional to the length of exposure.[7,21] A 4-year British study found a 27% lower caries incidence among children who were 12 years old when fluoridation began in their community, relative to the incidence in controls of the same age in non-fluoridated areas.[49] This well-conducted study clearly demonstrated the posteruptive effects of fluoride in the drinking water, and further evidence for weak preeruptive effects of fluoridated water has come from Okinawa and

Australia. In Okinawa, there was no difference in caries status among nursing students aged 18-22 years when those who had received fluoridated water only until 5-8 years of age (and none thereafter) were compared with those who had never received fluoridated water.[55] In Perth, Australia, the main factors associated with freedom from caries were early use of toothpaste and residence in a fluoridated area from 4 to 12 years of age, as opposed to birth to 4 years of age.[72]

Economics of fluoridation

It was stated at the beginning of this chapter that a major strength of water fluoridation, as a method of exposing a whole community to the benefits of fluoride, was its cost-effectiveness. The average annual cost of water fluoridation in the United States has been estimated as some 51 cents per person, though in any one community the range was from 12 cents to $5.41 per person.[71] Factors which influenced the per capita cost were determined to be:

- The size of the community: the bigger the population, the lower the per capita cost.

- The number of fluoride injection points required.

- The amount and type of equipment to be used.

- The amount and type of fluoride chemical used, its price, plus the cost of transportation and storage.

- Probably the expertise of water plant personnel.

The figures on fluoridation costs in USA were based on actual costs from water treatment plants, though of course they will soon become dated. Reviews of fluoridation costs in Europe have come from Kunzel[56] & Dowell,[40] and the subject was covered at a 1982 conference convened by the World Health Organization and the Fédération Dentaire Internationale.[66] These reviews all provided cost estimates for fluoridation that were low over a long period of time.

Perhaps more important than the actual costs of fluoridation were the estimates of its savings in treatment costs. The health economists at the 1989 Michigan workshop[71] concluded that water fluoridation was one of the very few public health measures to demonstrate true cost-savings: the measure actually saved more money than it cost to operate. Estimates from the workshop were that fluoridation cost $3.35 per carious surface saved, far less than the fee for any restoration.

Data on the cost-savings of fluoridation go back to the Newburgh-Kingston study, where initial dental care for 6-year-old children cost 58% less in fluoridated Newburgh than in non-fluoridated Kingston.[5] These savings came from fewer extractions needed, fewer restorations, and a smaller proportion of complex restorations. Similar findings came from British studies, which reported a 49% saving for children aged 4-5 years and 54% for children aged 11-12 years.[41,83] These savings were maintained even after the caries decline was recognized.[9,10]

These figures are impressive, but they do have to be kept in perspective. While it is clear, for example, that fluoridation reduces the costs of restorative care for children, its effect on costs of adult dental care is less clear. It could be argued, for example, that savings from childhood will be lost later because greater tooth retention will increase the need for periodontal and prosthetic treatment in later years. The greater the degree of tooth retention, the more that dental services are likely to be needed in the later years of life.[24] This line of argument applies only to monetary expenditures because the value of a healthy dentition throughout life will vary from one individual to another: virtually beyond price for some, of little consequence to others. On the other hand, since flu-

oride seems to reduce root caries experience, it could just as easily be argued that the savings seen in childhood are continued throughout life. The outcome of this argument will become clearer as today's generation of young adults with little caries grows older.

Another caveat concerns the provision of diagnostic and preventive services to children in a fluoridated area. If regular check-ups are routinely provided for many children who have little caries, these services will add to the treatment costs without providing many benefits. In an organized children's dental service where caries and the associated need for restorations are diminishing, diagnosis and prevention will assume a greater proportion of the cost of care if no adjustments are made for reduced need. In areas where dental needs are sharply reduced, new standards for the frequency of dental visits, and for services such as radiographs, topical fluoride applications, and sealants usually need to be established. In these instances, "reduced costs of care" usually means that fewer dental personnel are needed to maintain the same number of children in good dental health. But if dentists continue to see such children twice a year and apply the full battery of diagnostic and preventive services each time, the substantial savings in the cost of restorative treatment will be drastically reduced.

Water fluoridation as social policy

There is no doubt that water fluoridation is a highly effective means of reducing caries experience in a community, and it is equally clear that it is safe and presents no great technical difficulty when there are existing municipal water supplies. While it is just one of several methods of bringing fluoride exposure to a community, no other method can do this as economically or comprehensively when the infrastructure conditions are right (i.e. an exten-

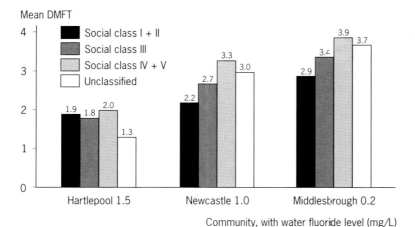

Fig. 15-5. Mean DMFT scores in 15-year-old children in three British communities with different water fluoride concentrations, stratified by four social class categories.[71]

sive water treatment system and people who drink the tap water, trained operators, availability of fluoride compounds). While socioeconomic status is a major determinant of caries experience, there is a smaller gradient in caries experience between socioeconomic groups in fluoridated areas than in those without fluoridation.[25,26,67,81] Fig. 15-5 shows that in naturally fluoridated Hartlepool (1.5-2.0 mg/L at the time), in Britain, there was virtually no difference in mean DMFT scores between the social classes, although some gradient was seen in Newcastle, with its water fluoridated at 1.0 mg/L, and in non-fluoridated Middlesbrough. (Newcastle had suffered considerable loss of fluoridation during the building of a new water treatment plant). Fluoridation reduces, though it does not eliminate, the social class gradient with caries, and it does this more cost-effectively than other fluoride methods. Where fluoridation is extensive in any one country, its effect on both caries and fluorosis is probably compounded because fluoride enters the food chain through the use of fluoridated water in processing foods and beverages.

The increase in fluorosis that has accompanied the caries decline in a number of countries has led to some rethinking of the role of fluorides in general, and of water fluoridation in particular. As one example, it has become clear that the guidelines developed years ago in the USA for the "optimum" concentration of fluoride in drinking water relative to ambient temperatures are too high for tropical regions.[59] Hong Kong has reduced its water fluoride levels on several occasions to its current level of 0.5 mg/L. This has been done because the fluorosis experience remained unacceptably high even with drinking water fluoridated at 0.6 to 0.8 mg/L.[45] In more temperate zones such moves have not yet been taken, but if fluorosis continues to increase, and particularly if mild and moderate forms of fluorosis become more prevalent, then it may have to be looked at carefully. Fluorosis would of course be more rationally controlled by reducing the extraneous sources of ingested fluoride, such as food and drink, inappropriate use of fluoride toothpaste in young children, and fluoride supplements. While that argument makes sense, political leaders may find it easier to reduce the level of fluoride in the drinking water. This would also reduce the "halo" effect, meaning the indirect effects of fluoridated water outside fluoridated areas through its use in processed foods and drinks. As an additional issue, if a community drinks water naturally fluoridated at, say, 0.4 mg/L, and is considering controlled fluoridation at 0.7 mg/L, then the cost-effectiveness of fluoridating at all would have to be examined carefully.

Whether to fluoridate or not comes down to the trade-off between caries and dental fluorosis. If there is a pressing need for caries control and a certain level of fluorosis can be tolerated, then water fluoridation is attractive policy because it is effective, cost-effective, and safe. If caries is seen as under control, and the tolerance for fluorosis is low, then it is not. Where the freedom-of-choice issue is not dominant, the future of water fluoridation as a measure for caries control will rest on how that balance is seen.

Summary

Fluoridation of public water supplies is a remarkably efficient method of controlling caries at the community level in economically developed countries. It grew, as a public health measure, from experiences some 50 or more years ago in naturally fluoridated areas where dental fluorosis was endemic and dental caries experience unusually low. Research since then has confirmed its status as a valuable public health measure in many countries. Its use results in reduced caries experience accompanied by some degree of fluorosis. Its main advantages, relative to other methods of using fluoride, are its cost-effectiveness, its continuing effects through life so long as individuals drink the water and the fact that it can benefit those members of the community who are hardest to reach through other public health programs.

Literature cited

1. Ainsworth NJ. Mottled teeth. Br Dent J 1933; 55: 233-50.

2. Arnold FA Jr, Dean HT, Knutson JW. Effect of fluoridated public water supplies on dental caries incidence. Results of the seventh year of study at Grand Rapids and Muskegon, Mich. Public Health Rep 1953; 68: 141-8.

3. Arnold FA Jr, Likins RC, Russell AL, Scott DB. Fifteenth year of the Grand Rapids fluoridation study. J Am Dent Assoc 1962; 65: 780-5.

4. Ast DB. The caries-fluorine hypothesis and a suggested study to test its application. Public Health Rep 1943; 58: 857-79.

5. Ast DB, Cons NC, Pollard ST, Garfinkel J. Time and cost factors to provide regular periodic dental care for children in a fluoridated and a non-fluoridated area: final report. J Am Dent Assoc 1970; 80: 770-6.

6. Ast DB, Finn SB, McCaffrey I. The Newburgh-Kingston caries-fluorine study. I. Dental findings after three years of water fluoridation. Am J Public Health 1950; 40: 716-24.

7. Ast DB, Fitzgerald B. Effectiveness of water fluoridation. J Am Dent Assoc 1962; 65: 581-8.

8. Ast DB, Smith DJ, Wachs B, Cantwell KT. The Newburgh-Kingston caries-fluorine study. XIV. Combined clinical and roentgenographic dental findings after ten years of fluoride experience. J Am Dent Assoc 1956; 52: 314-25.

9. Attwood D, Blinkhorn AS. Reassessment of the effect of fluoridation on cost of dental treatment among Scottish schoolchildren. Community Dent Oral Epidemiol 1989; 17: 79-82.

10. Attwood D, Blinkhorn AS. Dental health in schoolchildren 5 years after water fluoridation ceased in south-west Scotland. Int Dent J 1991; 41: 43-8.

11. Backer Dirks O. The relation between the fluoridation of water and dental caries experience. Int Dent J 1967; 17: 582-605.

12. Backer-Dirks O, Houwink B, Kwant GW. The results of 6-1/2 years of artificial drinking water in The Netherlands; the Tiel-Culemborg experiment. Arch Oral Biol 1961; 5: 284-300.

13. Black GV, McKay FS. Mottled teeth - an endemic developmental imperfection of the teeth heretofore unknown in the literature of dentistry. Dent Cosmos 1916; 58: 129-56.

14. Blayney JR, Hill IN. Fluorine and dental caries. J Am Dent Assoc 1967; 74 (Spec Iss): 233-302.

15. Blayney JR, Tucker WH. The Evanston dental caries study. J Dent Res 1948; 27: 279-86.

16. Blinkhorn AS, Attwood D, Gavin G, O'Hickey S. Joint epidemiological survey on dental health of 12-year-old school children in Dublin and Glasgow. Community Dent Oral Epidemiol 1992; 20: 307-8.

17. Booth JM, Mitropoulos CM, Worthington HV. A comparison between the dental health of 3-year-old children living in fluoridated Huddersfield and non-fluoridated Dewsbury in 1989. Community Dent Health 1992; 9: 151-7.

18. Bradnock G, Marchment MD, Anderson RJ. Social background, fluoridation and caries experience in a 5-year-old population in the West Midlands. Br Dent J 1984; 156: 127-31.

19. Brunelle JA, Carlos JP. Recent trends in dental caries in U.S. children and the effect of water fluoridation. J Dent Res 1990; 69 (Spec Iss): 723-7.

20. Burt BA. The changing patterns of systemic fluoride intake. J Dent Res 1992; 71: 1228-35.

21. Burt BA, Eklund SA, Loesche WJ. Dental benefits of limited exposure to fluoridated water in childhood. J Dent Res 1986; 61: 1322-5.

22. Burt BA, Ismail AI, Eklund SA. Root caries in an optimally fluoridated and a high fluoride community. J Dent Res 1986; 65: 1154-8.

23. Burt BA, Petterson EO. Fluoridation: developments in Sweden. Br Dent J 1972; 133: 57-9.

24. Burt BA, Warner KE. Prevention of oral disease; its potential for containing the cost of dental care. In: Kudrle RT, Meskin LH, eds. Opportunities for cost-containment in dentistry. Minneapolis, MN: University Minnesota Press 1980: 132-61.

25. Carmichael CL, French AD, Rugg-Gunn AJ, Furness JA. The relationship between social class and caries experience in five-year-old children in Newcastle and Northumberland after twelve years' fluoridation. Community Dent Health 1984; 1: 47-54.

26. Carmichael CL, Rugg-Gunn AJ, Ferrell RS. The relationship between fluoridation, social class and caries experience in 5-year-old children in Newcastle and Northumberland in 1987. Br Dent J 1989; 167: 57-61.

27. Churchill HV. Occurrence of fluorides in some waters of the United States. J Ind Eng Chem 1931; 23: 996-8.

28. Crisp P. Report of the Royal Commissioner into the fluoridation of public water supplies. Hobart, Australia. Government Printer, 1968: pp. 196-9.

29. Dean HT. Classification of mottled enamel diagnosis. J Am Dent Assoc 1934; 21: 1421-6.

30. Dean HT. The investigation of physiological effects by the epidemiological method. In: Moulton FR, ed. Fluorine and dental health. Washington, D.C.: American Association for the Advancement of Science 1942: 23-31.

31. Dean HT, Arnold FA Jr., Elvove E. Domestic water and dental caries. V. Additional studies of the relation of fluoride domestic waters to dental caries experience in 4,425 white children aged 12-14 years of 13 cities in 4 states. Public Health Rep 1942; 57: 1155-79.

32. Dean HT, Arnold FA Jr., Jay P, Knutson JW. Studies on mass control of dental caries through fluoridation of the public water supply. Public Health Rep 1950; 65: 1403-8.

33. Dean HT, Dixon RM, Cohen C. Mottled enamel in Texas. Public Health Rep 1935; 50: 424-42.

34. Dean HT, Elvove E. Studies on the minimal threshold of the dental sign of chronic endemic fluorosis (mottled enamel). Public Health Rep 1935; 50: 1719-29.

35. Dean HT, Elvove E. Further studies on the minimal threshold of chronic endemic dental fluorosis. Public Health Rep 1937; 52: 1249-64.

36. Dean HT, Elvove E, Poston RF. Mottled enamel in South Dakota. Public Health Rep 1939; 54: 212-28.

37. Dean HT, Jay P, Arnold FA Jr., Elvove E. Domestic water and dental caries. II. A study of 2,832 white children aged 12-14 years, of eight suburban Chicago communities, including L. acidophilus studies of 1,761 children. Public Health Rep 1941; 56: 761-92.

38. Dean HT, Jay P, Arnold FA Jr, McClure FJ, Elvove E. Domestic water and dental caries, including

certain epidemiological aspects of oral L. acidophilus. Public Health Rep 1939; 54: 862-88.

39. Department of Health and Social Security (Great Britain). The fluoridation studies in the United Kingdom and the results achieved after eleven years. London: Her Majesty's Stationery Office 1969: 33-44.

40. Dowell TB. The economics of fluoridation. Br Dent J 1976; 140: 103-6.

41. Downer MC, Blinkhorn AS, Attwood D. Effect of fluoridation on the cost of dental treatment among urban Scottish schoolchildren. Community Dent Oral Epidemiol 1981; 9: 112-6.

42. Duxbury JT, Lennon MA, Mitropoulos CM, Worthington HV. Differences in caries levels in 5-year-old children in Newcastle and North Manchester in 1985. Br Dent J 1987; 162: 457-8.

43. Eklund SA, Burt BA, Ismail AI, Calderone JJ. High-fluoride drinking water, fluorosis and dental caries in adults. J Am Dent Assoc 1987; 114: 324-8.

44. Englander HR, Wallace DA. Effects of naturally fluoridated water on dental caries in adults. Public Health Rep 1962; 77: 887-93.

45. Evans RW, Stamm JW. Dental fluorosis following downward adjustment of fluoride in drinking water. J Public Health Dent 1991; 51: 91-8.

46. Fédération Dentaire Internationale. Basic fact sheets. London: FDI 1987.

47. French AD, Carmichael CL, Rugg-Gunn AJ, Furness JA. Fluoridation and dental caries experience in 5-year-old children in Newcastle and Northumberland in 1981. Br Dent J 1984; 156: 54-7.

48. Groeneveld A, Van Eck AAMJ, Backer Dirks O. Fluoride in caries prevention: is the effect pre- or post-eruptive? J Dent Res 1990; 69 (Spec Issue): 751-5.

49. Hardwick JL, Teasdale J, Bloodworth G. Caries increments over 4 years in children aged 12 at the start of water fluoridation. Br Dent J 1982; 153: 217-22.

50. Hutton WL, Linscott BW, Williams DB. The Brantford fluorine experiment. Interim report after five years of water fluoridation. Canad J Public Health 1951; 42: 81-7.

51. Hutton WL, Linscott BW, Williams DB. Final report of local studies on water fluoridation in Brantford. Canad J Public Health 1956; 47: 89-92.

52. Ismail AI, Shoveller J, Langille D, MacInnis WA, McNally M. Should the drinking water of Truro, Nova Scotia, be fluoridated? Water fluoridation in the 1990s. Community Dent Oral Epidemiol 1993; 21: 118-25.

53. Jackson D, James PM, Thomas FD. Fluoridation in Anglesey 1983: a clinical study of dental caries. Br Dent J 1985; 158: 45-9.

54. Kalsbeek H, Kwant GW, Groeneveld A, Dirks OB, van Eck AA, Theuns HM. Caries experience of 15-year-old children in The Netherlands after discontinuation of water fluoridation. Caries Res 1993; 27: 201-5.

55. Kobayashi S, Kawasaki K, Takagi O, Nakamura M, Fujii N, Shinzato M, Maki Y, Takaesu Y. Caries experience in subjects 18-22 years of age after 13 years' discontinued water fluoridation in Okinawa. Community Dent Oral Epidemiol 1992; 20: 81-3.

56. Kunzel W. The cost and economic consequences of water fluoridation. Caries Res 1974; 8 (Suppl 1): 28-35.

57. Kunzel W. Effect of an interruption in water fluoridation on the caries prevalence of the primary and secondary dentition. Caries Res 1980; 14: 304-10.

58. Lemke CW, Doherty JM, Arra MC. Controlled fluoridation: the dental effects of discontinuation in Antigo, Wisconsin. J Am Dent Assoc 1970; 80: 782-6.

59. Manji F, Baelum V, Fejerskov O, Gemert W. Enamel changes in two low-fluoride areas in Kenya. Caries Res 1986; 20: 371-80.

60. McKay FS. The relation of mottled enamel to caries. J Am Dent Assoc 1928; 15: 1429-37.

61. McKay FS. Mottled enamel: the prevention of its further production through a change of water supply at Oakley, Idaho. J Am Dent Assoc 1933; 20: 1137-49.

62. McKay FS. Mass control of dental caries through the use of domestic water supplies containing fluorine. Am J Public Health 1948; 38: 828-32.

63. Mitropoulos CM, Lennon MA, Langford JW, Robinson DJ. Differences in dental caries experience in 14-year-old children in fluoridated South Birmingham and in Bolton in 1987. Br Dent J 1988; 164: 349-50.

64. Murray JJ. Adult dental health in fluoride and non-fluoride areas. Part 1. Mean DMF values by age. Br Dent J 1971; 131: 391-5.

65. Murray JJ. Adult dental health in fluoride and non-fluoride areas. Part 3. Tooth mortality by age. Br Dent J 1971; 131: 487-92.

66. Murray JJ, ed. Appropriate use of fluorides for human health. Geneva: WHO 1986.

67. Murray JJ, Breckon JA, Reynolds PJ, Tabari ED, Nunn JH. The effect of residence and social class on dental caries experience in 15-16-year-old children living in three towns (natural fluoride, adjusted fluoride and low fluoride) in the north east of England. Br Dent J 1991; 171: 319-22.

68. Murray JJ, Rugg-Gunn AJ, Jenkins GN. Fluorides in caries prevention. 3rd ed. London: Wright, 1992.

69. Myers HM. Dose-response relationship between water fluoride levels and the category of questionable dental fluorosis. Community Dent Oral Epidemiol 1983; 11: 109-12.

70. Newbrun E. Effectiveness of water fluoridation. J Public Health Dent 1989; 49 (Spec Issue): 279-89.

71. Results of the workshop. J Public Health Dent 1989; 49 (Spec Issue): 331-7.

72. Riordan PJ. Dental caries and fluoride exposure in Western Australia. J Dent Res 1991; 70: 1029-34.

73. Rugg-Gunn AJ, Carmichael CL, Ferrell RS. Effect of fluoridation and secular trend in caries in 5-year-old children living in Newcastle and Northumberland. Br Dent J 1988; 165: 359-64.

74. Russell AL. The inhibition of approximal caries in adults with lifelong fluoride exposure. J Dent Res 1953; 32: 138-43.

75. Russell AL. Dental fluorosis in Grand Rapids during the seventeeth year of fluoridation. J Am Dent Assoc 1962; 65: 608-12.

76. Russell AL, Elvove E. Domestic water and dental caries. VII. A study of the fluoride-dental caries relationship in an adult population. Public Health Rep 1951; 66: 1389-401.

77. Smith MC, Lantz EM, Smith HV. The cause of mottled enamel, a defect of human teeth. J Dent Res 1932 12:149-59. [Reprinted from: Tech Bull No 32. Tucson: University of Arizona College of Agriculture, 1931].

78. Stamm JS, Banting DW, Imrey PB. Adult root caries survey of two similar communities with contrasting natural fluoride levels. J Am Dent Assoc 1990; 120: 143-9.

79. Stephen KW, McCall DR, Tullis, JI. Caries prevalence in northern Scotland before, and 5 years after, water fluoridation. Br Dent J 1987; 163: 324-6.

80. Swedish Ministry of Health and Social Affairs. The use of fluoride in dental caries prevention; summary of a report by the Swedish Fluoride Commission. Stockholm: Ministry of Health and Social Affairs, 1981.

81. Treasure ET, Dever JG. The prevalence of caries in 5-year-old children living in fluoridated and non-fluoridated communities in New Zealand. N Z Dent J 1992; 88: 9-13.

82. Velu H, Balozet L. Darmous (dystrophic dentaire) du mouton et solubilité du principe actif des phosphates naturels qui le provique. Bull Soc Path Exot 1931; 24: 848-51.

83. Whittle JG, Downer MC. Dental health and treatment needs of Birmingham and Salford school children. Br Dent J 1979; 147: 67-71.

FLUORIDE TABLETS, SALT FLUORIDATION, AND MILK FLUORIDATION

B.A. Burt • T.M. Marthaler

Introduction – Fluoride tablets – Salt fluoridation – Milk fluoridation – Summary

Introduction

When water fluoridation was first introduced in the mid-1940s it was assumed that fluoride produced most of its cariostatic effects through preeruptive effects. Ingestion of fluoride in the early years of life was thus considered essential for the full benefits of fluoride to be realized, and the earlier in life this ingestion started, the more complete the benefits. It was natural, therefore, that alternative means of ingesting fluoride by infants and young children would be sought for those children who did not receive fluoridated water.

Scientific evidence now favors the primacy of fluoride's posteruptive effects in cariostasis, which has led to a rethinking of the "systemic" benefits of fluoride. This chapter reviews three means of providing ingestable fluoride which were originally developed to provide preeruptive benefits. One of them clearly still has a place in caries prevention in the modern world, while the other two have a more limited application.

Fluoride tablets

Fluoride dietary supplements were first introduced in the late 1940s, and were intended as a substitute for fluoridated water for children in non-fluoridated areas. Because they are manufactured as (a) tablets or drops, intended to be swallowed (some drops are in fluoride-vitamin combinations for infants); (b) tablets for chewing; or (c) lozenges intended to be sucked slowly or permitted to dissolve slowly in the mouth, the term "supplements" is used to refer generically to all forms.

Supplements contain a measured amount of fluoride, typically 0.25 mg, 0.5 mg, or 1.0 mg, usually as sodium fluoride, but sometimes as acidulated phosphate fluoride, potassium fluoride, or calcium fluoride. They were, and still are, intended for use only in areas where there is little or no fluoride in the drinking water, and where there is no other intentional use of ingested fluoride. There are few data on the extent to which these products are used, but they are known to have widespread use as a caries

Table 16-1
Recommended fluoride tablet schedules (mg F/day) for four countries in Europe

				Year of life			
	0-1*	1-2	2-3	3-4	4-5	5-6	6+
France	0.25	0.25	0.5	0.5	0.75	0.75	1.0
Switzerland	0.25	0.25	0.5	0.5	0.75	0.75	1.0
Germany	0.25	0.25	0.5	0.75	0.75	0.75	1.0
Austria	0.25	0.25	0.5	0.5	0.75	1.0	1.0

*In Switzerland and Austria, intake is recommended to start at 6 months, at birth in France and Germany.

preventive for children. In many countries, supplements are available only on prescription, though others permit over-the-counter sales. In some countries they were, and still are in some cases, distributed to children through public health programs.

Rationale for fluoride supplements

Supplements were introduced at a time when it was assumed that fluoride's cariostatic effects were principally preeruptive. A 1958 report from the American Dental Association, for example, stated unequivocally that prescription fluorides were not beneficial to adults. In that same report, the directions for use of supplements with children, in low water-fluoride areas, were that a 1.0 mg fluoride tablet should be dissolved in a quart (0.95 L) of water used for drinking purposes and food preparation for children up to 2 years old. For children between 2 and 3 years, a tablet (1.0 mg fluoride) was to be administered every other day in fruit juice or water to be consumed at one time. After 3 years of age, the recommendation was that the tablet be administered daily in fruit juice or water to be drunk at one time.[4]

Although the primacy of fluoride's posteruptive cariostatic effects has evolved in more recent years, recommended schedules for supplement use in many countries have been slow to respond to this change. Table 16-1, for example, shows the schedule for supplement use in four European countries at the end of 1993. Table 16-2 shows the schedule recommended by the American Dental Association from the mid-1970s until its modification in 1994, a perusal of which will show that it differs little from the 1958 recommendations mentioned earlier.

As will be discussed, the posteruptive efficacy of fluoride supplements has been demonstrated with school-age children, though the original rationale for their use, i.e. preeruptive uptake by developing enamel to form a "more resistant" tooth, is no longer tenable.

Efficacy of fluoride supplements in infants

Some of the earliest studies on the efficacy of fluoride supplements among infants were conducted in eastern Europe, and were summarized, favorably for the most part, in extensive reviews in the 1970s.[9,23] While it is recognized that good clinical trials in an infant population are inherently difficult, some of these studies were flawed to the extent that their results are questionable. Flaws included the use of selected groups of participants rather than random allocation, the absence of concurrent controls, non-blinded examiners, and severe attrition of participants. The conclusions from

Table 16-2
Fluoride supplement schedule (mg F/day) recommended by the American Dental Association from 1976 to 1994.
(now superseded, see Table 16-4)

Age	Fluoride concentration in drinking water (mg/L)		
	< 0.3	0.3-0.7	> 0.7
0-2 years	0.25	0	0
2-3 years	0.5	0.25	0
3-16 years	1.0	0.5	0

these reviews, that supplements led to caries reductions of 50-80% in the primary dentition and 20-40% in the permanent dentition when used from birth, are likely to overestimate efficacy. Several widely quoted studies in the United States also had design flaws that were serious enough to cast doubt on the results.[1,5,46]

Many dentists around the world hold firm beliefs about the value of fluoride supplements ingested from birth. As examples, the American Dental Association recommendations that supplements be taken from birth[24,27] remained in place until 1994, and France has not altered the supplement schedule shown in Table 16-1 despite the increasing availability of fluoridated salt. But the evidence to support the use of supplements from birth is clearly thin. If it is assumed that there is little preeruptive efficacy, a reasonable choice for supplement use is to start no earlier than the eruption of the primary molars, or during the third year of life.

Posteruptive efficacy of fluoride supplements
Well-conducted clinical trials have shown that fluoride supplements provide posteruptive cariostasis in school-age children. American studies in which the supplements were chewed, swished and swallowed by schoolchildren under supervision have reported caries reductions of 20-28% over 3-6 years.[22,26] Concurrent controls, placebos, and double-

blind conditions were part of the design of these studies. Caries reductions were higher for those teeth erupting during the period of the study, and in one of these studies, beneficial effects were still discernible 4 years later.[25] More spectacular results, an 81.3% reduction in caries incidence, were reported from a study in Glasgow, Scotland, in which children initially aged 5.5 years from lower socioeconomic groups sucked a 1.0 mg fluoride tablet, or a placebo, under supervision in schools every school day for 3 years.[81] The benefits were almost all seen in the erupting permanent first molars.

The results from retrospective analyses of supplement use provide weaker evidence than do clinical trials, and results of such studies have been mixed. Positive results from the use of supplements have been reported from Britain, New Zealand, The Netherlands, Australia, Switzerland, and Sweden.[2,19,21,33,48,92,93] Retrospective studies are easily biased by self-selection of supplement users, and such bias was evident in all of these studies. The problem that arises is that cause-and-effect cannot be judged. The favorable results may have come from use of the supplements, or they may have been seen anyway because of the dental awareness of the families choosing to use supplements. Even with the biasing effects of self-selection, there are other evaluatory studies which found no difference in caries experience between those children who reported using fluoride supplements and those who did not.[7,36,40,42,85]

There have been well-conducted clinical trials in which fluoride supplements were tested in combination with other fluoride therapies in school-based studies. Driscoll and colleagues[28] found that supplements used with the swish-and-swallow procedure over 8 years, gave slightly better results than fluoride mouthrinsing, though caries increments in all study groups were small. In Scotland, no difference in caries incidence could be found over 6 years between three groups of children using fluoride supplements, mouthrinse, and combinations of both with placebos.[82] A Swedish study comparing supplements, fluoride toothpaste, and fluoride varnish could find no difference between the groups.[70]

Evidence for the efficacy of any preventive procedure should come, as far as possible, from clinical trials which meet specific criteria for quality. Only a handful of fluoride supplement trials meet these standards. The evidence from these trials is that supplements are effective when used with school-age children, and when the supplement was used topically by chewing or permitting slow dissolution in the mouth. There is little satisfactory evidence for the efficacy of fluoride supplements when used from birth or early infancy.

Supplements and risk of fluorosis

What has come to be called the "critical period" for the development of fluorosis is the late secretion-early maturation period of preeruptive dental enamel. While fluorosis can develop at any stage of preeruptive development under certain conditions, in this critical period the developing enamel is especially sensitive to ingested fluoride.[20,32,45]

There have been some reports in which no association could be found between supplement use and the development of fluorosis.[7,83] The fluorosis found among the 322 children in one of these studies[83] was attributed to the swallowing of fluoride toothpaste rather than to the supplements. On the other hand, there is a substantial literature in which fluorosis has been associated with supplement use.[1,18,19,21,40,42,44,73,84,85,95,96] A number of case studies have also been reported on fluorosis among patients who ingested 0.5 mg or 1.0 mg fluoride supplements daily from infancy.[14,63,67]

Probably the strongest evidence to show that fluoride supplements are a risk factor for fluorosis, especially when ingested during the critical period of late secretion-early maturation, came from the case-control study of Pendrys & Katz.[68] Taken together, the evidence is clear that fluoride supplements, when ingested prior to tooth eruption, are a risk factor for dental fluorosis.

Intake of fluoride from all sources

The problem of ingested fluoride from multiple sources in the early years of life compounds the fluorosis problem. The amount of fluoride in early childhood which would lead to fluorosis was originally estimated to be 0.1 mg F/kg body weight/day.[35] Since then this estimate has been revised downward, with 0.03 F/kg body weight/day being the lowest limit suggested.[34] One report concluded that intakes around this level caused a "surprisingly high" severity of fluorosis in Kenyan children.[6]

At a time when the preeruptive intake of fluoride was considered the primary mode of fluoride action, the ingestion of fluoride in the range 0.05-0.07 mg F/kg body weight/day was considered "optimal" for preeruptive caries prevention.[66] In light of present knowledge that preeruptive fluoride has little preventive effect, this range has better application as an estimate of the maximum amount to be ingested by young children if fluorosis is to be kept to its lowest level. In modern North American conditions, when fluoride is being ingested from a number of sources (much of it inadvertent), it is likely that many young children are ingesting 0.4-0.6 mg F/day from foods,

Table 16-3

Fluoride supplement schedule (mg F/day) adopted by the Canadian Dental Association, 1992

Age	Fluoride concentration in drinking water 0.3 mg/L*
Birth-3 years	0
3-6 years	0.25
6+ years	1.0

* Supplements are not recommended when drinking water contains 0.3 mg F/L or more.

Table 16-4

Fluoride supplement schedule (mg F/day) recommended by the American Dental Association, 1994

Age	Fluoride concentration in drinking water (mg/L)		
	< 0.3	0.3-0.6	> 0.6
6 months-3 years	0.25	0	0
3-6 years	0.5	0.25	0
6-16 years	1.0	0.5	0

beverages, and toothpaste.[10] In some parts of Europe a similar situation may exists, for while the children may be ingesting less fluoride from food and drink because of the absence of fluoridated water in food processing, they may be getting more fluoride from high-concentration toothpastes, which are more common in Europe than in North America. Where 0.4-0.6 mg F/day is being ingested by a child under 3 years of age, regardless of the source of the fluoride, it is likely to be enough to cause fluorosis. Adding more fluoride from a supplement would only make the problem worse while adding no cariostatic benefits. When considering the risk:benefits of fluoride supplements, total

fluoride ingestion from all sources must be borne in mind.

Now that the problem of fluoride intake from multiple sources is generally recognized, there have been a number of recommendations for sharply-reduced fluoride supplement schedules in recent years. A group from the European Community (EC) in 1991 recommended that a supplement of 0.5 mg F should be used only for "at-risk" individuals from the age of 3 years on, and that supplements had no place as a public health measure.[13] These recommendations, however, cannot be enforced by the EC and individual countries still use their own schedules, as shown in Table 1. Canada decided in 1992 to retain a supplement schedule only for use in high-risk children (acknowledging that the definition of high-risk is elusive but leaving it to clinicians' judgment). This schedule is shown in Table 16-3, and like the European recommendations it does not advocate beginning supplements under the age of 3 years. In 1994, the American Dental Association recommended a reduced schedule for use in the USA – this schedule is shown in Table 16-4. Recommendations for change have also been made for Australia[71] and for Switzerland, where fluoridated salt is nationally available.[47]

Are fluoride supplements appropriate for caries prevention?

Fluoride supplements were introduced at a time when fluoridated water was the only source of fluoride. They predated fluoride toothpaste, mouthrinses and the widescale use of high-concentration gels. They also preceded the presence of fluoride in processed food and beverages in highly fluoridated countries. In view of the multiple sources of fluoride in the developed countries today, routine supplement use is likely to be inappropriate for most children. The argument is essentially one of risk:benefits: fluoride has little preeruptive impact on caries prevention, but presents a clear risk of fluorosis. Fluoride supplements, when ingested for a preeruptive effect by infants and young children, therefore carry more risk than benefit for children in countries where fluoride toothpastes and other topical fluorides are widely used.

Most fluorosis seen when young children use supplements is of the mildest variety, which many dentists claim is of no public health significance. These arguments date back to Dean's development of the Community Fluorosis Index (CFI), and his footnote that a CFI below 0.6 did not constitute a public health problem. [15] This personal view of Dean's may have been correct during the 1930s, when social deprivation and severe caries were common, but it may not be applicable in modern conditions, and it can be dangerous for dental professionals to make judgments as to what is or is not esthetic. There is now evidence that the public may be more aware of very mild fluorosis than had previously been imagined.[12,72,83]

It is possible that slow-dissolution fluoride lozenges may find a role in caries control in older children and adults, persons for whom the risk of enamel fluorosis is no longer present. The intent is that the supplements will help maintain levels of fluoride in the oral cavity, a goal which is the basis of fluoride use in caries prevention. The benefit of fluoride supplements used in this way still remains to be tested, and there are other existing methods, mostly through fluoride in the drinking water and in toothpaste, of maintaining the fluoride level in the oral cavity. Fluoride supplements are inappropriate for public health use in most countries, and if used at all should be restricted to individual patients older than 7 years with severe caries.

Salt fluoridation

Salt fluoridation is the controlled addition of fluoride, usually as sodium or potassium fluoride, during the manufacture of salt for human consumption. As mentioned earlier, when salt fluoridation was first adopted in Switzerland in the early 1950s, the prevailing view was that ingestion of fluoride was necessary for cariostatic effects. With the current acceptance of fluoride's essentially topical effects, fluoridated salt controls caries through helping to maintain a constant, low level of fluoride in the intraoral environment. The more that the various sources of salt contain fluoride (i.e. salt for domestic use, salt used in restaurants, bakeries, food processing, and other institutional food providers such as hospitals), the more effectively will the ambient levels of intraoral fluoride be maintained and the more effective will fluoridated salt be in caries control.

Fluoridated salt as a means of preventing caries was first suggested by Wespi,[89,90] who was actually a gynecologist. Wespi had firsthand knowledge of the success of iodized salt, which had been initiated in Switzerland in 1922 to prevent goiter, an endemic condition in many parts of the Alpine region through the first half of this century. Aided by his reputation as an expert on iodized salt and with a strong commitment to public health, Wespi suggested to the Board of Cantonal Health Directors in Switzerland that fluoride should join iodine as a salt additive. The Canton of Zurich was the first to act on this suggestion, and authorized the sale of fluoridated domestic salt in 1955. This salt contained 90 mg F/kg, and was prepared by Switzerland's constitutional monopoly salt producer. Most other cantons followed Zurich's lead within 10 years, and as early as 1966 the sales figures showed that fluoridated salt accounted for 65% of the domestic salt market.

In 1970 the Canton of Vaud, in western (French-speaking) Switzerland, began its manufacture of fluoridated salt at 250 mg F/kg. This concentration had been suggested by Wespi and by Muhlemann,[64] because earlier

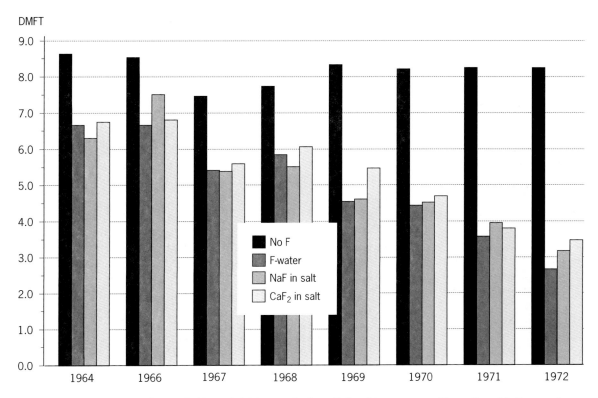

Fig. 16-1. Mean DMF teeth per child aged 6-14 years in four Colombian towns with no fluoridation, water fluoridation or salt fluoridation. The fluoridation programs began in Summer 1965. Source: Gillespie & Roviralta[37]

research[54] had shown that the initial concentration (90 mg F/kg) was too low for the most effective cariostasis. Vaud went even further, and required the bulk salt delivered to bakeries, restaurants, hospitals, and other institutions providing food to contain 250 mg F/kg. This was in addition to the existing program of fluoridating all domestic salt.

By 1983, the initial concentration of 90 mg F/kg was raised to 250 mg F/kg for salt distributed everywhere in Switzerland except for the Canton of Basel, which has had fluoridated water since 1962. Other countries have since followed Switzerland's lead and adopted salt fluoridation: France in 1986, Germany in 1991,

Costa Rica and Jamaica in 1987. This list is likely to grow since other countries are considering the measure.

Effectiveness of fluoridated salt

In 1960, evaluations of salt fluoridation in the Canton of Zurich (90 mg F/kg at the time) found that children from families reporting use of fluoridated salt, when compared to children whose families reported not using it, had significantly lower caries prevalence.[51,54] The World Health Organization soon became interested in salt fluoridation as a method of caries control in third world countries, and in collaboration with the National Institute of Dental Research

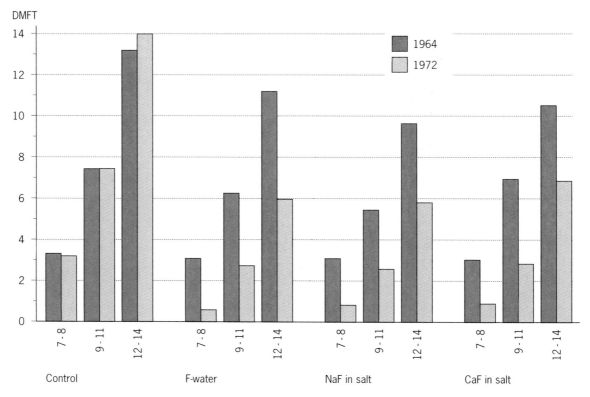

Fig. 16-2. Mean DMF teeth per child in the four Colombian towns with no fluoridation, water fluoridation, or salt fluoridation in 1964 and 1972. Children's agegroups were 7-8, 9-11, and 12-14. Source: Gillespie & Roviralta[37]

in the United States promoted trials of the procedure in Colombia, beginning in 1965.[37,52] In these trials, three Colombian towns adopted a fluoride regimen; two of them introduced fluoridated salt at 200 mg F/kg and the third fluoridated its drinking water. A fourth town with no fluoride regimen was included in the study as a control. After 7 years, DMFT scores in children fell in all three towns using the fluoride regimens, while they remained unchanged in the control community. These results are depicted in Fig. 16-1. Fig. 16-2 shows the caries reductions for three different agegroups over the same period. It can be seen that there were substantial benefits even among the

12-14-year-olds, who were 5-7 years old when the fluoride programs started.

Studies with fluoridated salt also began in four Hungarian communities in the mid-1960s, originally using salt fluoridated at 200-250 mg F/kg and later salt with 350 mg F/kg. Three other comparison villages were included in these trials; no village had drinking water with fluoride above 0.2 mg/L.[86] Clear though the results were (Tables 16-5 and 16-6), it was of interest that after 10 years of salt fluoridation, the caries experience of children in the test villages was still not as favorable as that in a comparable Hungarian town where drinking water is naturally fluoridated at 1.0 mg/L. Adults

Table 16-5
Mean DMFT in young adults of Deszk, Hungary, 250 mg F/kg in the domestic salt, 1966-1981 (Toth[86])

	Age 15-20	Age 21-25	Age 26-30
1966	10.73	17.00	18.84
1971	11.80	15.26	17.50
1979	7.56	11.20	15.84
Difference 1971-1979	4.24	4.06	
Confidence limits	2.0-6.4	1.1-7.1	
Reduction 1971-79	36%	27%	

Table 16-6
Mean dmft (age 5-6) and DMFT (age 13-14) per child in the Hungarian salt fluoridation trials, 1982 (Toth[86])

	Age 5-6		Age 13-14	
	n	Mean	n	Mean
Fluoridated Salt				
1966	19	6.78	47	8.21
1982	91	3.16	78	3.29
Control				
1982	52	6.70	73	10.27
Percent reduction 1982	53%		68%	

were examined in one of the test villages in 1966, 1971 and 1979. There was a slight decrease in mean DMFT scores from 1966 to 1971, and more noticeable decreases from 1971 to 1979.[86] These data are shown in Table 16-5, though they would have been of more value if caries had been studied among adults in the control communities.

Because Toth's studies in Hungary found that average discretionary salt consumption of persons aged 7 to over more than 60 was 3.34 g/person/day, all test communities in the Hungarian studies were provided with salt containing 350 mg F/kg after 1981. The last available Hungarian data were collected in 1982-83,[86] and are summarized for children in Table 16-6. By 1982, it can be seen that children aged 12-14 years in the control communities averaged 10.3 DMF teeth, while those in the villages with fluoridated salt averaged only 3.3 DMF teeth.

In Switzerland, studies with salt containing 250 mg F/kg began in 1970 in the Canton of Vaud and in 1974 in the eastern Canton of Glarus. At this time, the generalized decline in caries experience among children was already

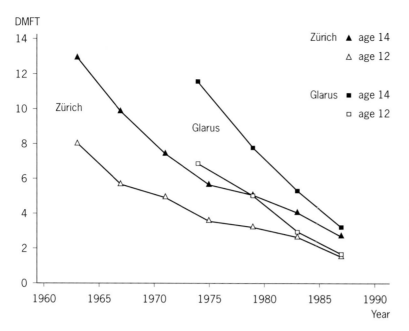

Fig. 16-3. Mean DMF teeth per child aged 12 or 14 in the Canton of Zurich 1963-87 and in the Canton of Glarus 1974-87. Glarus uses fluoridated salt in households and in bakeries. Source: Marthaler et al [56]; Steiner et al.[78,79]

detectable,[49,50,58] and this complicated the interpretation of the Swiss results. However, mean caries scores from the Vaud schoolchildren examined every 4 years since 1970 were consistently lower than those from the two adjacent control cantons.[16,17,57]

The caries decline in the Canton of Glarus has been particularly steep since the introduction of fluoridated salt. It is likely that fluoridated salt has played a part in this decline, though cause-and-effect relationships cannot be concluded from the observational data. Both domestic salt and salt for bakeries (but not other institutions) in Glarus has contained 250 mg F/kg since 1975-76. Fluoride toothpaste was reported to be used regularly in 1974 by 45% of the examined children and intermittently by 37%,[79] compared with the 67% (estimated from sales figures) of all Swiss people at that time. By 1987 the use of fluoride toothpaste among Glarus children was up to 93%, close to the Swiss average. The school-based program

of brushing with a fluoride gel (12,500 mg F/L) six times per year, common in Switzerland since 1970, started in Glarus only in 1982 and reached fewer than half the schools under study.

During the period from the first introduction of fluoridated salt in the Canton of Glarus in 1974 up to 1983, mean DMFT scores in 14-year-old children dropped 53%.[78,79] This rate of decrease is faster than that seen in the first 10 years of water fluoridation in Basel,[38] and was also faster than that seen in the Canton of Zurich, where the school-based fluoride toothbrushing program has been carried out regularly since 1963. The caries declines in Glarus and Zurich are compared in Fig. 16-3. The marked reduction among the Glarus children can be attributed largely to the effects of fluoride in toothpaste, salt, and probably other environmental sources. While the precise role of any one form of fluoride cannot be stated, it is likely that the steeper decline in Glarus, com-

Table 16-7
DMF experience and gingival bleeding in 20-year-old Swiss military recruits, 1985 (Menghini et al.[62])

	n	DMFT	DFSr*	Bleeding**
Western Switzerland				
Without salt fluoridation	153	10.2	7.7	1.7
Fluoridated salt since age 5 (Canton of Vaud)	56	7.1	4.8	1.7
Northern Switzerland, salt fluoridation only since 1983				
Little or no prevention	342	11.0	9.7	1.2
With prevention***	87	9.8	8.3	1.0

*   DFSr: mean DF approximal surfaces per recruit on lateral bitewing radiographs;
the radiolucencies limited to the enamel not included.

**   Bleeding: mean number of bleeding gingival units of six which were probed gently,
located on the right molars and incisors.

*** Prevention was based on six toothbrushing exercises per year at school with a fluoride product,
and dental health education. These school-based programs reached children from age 5 or 6 up to the age of 12-15; the
low fluoride salt (only 90 ppm F until 1983) had little effect on caries experience in Northern Switzerland.

pared to Zurich, is at least partly a result of the use of fluoridated salt in bakeries as well as in domestic salt.

Distribution of fluoride tablets ended in Swiss schools in 1983 with the universal introduction of fluoridated salt, but caries experience has continued to decline among schoolchildren since then.[50,55,60,79] Further evidence for the efficacy of fluoridated salt came from examinations of 20-year-old Swiss military recruits in 1985,[62] summarized in Table 16-7. Those from the Canton of Vaud, where both domestic and institutional salt has contained 250 mg F/kg since 1970, had considerably lower mean DMFT scores than did those from other parts of French-speaking Switzerland.

The evidence for the efficacy of salt fluoridation is thus based on a limited number of field trials and observational studies. Like water fluoridation, the nature of the procedure does not lend itself to randomized, double-blind clinical trials. While the field trial design (i.e. where a whole community knowingly adopts a procedure) is scientifically weaker than a clinical trial, the evidence for salt fluoridation is consistent and plausible.

Individual choice or full coverage?

Water fluoridation reaches everybody, a major advantage in terms of oral health and a problem in terms of social policy for those who dislike the overtones of compulsion. When domestic salt with added fluoride appears alongside non-fluoridated salt on the supermarket shelves, consumers have a choice. This makes fluoridated salt more palatable from the social policy viewpoint, but weakens its caries-preventive impact across the whole population. With the "full coverage" policy used by the Swiss Canton of Vaud, namely that of flu-

Table 16-8
Various levels of coverage with fluoridated salt, 1994.
For different cantons of Switzerland and three other countries

Type of salt fluoridated	Vaud (Cantons of Switzerland)	Glarns	France	Costa Rica	Colombia
Domestic	+ *	+	+	+	+
Bread	+	+	–	–	+
Restaurants, hospitals, canteens	+	–	–	+	+
School meals for children	+	–	– **	+	+
Prepackaged industrial products	–	–	–	–	– ?
mg F/kg in salt	250	250	250	250	200

*   The table salt is not fluoridated (for technical reasons); it constitutes approximately 12% of all domestic salt.
** Authorized in France since July 1983, used also in the Swiss Canton of Ticino.

oridating all salt on the supermarket shelves as well as the salt delivered in bulk to restaurants, bakeries, food processors, hospitals and other institutions, oral health will benefit but consumer choice will be curtailed. (Vaud still permits "natural" salt to be sold in specialty health food shops, but this market is small. It is interesting that the Vaud government received few complaints about its virtually compulsory plan for fluoridated salt, whereas the fluoridated city of Basel has to deal constantly with such opposition. Presumably the small market for "natural" salt is sufficient to blunt any concerns about compulsory fluoridation).

A full-coverage program like that in Vaud thus effectively puts fluoridated salt in the same social category as fluoridated water. Social policy with fluoridated salt therefore has to balance the trade-off between public health and consumer choice, a trade-off which takes different forms in different countries.

In Switzerland, fluoridated salt claimed 75% of the national domestic salt market in 1987-91.

Nearly all domestic salt is iodized, though salt without either iodine or fluoride is still available as a third choice in about one-third of Swiss supermarkets and other food shops. From 1994, fluoridated salt was the only domestic salt offered in 500 g and 1000 g packages, while the other types was available only in 500 g packages. The price for all 500 g packages was the same. It is expected that this policy will raise the market share of fluoridated salt above 80% after a setback in 1992-93, when all forms of salt were available in the more economic 1000 g packages.

In France and Germany the fluoridated salt program is limited to domestic salt, which is available alongside non-fluoridated salt. Non-iodized domestic salt is also available in those countries. In both Costa Rica and Jamaica all domestic and institutional salt, except that for bakeries, is fluoridated. The exclusion of bakeries is a result of the distribution systems in Costa Rica and Jamaica; bakeries in those countries use an unusually fine grade of salt which is distributed through channels separate from other bulk distributions. Despite the extensive studies carried out in Colombia and Hungary, various political and logistic problems have precluded salt fluoridation from becoming established in those countries. Table 16-8 summarizes the distribution of fluoridated salt in various countries and in different regions of Switzerland.

It can be seen that the term "salt fluoridation" covers several types of availability and distribution of the product. It is politically easier to permit choice among different kinds of domestic salt, while public health authorities often prefer to see fewer options for choosing non-fluoridated salt. The more favorable attitude of European governments toward fluoridated salt, relative to water fluoridation, is largely based on the availability of choice. The more comprehensive the use of fluoridated salt becomes,the less choice consumers have, but the more oral health is likely to improve. As in other areas, the use of fluoridated salt presents trade-off decisions to be made.

The ideal fluoride concentration in salt

The concentration of fluoride in salt is largely based on average salt consumption. The daily intake of domestic salt in European populations has been estimated to range from 1.5 to 3.34 g/day,[3,87] so that a person consuming 2.25 g of the salt initially fluoridated at 90 mg F/kg would ingest only 0.2 mg fluoride from it.

Salt consumption is commonly assessed from urinary sodium excretion. This method was used in the Intersalt Cooperative Research Group study, usually called the Intersalt study, which comprised 52 centers in 32 countries.[41] When the outliers were excluded from the results, median sodium excretion for adults aged 20-59 years ranged from 96 to 194 mM/24 hours, which corresponds to 5.6-11.3 g salt/24 hours. It is pertinent to note that in this range there were no consistent relationships between sodium intake and hypertension. In the United

Table 16-9
Approximate salt intake from various sources in Switzerland[3,59]

	g/day
Salt added in the household: Domestic salt	1.5- 2
Salt contained in glutamate shakers, bouillon cubes, etc.	2 - 3
Salt in bread	2 - 3
Salt in other food (cheese and industrially prepared food)	2.5- 4
Total	8.4-10.3

States, the second National Health and Nutrition Examination Survey of 1976-80 found that after the first year of life, salt intake remained fairly constant at 3.5 g per 4.2 MJ/day (1000 calories) of energy intake, independent of age.[11] This means that an adult ingesting 8.4 MJ/day (2000 calories) per day would take in 7 g of salt. These results are likely to be underestimates, however, because they do not account for added discretionary salt. Recent estimates in the developed countries suggest that daily discretionary salt consumption is now more in the order of 1.5-2.0 g/day,[3] and that salt from bread and other processed foods makes up the remainder of the daily intake of 5.6-11.3 g. Table 16-9 shows the data for Switzerland, where daily adult intake was estimated at 8.4-10.3 g. Discretionary salt consumption appears to be higher in Latin America, but specific data are not available.

Using salt containing 250 mg F/kg, the summarized results of Swiss studies estimating fluoride intake of children under various conditions are shown in Table 16-10. Total fluoride intake is at the lower limit of recommended

303

Table 16-10
Fluoride intake (mg per day) and excretion (µg F/h) by children
at aged 10-14 in Switzerland and France (Strasbourg)

Source of fluoride	Zurich 1983, Geneva 1984, low-F	Geneva 1988, domestic F-salt	Glarus, Vaud, F-salt, domest and for bread	Strasbourg, 1992, low-F (groups II & IV)	Strasbourg, domestic F-salt (I)	Strasbourg, 1 mg F daily in tablets (III)
Food and water	0.2-0.5	0.2-0.5	0.2-0.5	0.2-0.5		0.2-0.5
Domestic salt*	0.1**	0.4	0.4	negligible	?	–
Salt in bread*	–	–	0.4	–	–	–
Dentifrices	0.18	0.18	0.18	0.1	0.1	0.1
F-Tablets	–	–	–	–	–	1.0
Total	0.38-0.78	0.78-1.08	1.18-1.48	0.3-0.6	?	1.3-1.6

Fluoride excretions (no nocturnal data from Glarus)

24-urine	–	–	–	8.7-11.5	21.1	26.3
Morning	8.6-11.1	13.8-16.7	18.5-26.1	7.3- 7.6	19.2	28.3
Afternoon	13.5-16.0	40.1-48.1	31.2-47.8	9.5-20.0	25.7	23.6
Night	8.8	16.4-19.2	24.6	8.8-12.9	19.2	27.0

Excretion averages in Strasbourg, France, from Obry-Musset et al.[65]
* with 250 ppm fluoride whether domestic or in bread
**from salt containing 90 ppm F used by 66% of the children in Zurich (later in 1983 changed to 250 ppm F)

intake when adjusted for age of the children.[47] Table 16-10 also includes the summarized results of urinary excretion studies in Switzerland. Urinary fluoride concentrations are usually determined from 24-hour urine collections.[39,69] In studies using salt with 200-350 mg F/kg, average urinary concentrations of 0.69-1.24 mg F/L were reported.[52] Other studies[61,77] collected urine under supervision at school and obtained night samples from some children. Obry-Musset and colleagues[65] collected 24-hour urine from the children in their study.

Urine collections covering 24 hours are difficult to get and cumbersome to study, but on the basis of a morning and afternoon collection at school and one at night, 24-hour urine excretion can be extrapolated accurately enough to estimate fluoride excretion.[53] While fluoride intake is the main factor influencing fluoride excretion, less fluoride than average is excreted when the urinary flow is slow[29] and when urinary pH is below approximately 6.5.[91]

Additional studies of fluoride excretion, using 24-hour urine collections, were conducted in Sri Lanka and England.[74] The 4-year-olds in Sri Lanka, with drinking waters ranging from 0.1 to 1.1 mg F/L, excreted 23 µg F/hour, while children of the same age in England, with drinking waters 0.8-1.0 mg F/L, excreted 18 µg F/hour. When the lower water intake of 4-year-old children and the urinary fluoride concentrations of 1.19 mg/L in Sri Lanka and 1.02 mg/L in England are accounted for, these results agree with those in Table 16-10.

304

Based on data from these studies, part of which are shown in Table 16-10, provisional guidelines on fluoride excretion can be used as estimates of total fluoride intake. Children aged 9-14 years with low fluoride intake tend to excrete some 10 µg F/hours, except for a few hours after main meals, when it can rise to 15 µg F/hour. In children consuming water with 1.0 mg F/L, or taking a 1.0 mg fluoride tablet per day, fluoride excretion ranges from 25 to 35 µg F/hour. Swiss children who had been consuming salt with 250 mg F/kg for at least 3 years excreted 31-48 µg F/hour after the main meal. These levels correspond to the elevated plasma levels after meals which have been previously reported.[31] Morning and nighttime urinary excretion by children who also ate bread made with fluoridated salt ranged between 18 and 26 µg F/hour, whereas those eating bread made with non-fluoridated salt excreted 14-19 µg F/hour. These ranges need to be validated in groups who consume different diets.

Milk fluoridation

Milk fluoridation is the addition of a measured quantity of fluoride to bottled or packaged milk to be drunk by children. Strongly promoted by Ziegler, an influential pediatrician, the first project with fluoridated milk began in the Swiss city of Winterthur in 1955. Milk containing fluoride at 1.0 mg/L was provided to 749 children aged 9-44 months, and another 553 children were included as controls. After 6 years, substantial reductions in caries were reported for both the primary and permanent dentitions.[94]

The rationale for adding fluoride to milk is that this procedure "targets" fluoride directly to children, and thus would be less expensive than fluoridating the drinking water. Having both fluoridated and non-fluoridated milk available also maintains consumer choice.

However, despite considerable interest in many quarters, the choice of milk as a vehicle for fluoride raises questions. The first concerns absorption, for it was shown a long time ago that while fluoride is absorbed almost as completely from milk as it is from water, the process takes considerably longer.[30] If fluoride acted preeruptively to prevent caries that would not matter much, but in the current model of fluoride cariostasis it means that virtually no topical effect take place. There are also practical concerns, such as the considerable number of children in most countries who do not drink milk for one reason or another.

There have been only a few studies on the cariostatic efficacy of fluoridated milk, and some of them were flawed in design or operation.[75,97] These and other studies[8,80] reported favorable results, and increases in the fluoride content of enamel have been reported in children who consumed fluoridated milk for a year.[88] The study in Scotland[80] provided 1.5 mg F in 200 mL of milk to the children on each school day.

Few public health programs using fluoridated milk have become established, though there are reports of such programs in Bulgaria and another to begin in St. Helens, near Liverpool, in England.[43] However, it is hard to recommend further research into milk fluoridation in view of the large number of fluoride vehicles available today and the restricted topical effects from fluoride in milk. In 1972, Stamm[76] summarized the following four criticisms of milk fluoridation as a public health measure:

- Since children from the lower socioeconomic groups tend to drink the lowest amount of fresh milk, they would benefit least;
- Any benefit ceases as an individual matures and drinks less milk;
- Slow absorption means no topical effect, and

- Figures show that the procedure can be relatively costly, despite proponents' claims to the contrary.

These criticisms still appear valid today.

Summary

While the original rationale for ingested fluoride no longer holds, there are several ways of making fluoride available to a population by ingestable means which can be effective and relatively cheap. Because any ingestable fluoride carries the risk of fluorosis, it is axiomatic that only one form of ingestable fluoride should be available in a community at any one time. This means that supplements should not be used in a fluoridated community, nor in a region where fluoridated salt is widely used.

The evidence for the effectiveness of salt fluoridation, while not overwhelming, is consistent and entirely plausible. It has been successful in Switzerland, where a technically advanced society and a single salt distributor are major factors in this success. Salt fluoridation is likely to carry greater benefits in terms of oral health where it is universally used in all food preparation than where it is simply made available for domestic use. The greater the oral health benefit, the less the degree of consumer choice. Determination of the right degree of trade-off between oral health and individual choice is essentially a social and political decision.

Fluoride supplements have a long tradition, but while they are effective in school-age children, their use among infants and young children cannot be encouraged. Even if there are some preeruptive benefits from their use, these benefits are likely to be marginal in those countries where fluoride is readily available from toothpaste, mouthrinses, and gels. Any benefit from preeruptive ingestion is outweighed by the risk of fluorosis. As mentioned, supplements should never be used in circumstances where either water or salt is fluoridated. It is hard to recommend the use of fluoridated milk in view of the inherent difficulties in the procedure.

Literature cited

1. Aasenden R, Peebles TC. Effects of fluoride supplementation from birth on deciduous and permanent teeth. Arch Oral Biol 1974; 19: 321-6.

2. Allmark C, Green HP, Linney AD, Wills DJ, Picton DC. A community study of fluoride tablets for school children in Portsmouth. Results after six years. Br Dent J 1982; 153: 426-30.

3. Altherr D. Studie über den Salzkonsum und die Fluoridausscheidung im Urin. Med Diss, Zürich 1992.

4. American Dental Association, Council on Dental Therapeutics. Prescribing supplements of dietary fluorides. J Am Dent Assoc 1958; 56: 589-91.

5. Arnold FA Jr, McClure FJ, White CL. Sodium fluoride tablets for children. Dent Progress 1960; 1: 8-12.

6. Baelum V, Fejerskov O, Manji F, Larsen MJ. Daily dose of fluoride and dental fluorosis. Tandlaegebladet 1987; 91: 452-6.

7. Bagramian RA, Narendran S, Ward M. Relationship of dental caries and fluorosis to fluoride supplement history in a non- fluoridated sample of schoolchildren. Adv Dent Res 1989; 3: 161-7.

8. Banoczy J, Zimmermann P, Hadas E, Pinter A, Bruszt V. Effect of fluoridated milk on caries: 5 year results. J Roy Soc Health 1985; 105: 99-103.

9. Binder K, Driscoll WS, Schutzmannsky G. Caries-preventive fluoride tablet programs. Caries Res 1978; 12: 22-30.

10. Burt BA. The changing patterns of systemic fluoride intake. J Dent Res 1992; 71 (Spec Issue):1228-37.

11. Carroll MD, Abraham S, Dresser CM. Dietary intake source data: United States, 1976-80. National Center for Health Statistics, National Health Survey Series 11, No. 231, 1983.

12. Clark DC, Hann HJ, Williamson MF, Berkowitz J. Aesthetic concerns of children and parents in relation to different classifications of the Tooth Surface Index of Fluorosis. Community Dent Oral Epidemiol 1993; 21: 360-4.

13. Clarkson J. A European view of fluoride supplementation. Br Dent J 1992; 172: 357.

14. Corpron RE, Burt BA. Fluorosis from supplementation with fluoride tablets: a case report. J Mich Dent Assoc 1978; 60: 615-8.

15. Dean HT. Epidemiological studies in the United States. In: Moulton FR, ed. Dental caries and fluorine. Washington, DC: AAAS 1946: 5-31.

16. De Crousaz P, Marthaler TM, Weisner V, Bandi A, Steiner M, Robert A, Meyer R. Caries prevalence of children after 12 years of salt fluoridation in a canton of Switzerland. Helv Odont Acta 1985; 29: 21-31.

17. De Crousaz P, Marthaler TM, Menghini GM, Steiner M. Fluoration du sel alimentaire en Suisse. Rev Euro d'Ontol Real Clin 1993; 4: 343-50.

18. de Liefde B, Herbison GP. Prevalence of developmental defects of enamel and dental caries in New Zealand children receiving differing fluoride supplementation. Community Dent Oral Epidemiol 1985; 13: 164-7.

19. de Liefde B, Herbison GP. The prevalence of development defects of enamel and dental caries in New Zealand children receiving differing fluoride supplementation, in 1982 and 1985. N Z Dent J 1989; 85:2-8.

20. DenBesten PK, Thariani H. Biological mechanisms of fluorosis and level and timing of systemic exposure to fluoride with respect to fluorosis. J Dent Res 1992; 71: 1238-43.

21. D'Hoore W, Van Nieuwenhuysen JP. Benefits and risks of fluoride supplementation: caries prevention versus dental fluorosis. Eur J Pediatr 1992; 151: 613-6.

22. DePaola PF, Lax M. The caries-inhibiting effect of acidulated phosphate-fluoride chewable tablets: a two-year double-blind study. J Am Dent Assoc 1968; 76: 554-7.

23. Driscoll WS. The use of fluoride tablets for the prevention of dental caries. In: Forrester DJ, Schulz EM, Jr, eds. International Workshop on Fluorides and Dental Caries Reductions. Baltimore: University of Maryland School of Dentistry 1974: 25-93.

24. Driscoll WS. What we know and don't know about dietary fluoride supplements – the research basis. J Dent Child 1985; 52: 259-64.

25. Driscoll WS, Heifetz SB, Brunelle JA. Caries-preventive effects of fluoride tablets in school-children four years after discontinuation of treatments. J Am Dent Assoc 1981; 103: 878-81.

26. Driscoll WS, Heifetz SB, Korts DC. Effect of chewable fluoride tablets on dental caries in schoolchildren: results after six years of use. J Am Dent Assoc 1978; 97: 820-4.

27. Driscoll WS, Horowitz HS. A discussion of optimal dosage for dietary fluoride supplementation. J Am Dent Assoc 1978; 96: 1050-3.

28. Driscoll WS, Nowjack-Raymer R, Selwitz RH, Li SH, Heifetz SB. A comparison of the caries-preventive effects of fluoride mouthrinsing, fluoride tablets, and both procedures combined: final results after eight years. J Public Health Dent 1992; 52: 111-6.

29. Ekstrand J, Ehrnebo M, Boreus LO. Fluoride bio-availability after intravenous and oral administration: importance of renal clearance and urine flow. Clin Pharmacol Thera 1978; 223: 329-37.

30. Ericsson Y. State of fluorine in milk and its absorption and retention when administered in milk. Investigations with radio-active fluorine. Acta Odont Scand 1958; 16: 51-72.

31. Ericsson Y, Andersson R. Fluoride ingestion with fluoridated domestic salt under Swedish dietary conditions. Caries Res 1983; 17: 277-88.

32. Evans RW, Stamm JW. An epidemiologic estimate of the critical period during which human maxillary central incisors are most susceptible to fluorosis. J Public Health Dent 1991; 51: 251-9.

33. Fanning EA, Cellier KM, Somerville CM. South Australian kindergarten children: effects of flu-

307

oride tablets and fluoridated water on dental caries in primary teeth. Aust Dent J 1980; 25: 259-63.

34. Fejerskov O, Stephen KW, Richards A, Speirs R. Combined effect of systemic and topical fluoride treatments on human deciduous teeth – case studies. Caries Res 1987; 21: 452-9.

35. Forsman B. Early supply of fluoride and enamel fluorosis. Scand J Dent Res 1977; 85: 22-30.

36. Friis-Hasche E, Bergmann J, Wenzel A, Thylstrup A, Pedersen KM, Petersen PE. Dental health status and attitudes to dental care in families participating in a Danish fluoride tablet program. Community Dent Oral Epidemiol 1984; 12: 303-7.

37. Gillespie GM, Roviralta G, eds. Salt fluoridation. Scientific Publication no. 501, Washington, DC: Pan American Health Organization (WHO-AMRO) 1985.

38. Gülzow HJ, Maeglin B, Mühlemann HR, Ritzel G, Stäheli D. Kariesbefall und Kariesfrequenz bei 7-15 jährigen Basler Schulkindern im Jahre 1977, nach 15jähriger Trinkwasserfluoridierung. Schweiz Monatsschr Zahnheilk 1982; 9: 255-62.

39. Hefti A, Wespi HJ, Regolati B, Marthaler TM. 24-Stunden-Ausscheidung von Fluorid im Urin bei Salz- und Trinkwasserfluoridierung. Schweiz Monatsschr Zahnheilk 1981; 91: 559-65.

40. Holm AK, Andersson R. Enamel mineralization disturbances in 12-year-old children with known early exposure to fluorides. Community Dent Oral Epidemiol 1982; 10: 335-9.

41. Intersalt Cooperative Research Group. Intersalt: an international study of electrolyte excretion and blood pressure. Results for 24 hour urinary sodium and potassium excretion. Br Med J 1988; 297: 319-28.

42. Kalsbeek H, Verrips E, Dirks OB. Use of fluoride tablets and effect on prevalence of dental caries and dental fluorosis. Community Dent Oral Epidemiol 1992; 20: 241-5.

43. Jones S, Crawford AC, Jenner AM, Roberts JT, Lennon MA. The possibility of school milk as a vehicle for fluoride: epidemiological, organisational and legal considerations. Community Dent Health 1992; 9: 335-42.

44. Larsen MJ, Kirkegaard E, Poulsen S, Fejerskov O Dental fluorosis among participants in a non-supervised fluoride tablet program. Community Dent Oral Epidemiol 1989; 17: 204-6.

45. Larsen MJ, Richards A, Fejerskov O. Development of dental fluorosis according to age at start of fluoride administration. Caries Res 1985; 19: 519-27.

46. Margolis FJ, Reames HR, Freshman E, Macauley JC, Mehaffey H. Fluoride: ten-year prospective study of deciduous and permanent dentition. Am J Dis Child 1975; 130: 794-800.

47. Marthaler TM. Age-adjusted limits of fluoride intake to minimize the prevalence of fluorosis. J Biol Buccale 1992; 20: 121-7.

48. Marthaler TM. Caries inhibiting effect of fluoride tablets. Helv Odont Acta 1969; 13: 1-13.

49. Marthaler TM. Programme der präventiven Zahnmedizin in der Schule. Soz präv ued 1978; 23: 177-80.

50. Marthaler TM. Results obtained and methods used in caries prevention in Switzerland. In: Frank RM, O'Hickey S, eds. Strategy for dental caries prevention in European countries according to their laws and regulations. Oxford: IRL Press 1987: 159-72.

51. Marthaler TM. Zur Frage des Fluorvollsalzes; erste klinische Resultate. Schweiz Monatsschr Zahnheilk 1961; 71: 671-82.

52. Marthaler TM, Mejia R, Toth K, Vines JJ. Caries preventive salt fluoridation. Caries Res 1978; 12 (Suppl 1): 15-21.

53. Marthaler TM, Menghini GD, Steiner M, Sener-Zanola B, de Crousaz P. Excrecion urinaria de fluoruro en ninos suizos que consumen suplementos de fluoruro en la sal o el agua (urinary fluoride excretions in Swiss children consuming supplemental fluoride in salt or drinking water). Archiv Odontoestomatol Prev Comunitaria 1992; 4: 27-35.

54. Marthaler TM, Schenardi C. Inhibition of caries in children after 5 1/2 years' use of fluoridated table salt. Helv Odont Acta 1962; 6: 1-6.

55. Marthaler TM, Scheiwiler A, Steiner M, Menghini GD. Kariesvorbeugung bei der Schuljugend von Wil SG 1963 bis 1990: Vorgehen und Ergebnisse. Schweiz Monatsschr Zahnmed 1992a; 102: 930-3.

56. Marthaler TM, Steiner M, Menghini G, Bandi A. Kariesprävalenz bei Schülern im Kanton Zürich,

Resultate aus dem Zeitraum 1963 bis 1987. Schweiz Monatsschr Zahnmed 1988; 98: 1309-15.

57. Marthaler TM, Steiner M, Menghini G, de Crousaz P. DMF teeth in schoolchildren after 18 years of collective salt fluoridation. Caries Res 1989; 23: 428.

58. Marthaler TM, Weisner V, Menghini G, Steiner M. Zur Epidemiologie der Zahnkaries: Resultate von Einzelerhebungen in verschiedenen Gebieten der Schweiz 1972-1985. Schweiz Monatsschr Zahnheilk 1986; 96: 1441-50.

59. Matt M. Studie über den Speisesalzkonsum und die Fluoridausscheidung im Urin im Fürstentum Liechtenstein. Med Diss, Zürich, 1990.

60. Menghini G, Steiner M, Marthaler TM, Bandi A. Prevalenza della carie dentaria presso gli scolari di tre comuni del Canton Ticino, evoluzione dal 1983 al 1987. Boll Informazione Med Dent Cantone Ticino 1989; 26: 25-33.

61. Menghini G, de Crousaz P, Steiner M, Helfenstein U, Sener B. Excretion urinaire de fluorures chez des ecoliers de Geneve et Lausanne, en relation avec la fluoration du sel. Schweiz Monatssch Zahnmed 1989; 99: 292-8.

62. Menghini GD, Marthaler TM, Steiner M, Bandi A, Schürch E Jr. Kariesprävalenz und gingivale Verhältnisse bei Rekruten im Jahre 1985, Einfluss der Vorbeugung. Schweiz Monatsschr Zahnmed 1991; 101/9: 1119-26.

63. Messer LB, Walton JL. Fluorosis and caries experience following early post-natal fluoride supplementation: a report of 19 cases. Pediatr Dent 1980; 2: 267-74.

64. Mühlemann HR. Fluoridated domestic salt. A discussion of dosage. Int Dent J 1967; 17: 10-7.

65. Obry-Musset AM, Bettembourg D, Cahen PM, Voegel JC, Frank RM. Urinary fluoride excretion in children using potassium fluoride containing salt or sodium fluoride supplements. Caries Res 1992; 26: 367-70.

66. Ophaug RH, Singer L, Harland BF. Estimated fluoride intake of average two-year-old children in four dietary regions of the United States. J Dent Res 1980; 59: 777-81.

67. Osuji OO, Nikiforuk G. Fluoride supplement-induced dental fluorosis: case reports. Pediatr Dent 1988; 10: 48-52.

68. Pendrys DG, Katz RV. Risk of enamel fluorosis associated with fluoride supplementation, infant formula, and fluoride dentifrice use. Am J Epidemiol 1989; 130: 1199-208.

69. Peters G, Peters-Haefeli L, Marthaler TM, Michod J, Joel M, Robert A. L'excretion urinaire de fluorures chez des habitants du Canton Vaud ingerant uniquement du sel fluore compare a celle d'habitants de communes limitrophes ingerant du sel non-fluore. Soz Prav Med 1975; 20: 263-71.

70. Petersson LG, Koch G, Rasmusson CG, Stanke H. Effect on caries of different fluoride prophylactic programs in preschool children. A two year clinical study. Swed Dent J 1985; 9: 97-104.

71. Riordan PJ. Fluoride supplements in caries prevention: a literature review and proposal for a new dosage schedule. J Public Health Dent 1993; 53: 174-89.

72. Riordan PJ. Perceptions of dental fluorosis. J Dent Res 1993; 72: 1268-74.

73. Riordan PJ, Banks JA. Dental fluorosis and fluoride exposure in Western Australia. J Dent Res 1991; 70: 1022-8.

74. Rugg-Gunn AJ, Nunn JH, Ekanajake L, Saparamadu KDG, Wright WG. Urinary fluoride in 4-year-old children in Sri Lanka and England. Caries Res 1993; 27: 478-83.

75. Rusoff LL, Konikoff BS, Frye JB, Johnston JE, Frye WW. Fluoride addition to milk and its effect on dental caries in school children. Am J Clin Nutr 1962; 11: 94-101.

76. Stamm JW. Milk fluoridation as a public health measure. J Canad Dent Assoc 1972; 38: 446-8.

77. Steiner M, Marthaler TM, Menghini G, Helfenstein U. Fluoridausscheidung im Urin von Schulkindern im Zusammenhang mit der Speisesalzfluoridierung. Schweiz Monatsschr Zahnmed 1985; 95: 1109-17.

78. Steiner M, Marthaler TM, Wiesner V, Menghini G. Kariesbefall bei Schulkindern des Kantons Glarus, 9 Jahre nach Einführung des höher fluoridierten Salzes (250 mg F/kg). Schweiz Monatsschr Zahnmed 1986; 96: 688-99.

79. Steiner M, Menghini G, Marthaler TM. Kariesbefall bei Schulkindern des Kantons Glarus, 13 jahre nach der Einführung des höher fluoridierten Salzes. Schweiz Monatsschr Zahnmed 1989; 99: 897-906.

80. Stephen KW, Boyle IT, Campbell D, McNee S, Boyle P. Five-year double-blind fluoridated milk

study in Scotland. Community Dent Oral Epidemiol 1984; 12: 223-9.

81. Stephen KW, Campbell D. Caries reduction and cost benefit after 3 years of sucking fluoride tablets daily at school. A double-blind trial. Br Dent J 1978; 144: 202-6.

82. Stephen KW, Kay EJ, Tullis JI. Combined fluoride therapies. A 6-year double-blind school-based preventive dentistry study in Inverness, Scotland. Community Dent Oral Epidemiol 1990; 18: 244-8.

83. Stephen KW, McCall DR, Gilmour WH. Incisor enamel mottling prevalence in child cohorts which had or had not taken fluoride supplements from 0-12 years of age. Proc Finn Dent Soc 1991; 87: 595-605.

84. Suckling GW, Pearce EI. Developmental defects of enamel in a group of New Zealand children: their prevalence and some associated etiological factors. Community Dent Oral Epidemiol 1984; 12: 177-84.

85. Thylstrup A, Fejerskov O, Bruun C, Kann J. Enamel changes and dental caries in 7-year-old children given fluoride tablets from shortly after birth. Caries Res 1979; 13: 265-76.

86. Toth K. Caries prevention by domestic salt fluoridation. Budapest: Akademiai Kiado 1984.

87. Toth K, Sugar E. Ueber den täglichen auf das Körpergewicht bezogenen Verbrauch von Speisesalz. Dtsch Zahnärztl Z 1975; 30: 231-6.

88. Toth Z, Zimmermann P, Gintner Z, Banoczy J. Changes of acid solubility and fluoride content of the enamel surface in children consuming fluoridated milk. Acta Physiol Hung 1989; 74: 135-40.

89. Wespi HJ. Gedanken zur Frage der optimalen Ernährung in der Schwangerschaft. Schweiz Med Wochenschr 1948; 7: 153-5.

90. Wespi HJ. Fluoridiertes Kochsalz zur Kariesprophylaxe. Schweiz Med Wschr 1950; 80: 561-4.

91. Whitford GM. The metabolism and toxicity of fluoride. In: Myers HM, ed. Monographs in oral science, Vol 13. Zurich: Karger 1989.

92. Widenheim J, Birkhed D. Caries-preventive effect on primary and permanent teeth and cost-effectiveness of an NaF tablet preschool program. Community Dent Oral Epidemiol 1991; 19: 88-92.

93. Widenheim J, Birkhed D, Granath L, Lindgren G. Preeruptive effect of NaF tablets on caries in children from 12 to 17 years of age. Community Dent Oral Epidemiol 1986; 14: 1-4.

94. Wirz R. Ergebnisse eines Grossversuches mit fluoridierter Milch in Winterthur von 1958 bis 1964. Schweiz Monatsschr Zahnheilk 1964; 4: 767-84.

95. Woltgens JH, Etty EJ, Nieuwland WM. Prevalence of mottled enamel in permanent dentition of children participating in a fluoride programme at the Amsterdam dental school. J Biol Buccale 1989; 17: 15-20.

96. Woolfolk MW, Faja BW, Bagramian RA. Relation of sources of systemic fluoride to prevalence of dental fluorosis. J Public Health Dent 1989; 49: 78-82.

97. Zahlaka M, Mitri O, Munder H, Mann J, Kaldavi A, Galon H, Gedalia I. The effect of fluoridated milk on caries in Arab children. Results after 3 years. Clin Prev Dent 1987; 9(4): 23-5.

Chapter 17

TOPICAL FLUORIDES IN CARIES PREVENTION

H.S. Horowitz • A.I. Ismail

Introduction – Professionally applied fluorides – Self-applied fluorides – Slow-release systems
Combinations of fluoride – Recommendations for use of topical fluorides

Introduction

Topical fluorides for the prevention of dental decay are the most widely used dental products at home and in dental offices. Strong scientific evidence exists to support the efficacy of many topical fluorides in caries prevention. An efficacious product produces a statistically and clinically significant benefit under ideal testing conditions in carefully controlled clinical trials. In contrast, an effective product produces a statistically and clinically significant benefit when evaluated under realistic field conditions, as found in typical communities. For example, community clinical trials in the 1990s should be done in Western countries in individuals who regularly use fluoride dentifrices, in as much as these products are used by most persons in those countries. The distinction between efficacy and effectiveness is important in deciding what impact a topically applied fluoride agent has in reducing dental decay in a target population.[34]

The concentrations of fluoride contained in agents designed primarily for topical applica-

tion vary greatly, ranging nearly 100-fold from about 225 parts per million (ppm) in 0.05% sodium fluoride mouthrinses sold over-the-counter to almost 20,000 ppm in an 8% stannous fluoride solution, intended for professional application. The topical effect of salivary-secreted fluoride is discussed in Chapter 12.

Topical fluorides may be applied by dental health personnel in dental offices or clinics or may be self-applied. Although some exceptions exist, in general, high-fluoride concentration agents are applied professionally and low-fluoride concentration agents or products are applied by the individuals themselves. Topically applied fluorides do not increase the fluoride concentration of enamel greatly; rather, they tend to provide local protection at or near the tooth surface by incorporating and concentrating fluoride in plaque and the oral mucosa.[50] This fluoride serves as a reservoir of available fluoride ions. During a cariogenic challenge, fluoride from these sources is mobilized to assist remineralization. Recent research has shown that fluoride in high concentrations deposits a calcium fluoride-like material on tooth enamel or in plaque, which releases fluoride during cariogenic challenges.[40]

Professionally applied fluorides

Dental personnel have been applying fluoride agents to the teeth since the early 1940s. After fluoride was identified as an element with cariostatic properties, it was surmised that fluoride applied to the teeth would be deposited in the outer enamel, making it more resistant to dissolution by acids. Although it is now known that the mechanisms of action of fluoride are more complex and that frequency and availability of low concentrations of fluoride are more important in caries prevention than is concentration, there is abundant scientific evidence from well-conducted studies to support the value of infrequent professional applications of fluoride agents for prevention of dental caries. Currently recognized agents include various fluoride solutions, gels and varnishes.

Fluoride solutions

Neutral sodium fluoride – Neutral sodium fluoride (NaF) solutions were the first agents studied for effectiveness in preventing dental caries. Bibby[4] and Knutson & Armstrong[27] published some of the earliest studies of NaF solutions in the early 1940s. In 1948, the USA Public Health Service (USPHS) recommended [26] that a series of 4-weekly applications of 2% NaF be given at ages 3, 7, 11 and 13. The teeth were given a coronal cleaning only before the first application of each series. At each application, teeth were wet with the solution, which was allowed to dry on the teeth for about 3 minutes.

The ages for application were selected so that fluoride would be applied after groups of teeth erupted into the mouth, which would minimize the amount of time that teeth were at risk to caries attack before preventive treat-

ments were given. The USPHS-suggested regimen for NaF applications was designed for public health programs in which a single clinician could treat a few children simultaneously. Because the NaF solution was allowed to dry on the teeth for 3 minutes, a clinician theoretically could apply fluoride to other children during the drying period. Because the series of four treatments was provided only four times between the ages of 3 and 13, different groups of children could be treated each year. The USPHS regimen, however, was not convenient for private practitioners, who tend to recall patients for check-ups at 6–12-month intervals.

Many studies conducted throughout the world have confirmed the effectiveness of solutions of NaF in preventing caries. Reductions in caries increments in permanent teeth averaging about 30% have been reported among children living in communities with fluoride-deficient water supplies.[39] Fewer studies of 2% NaF solutions applied to primary teeth have been conducted. The majority of these have shown reductions in the incidence of dental decay, although to a smaller degree than in permanent teeth.

Stannous fluoride – Dudding & Muhler[11] first described a method for applying a stannous fluoride (SnF_2) solution to the teeth for caries prevention in 1962. The important differences from the technique for NaF were that a thorough prophylaxis was to precede the SnF_2 application, the teeth were kept wet with the solution for 4 minutes, making a saliva ejector essential, and treatments were recommended at 6-month intervals. Because SnF_2 is relatively unstable, a freshly prepared solution is recommended for each patient. Both 8% and 10% SnF_2 solutions have been tested, with little difference observed in the effectiveness between the two concentrations.

Although Muhler and his associates at Indiana University reported consistently high reductions in dental caries increments with stan-

Table 17-1
Characteristics and effectiveness of NaF, SnF$_2$ and APF

Characteristic	NaF	SnF$_2$	APF
Percent and ppm F$^-$	2% 9,200	8% 19,500	1.23% F$^-$ 12,300
Frequency of application	4 at weekly intervals at ages 3, 7, 10 & 13	1 or 2/year	1 or 2/year
Taste	Bland	Disagreeable	Acidic
Stability	Stable	Unstable	Stable in plastic container
Tooth pigmentation	No	Yes	No
Gingival irritation	No	Occasional, transient	No
Average effectiveness	29%	32%	28%

nous fluoride and showed it to be superior to sodium fluoride, other investigators have failed to substantiate these results. Overall, studies have shown a reduction in dental caries of just over 30% with the use of 8% SnF$_2$ in unfluoridated communities.[39]

Acidulated phosphate-fluoride – In 1963, researchers at the Forsyth Dental Center introduced an acidified sodium fluoride solution, based on the premise that greater fluoride uptake by enamel occurs under acidic conditions.[49] Acidulated phosphate-fluoride (APF) has a pH of approximately 3.0, is buffered with 0.1 M phosphoric acid and contains a fluoride ion concentration of 1.23%.[49] The same technique is used to apply APF solutions and SnF$_2$. APF is stable when kept in a plastic container; a fresh solution need not be prepared for each patient. Although initial studies of solutions of APF indicated that it might be superior to neutral NaF and SnF$_2$, the entire body of literature on the agent indicates comparable effectiveness. Benefits have averaged about 28% in non-fluoridated communities.[39]

Comparative clinical characteristics of fluoride solutions
Table 17-1 compares the characteristics and effectiveness of the three principal fluoride agents used for professional application, neutral sodium fluoride, stannous fluoride and acidulated phosphate-fluoride. The USPHS-recommended and most widely tested regimen for applying sodium fluoride solutions, i.e. a series of four applications at weekly intervals,[26] is not convenient for private dental practitioners. Although the USPHS-recommended regimen was used fairly widely in the past in public health programs, few such programs exist today. However, there is little reason to believe that NaF, if applied at 6–12-month intervals as is recommended for SnF$_2$ and APF, would not produce similar benefits. The traditional regimen for NaF also has become inconsistent with current scientific knowledge that frequency of fluoride application is more important than concentration of the agent. The interval of up to 4 years between series of NaF applications may be too long for maximal cariostatic protection.

An aqueous solution of SnF_2 undergoes rapid hydrolysis and oxidation, which reduce or eliminate its effectiveness; consequently, a fresh solution is required for each treatment. It is astringent and has a disagreeable taste, but because SnF_2 is so reactive, flavoring to mask the taste is contraindicated. Persons with poor gingival health may experience a reversible gingival tissue irritation. Staining of the teeth with the use of SnF_2 has frequently been reported, probably from the tin component. The problem seems to be worse in patients with poor oral hygiene.

Because of its low pH, acidulated phosphate-fluoride has an acidic taste; flavoring this agent, however, does not present a problem. APF is stable when stored in a plastic container. It should not be stored in a glass container because it may remove minerals from (etch) the glass. Repeated or prolonged exposures of porcelain or composite restorations to APF can result in the loss of material, surface roughening and possible cosmetic changes. The American Dental Association has suggested, therefore, that it may be prudent not to use an acidic topical fluoride agent in patients with these types of restorations.[7]

Ammonium fluoride and titanium tetrafluoride have been tested *in vitro*. Results show that these agents deposit fluoride in enamel. Only a few clinical studies, however, have been done with these agents; results do not indicate their superiority to conventional fluoride agents. Ammonium fluoride has an unpleasant taste.

Amine fluorides

Amine fluorides have been used widely in Europe.[30] They are compounds in which fluoride ions are attached to amine radicals of organic carbon compounds. Amine fluorides have been used in toothpastes, mouthrinses and gels, occasionally in combination with other caries-preventive agents.[2] Amine fluorides have been reported to hold fluoride in contact with tooth surfaces for longer periods and to reduce the solubility of enamel better than do inorganic fluorides, as well as having bactericidal properties, which reduce dental plaque.[29] Although amine fluorides have been shown to be effective cariostatic agents, comparative data do not exist to show that they provide better decay-preventive effects than do inorganic fluoride agents, despite their superior surfactant and antibacterial properties.

Fluoride gels

Fluoride gels were developed because it was apparent that their viscosity would make them easier to work with and would readily permit their application in trays, so that the entire dentition could be treated at one time. NaF and APF gels contain the same concentrations of fluoride and pH as their respective aqueous solutions. In addition, the gels contain cellulose compounds for viscosity. Some gels are formulated to be thixotropic, that is, they tend to flow when under pressure but remain viscous when not. Theoretically, thixotropic gels may penetrate better interproximally and not drip from a tray as readily as non-thixotropic gels, but studies have not been done to confirm these attributes.

Fluoride gels may be considered to be as effective as their solution counterparts.[23] Two studies have shown that caries-preventive effects have persisted for 2 years after discontinuation of applications of APF gels. Fluoride gel products have dominated the market for many years in the United States because of their desirable working characteristics compared with fluoride solutions.

A fluoride foam with a pH of 6 is marketed in some countries. Less fluoride retention may result following use of the foam than from a traditional gel, but efficacy of the foam has not been investigated.

Fluoride prophylactic pastes

Until the mid-1980s, it was usual for professional fluoride applications to be preceded by a dental prophylaxis or toothcleaning. Consequently, it was logical to evaluate whether added effectiveness occurred when a fluoride prophylactic paste was used prior to a fluoride solution or gel application and whether a fluoride prophylactic paste could be considered an equally effective substitute for a traditional fluoride application. Although studies of sodium fluoride prophylaxis pastes date from 1946, serious interest in these products did not occur until the early 1960s. The United States Air Force[35] and Indiana University[5] both developed stannous fluoride prophylaxis pastes; the former used silex as an abrasive[35] and the latter, pumice.[5] Two other fluoride prophylaxis pastes have been sold commercially; one is an APF-silicone dioxide paste and the other a SnF_2-zirconium silicate paste.

The overall findings of studies that have evaluated the effectiveness of fluoride prophylaxis pastes are inconsistent or equivocal; therefore, their use alone cannot be considered an effective cariostatic method. Toothcleaning with a fluoride prophylactic paste should not supplant topical fluoride application with fluoride solutions or gels for children who require professional fluoride applications.

A thorough polishing of the teeth with a rubber cup or bristle brush may remove a thin, but highly mineralized, outer layer of enamel. Consequently, zealous polishing of the teeth should be avoided. If a prophylaxis is required for cosmetic purposes or as part of periodontal tissue therapy and a fluoride agent is not scheduled to follow the prophylaxis, then a fluoride prophylactic paste should definitely be used, which may help to replenish the minerals that are abraded during polishing. With respect to the need for cleaning the teeth prior to professional fluoride applications, at least five studies have shown that such cleanings do not enhance the cariostatic effectiveness of the applications.

Ripa[38] reviewed the literature on the need for toothcleaning prior to fluoride applications and has recommended that is be eliminated. Dental pellicle and plaque are not barriers to fluoride penetration from professional topical fluoride applications.

Fluoride varnishes

Fluoride varnishes were first developed in Europe in the 1960s in an attempt to increase the uptake of topically applied fluoride into enamel.[37] Although there is evidence that varnishes result in a higher concentration of fluoride in enamel compared with other topical fluorides, this increase does not necessarily lead to greater effectiveness. The use of a fluoride varnish, however, increases the fluoride concentration in saliva, which remains significantly higher 2 hours after its application than after the use of other fluoride agents.

The first fluoride varnish tested was Duraphat® (Woelm Pharma Co. Eschwege, Germany). Duraphat contains 5% wt sodium fluoride or 2.26% fluoride. It is a viscous, resinous lacquer which should be applied to dry, clean teeth. Duraphat hardens into a yellowish-brown coating in the presence of saliva. Another varnish developed in the 1970s was Fluor Protector® (Vivadent, Schaan, Liechtenstein) which contains silane fluoride (0.7% fluoride ion) in a polyurethane-based lacquer. Fluor Protector leaves a clear transparent film on the teeth. A new varnish product that has been recently tested in Norway, under the name of Carex, contains a lower fluoride concentration than Duraphat (1.8% fluoride).[20] The efficacy of this new varnish as a caries-preventive agent was found equivalent to that of Duraphat.[20]

Fluoride varnishes are widely used in Europe where most of the clinical trials, except for one Canadian study, were carried out. Fluoride varnishes have not been accepted by the American or Canadian Dental Associations, although they have been available in Canada for several years. In 1994, the US Food and Drug

Administration approved the marketing of DuraFlor®, a new name for Duraphat. The majority of studies of Duraphat have reported caries reductions in the permanent dentition of between 30% and 40%.[42] In the primary dentition, Duraphat has an efficacy ranging between 7% and 44%.[36] Fluor Protector has a range of efficacy between 1% and 17%, but its clinical effectiveness in caries prevention is questionable. Fluor Protector is approved for use in the USA as a cavity varnish.

Fluoride varnishes are particularly useful in handicapped children or for application after restorative treatment is completed under general anesthesia. They also may be used to target fluoride to specific tooth surfaces, e.g. roots, incipient carious lesions or the margins of restorations. Fluoride varnishes are safe because the amount of varnish usually used is 0.3-0.5 mL, which delivers only 3-6 mg fluoride. Patients should be instructed not to chew or brush for at least 4 hours after varnish application. Biannual applications of varnish are the most widely recommended.

Clinical considerations

The rigorous protocols required for clinical trials require that professional applications of fluoride be given at stipulated intervals, usually annually or semi-annually for as long as the study is scheduled to be continued – usually from 1-3 years. However, there is nothing inherently correct about these intervals. Fluoride treatments in dental office settings, in fact, should be tailored to the needs of individual patients.

If patients appear to be at high current risk to caries, as manifested by bacteriologic findings or the development of several new cavities or areas of demineralization because of dental caries since a previous examination, then rigorous fluoride therapy is warranted. The same holds true for patients with xerostomia that may be caused by medications, metabolic disturbances, such as Sjögren's Syndrome or radiation treatment. Such patients should be scheduled to receive frequent professional fluoride treatments and to use supplemental, self-applied topical fluoride methods at home.

In contrast, it is appropriate to question the need for routine professionally applied fluorides for patients who apparently are at low-risk to dental caries. Older teenagers or young adults who are caries-free or have only a few restorations confined to the pits and fissures of molars, the most caries-susceptible tooth surfaces, are unlikely to benefit from continued regular professional applications of concentrated fluoride agents. In essence, then, a regimen for professional fluoride applications should be tailored to the needs of each individual patient, as perceived by the dentist, rather than using the same regimen for all patients. Although there are not serious risks in giving routine fluoride applications, one must question the procedure from the standpoint of cost-effectiveness.

Newly erupted teeth are particularly susceptible to caries in high-risk patients because these teeth are relatively immature and not as highly mineralized as those that have been in the mouth for a few years. Newly erupted teeth absorb relatively larger amounts of fluoride than do teeth that have been in the mouth for several years. For that reason, professional fluoride applications should be provided to high-risk patients after the full complement of primary teeth have erupted, as soon after age 2 as possible, consistent with a child's ability to cooperate with the procedure. Ages 6-8, after permanent first molars and incisors have erupted, are another prime age grouping for professional fluoride applications, and then again at ages 11-14 to protect erupted permanent canines, premolars and second molars.

The data in Table 17-2 emphasize the importance of applying concentrated fluorides shortly after teeth erupt. The table shows the results of several studies in which different fluoride agents were evaluated among teeth that were

Table 17-2
Comparative effectiveness of professional fluoride treatments
according to status of tooth eruption at a study's initiation

Study	Fluoride agent	Caries reduction (%)	
		Previously erupted teeth	Newly erupted teeth
1. Averill HM, Averill JE, Ritz AG. J Am Dent Assoc 1967; 74: 996-1001	NaF	19	43
2. DePaola PF, Melberg JR. J Am Dent Assoc 1973; 87: 155-9	APF	21	36
3. Downer MC, Holloway PJ, Davies TGH. Brit Dent J 1976; 141: 242-7	APF	31	56
4. Horowitz HS, Heifetz SB. J Dent Child 1969; 26: 355-61	SnF_2	21	61
5. Muhler JC. J Dent Child 1960; 27: 157-61	SnF_2	44	84
6. Szwejda LF. J Public Health Dent 1972; 32: 110-8	APF	22	63

already erupted when the study was initiated and those that erupted during the investigation. These and other studies show that relative benefits were sizably greater among the newly erupted teeth.

Teeth should be dried before concentrated fluoride agents are applied, mainly to avoid dilution by saliva.[19] If stock trays are used for gel applications, a proper size should be selected to avoid incomplete coverage of the teeth when the trays are inserted. Enamel fluoride uptake from concentrated fluoride gels after 4 minutes is significantly greater than after 2 minutes or 1 minute.[48] Practitioners, therefore, should resist the temptation to decrease treatment time by shortening the period that gel-trays remain in a patient's mouth; a 4-minute application should continue to be used. Furthermore, for maximal fluoride uptake, patients should be advised not to rinse, eat or drink for 30 minutes after a professionally applied topical APF application, inasmuch as *in vivo* uptake of fluoride by artificially induced incipient lesions is reduced by about one-half when rinsing occurs immediately after an application.[45]

Only a few studies have been conducted on the cariostatic effects of topically applied fluorides in adults, mainly because, until recently, caries was considered a disease that primarily affected children. With the decline in caries prevalence that has occurred among school-age children in many Western countries, more and more younger adults have teeth that are caries-free. These teeth remain susceptible to caries throughout life, when cariogenic conditions prevail. Topically applied fluorides are likely to be effective in preventing caries in susceptible patients of any age. Professional fluoride applications should be given to adults who present evidence of developing new caries lesions in both coronal and exposed root surfaces of teeth and around the margins of existing restorations. Professional fluoride treatments are especially recommended for adults with known risk factors, such as xerostomia.

Toxicity considerations

Professional fluoride solutions and gels contain high concentrations of fluoride. Even small 5-mL volumes of 2% NaF, 8% SnF_2 and APF have 46, 98 and 62 mg fluoride, respectively, which exceed safely tolerated amounts in young children. Therefore, great care should be taken

Table 17-3

Recommended procedures for reducing amounts of ingested fluoride from gel-tray applications

- Place patient in an upright position.
- Advise patient about importance of not swallowing the gel.
- Use no more than 2 ½ ml of gel per tray.
- Use custom-fitted or proper size stock trays with absorptive liners.
- Use suction device during and following treatment.
- Remove excess gel from teeth with gauze following tray removal.
- Have patient expectorate repeatedly and thoroughly following treatment.

Table 17-4

Methods of self-application of fluorides used in supervised programs

1. Toothbrushing with dentifrices
2. Toothbrushing with solutions or gels
3. Toothbrushing with prophylaxis pastes
4. Applying gels in trays
5. Mounthrinsing with solutions
6. Using dietary supplements

to ensure that these agents are handled properly, especially among youngsters.[12] Nausea, vomiting, abdominal pain and hypersalivation occasionally occur in youngsters given professional applications of fluoride. Practitioners sometimes attribute such reactions to apprehension of the patient or to the child's being a "gagger"; however, many of these reactions may result from the child's ingesting excessive amounts of fluoride.

Procedures for reducing the ingestion of fluoride during professional gel-tray applications are shown in Table 17-3.[28] These recommendations pertain to patients of all ages, but particularly to young children, who can safely tolerate only smaller amounts of fluoride.

Self-applied fluorides

Professionally applied fluoride treatments are well-suited to private practice settings or clinics, but they are inherently expensive because they depend upon one professionally trained person treating one patient at a time, frequently with expensive equipment or supplies. To circumvent the high costs and inefficiency associated with professionally applied fluoride treatments, various methods of supervised, self-application methods of fluoride delivery have been developed and evaluated in community and school settings since the mid-1940s.

Self-application of fluoride is usually carried out with groups of persons, usually children, at one time, under only general supervision. Methods of self-application of fluoride must, first and foremost, be completely safe. Further, they must be known to be effective for preventing caries in groups of individuals. The methods must be suitable for use by large groups and at reasonably low costs. In order to gain acceptance, a method must be acceptable to participants and easy to use in order to ensure compliance. To keep costs to a minimum, the methods should require few professional personnel and should be able to be supervised by non-dental personnel after short periods of in-service training.

Table 17-4 lists the principal methods that have been evaluated and used in programs for the self-application of fluorides. The first of the listed methods, toothbrushing with fluoride dentifrices. is discussed in Chapter 18.

Toothbrushing with solutions or gels

Studies in the early 1960s, in which Scandinavian children brushed their teeth five times a year with solutions of sodium zirconium fluoride or ferric fluoride, showed modest to moderate reductions in the incidence of dental caries.[3] In these studies, approximately 200 children per day could administer preventive treatments themselves under general supervision. These studies led investigators in other countries to evaluate various self-applied fluoride solutions and gels applied with a toothbrush for their cariostatic properties.[6,24] Frequencies of application varied in these studies, but the regimen most often tested entailed brushing four or five times each school year or approximately once every 2 months. In these studies, treatments of eight to ten children at a time were supervised by professional or lay personnel.

Although the majority of these studies showed that toothbrushing with solutions or gels could reduce the incidence of dental decay, the method required many paper supplies and toothbrushes and convenient areas for expectoration. Moreover, participants in some of these studies did not readily find the procedures acceptable. Today, few programs using this regimen exist because other methods have more desirable administrative and acceptance characteristics.

Toothbrushing with prophylactic pastes

School-based toothbrushing programs with fluoride- containing prophylactic pastes were evaluated in the 1970s, primarily in the United States. Several localities, both fluoridated and unfluoridated, implemented preventive programs with this regimen. Although APF-silicon dioxide pastes (0.4%F) were tested, the most popular agent for programs was 9% SnF_2 with a zirconium silicate abrasive.[17] The frequency of application varied from one to four times a year, but most evaluations were of a single application each year. Results of studies conducted by investigators at Indiana University tended to be highly positive, but other investigators failed to replicate these findings.[18]

This type of preventive program had inherent appeal because very large groups of children, sometimes entire school populations, would simultaneously treat themselves, under the general supervision of roving professional or trained volunteer supervisors. The advocates of the regimen claimed that the brushing programs not only provided cariostatic benefits, but improved toothbrushing ability, which would result in improved gingival health for participants, their teachers, parents and, because of the publicity associated with these programs, for entire communities as well.[17] Scientific support for these adjunctive claims has never been provided.

Applying gels in trays

The use of either APF or NaF gels with 5000 ppm fluoride ion concentration in custom-made trays, applied by children for 2 school years in a fluoride-deficient community showed profound reductions (75-80%) in the increment of dental caries.[15] Subsequent to the cessation of treatments, children formerly treated with the fluoride gels continued to derive sizable caries protection during the next 23 months.[14] A similar regimen in a fluoridated community, in which preventive treatments were given only three times a week for 3 years, showed only modest reductions in dental caries.[16]

Despite the dramatic caries protection observed in the fluoride-deficient community, programs using this regimen have not been adopted in school- or community-based programs, primarily because of the high costs of fabricating custom-fitted trays for the participants and of the fluoride agents themselves. Other investigators have tested the same methods but with less frequent applications, and have observed only modest caries-preventive effects.

319

The same agents are available by prescription for use at home. These gels contain 1.1% NaF or about one-half the concentration of fluoride gels used for professional applications in dental operatories, and are either neutral or are acidulated to a pH of 4.5. Thermoplastic custom trays to hold the gel may be fabricated in dental offices. An advantage of the gel-tray method is that the concentrated fluoride is applied, without dilution, directly to the teeth for a relatively long period; a minimum of 5 minutes is recommended. These gel-tray products have high fluoride concentrations. Consequently, they should be reserved only for children with rampant dental caries and only after they and their parents have been instructed in their proper use. Their use is contraindicated by any children younger than school age.

Because salivary flow is reduced during sleep, self-applied fluoride gels should be used, if possible, just before bedtime. Whenever they are applied, however, the user should refrain from eating or drinking afterwards for 30 minutes.

These products may be particularly advantageous for adults who have xerostomia or seem to be developing caries in exposed root surfaces. DePaola[8] reported, in 1993, that a small group (n=35) of older adults with one or more active non-cavitated buccal surface root caries lesions, who used a 5000 ppm neutral NaF gel daily, self-applied by toothbrush at home, and also received three professional applications of a 12,000 ppm neutral NaF gel at 4-month intervals, experienced arrestment of 91% of the lesions after 1 year. A comparable placebo control group (n=36) experienced a 40% arrestment of their non-cavitated root lesions. (All subjects received a fluoride toothpaste recognized as effective, toothbrushes and instruction on proper toothbrushing, flossing and use of materials.) The corresponding findings among cavitated root surface lesions showed a 57% arrestment in the treatment group after 12 months,

whereas only 8% of the cavitated root lesions in the control group were arrested during the same period.[8]

Now that the demand for preventing dental caries and repairing lesions caused by the disease has diminished among children in many countries, greater emphasis should be placed on investigating ways to prevent caries in adults. The numbers of older adults are increasing in many countries, and more of them are retaining their own teeth. Studies are underway to investigate various methods of applying fluoride to prevent coronal caries, root surface caries and recurrent caries around restorations in older adults.

Mouthrinsing with solutions

In the 1960s, several studies were done in Scandinavia to evaluate fluoride-containing mouthrinses as a method of caries prevention with promising results.[46] Additional studies in other countries confirmed the value of fluoride mouthrinsing.[22,41] Although other compounds have been tested, solutions of NaF in concentrations of 0.2% (909 ppm F) for rinsing fortnightly or once a week or of 0.05% (227 ppm F) for rinsing daily have been the ones most frequently evaluated and used. Usually, 10 mL of solution is used for mouthrinsing by swishing vigorously for 1 minute. Frequent mouthrinsing is congruent with current knowledge that remineralization of early caries lesions is enhanced by the frequent application and availability of low concentrations of fluoride in the immediate fluid environment of the teeth.

School-based fluoride mouthrinsing programs were evaluated in a series of demonstrations sponsored by the National Institute of Dental Research in the USA,[31] and, subsequently, many states and localities adopted such programs for communities, particularly in non-fluoridated areas. These programs had appeal because costs for supplies were low and the regimen could be supervised readily by school teachers, teacher aides or volunteers after minimal in-service training.

Two studies have been done to compare the effectiveness of weekly mouthrinsing in school with 0.2% sodium fluoride and daily rinsing with 0.05% sodium fluoride; one of the studies was done in a non-fluoridated community[21] and the other in a fluoridated community.[10] In each location, both regimens were shown to be effective in caries prevention, and, although the daily regimen tended to be slightly better, the difference in effectiveness was not statistically significant. Because a daily mouthrinsing program costs about four times as much as a weekly program, the daily regimen was not considered to be sufficiently more cost-effective. Consequently, weekly fluoride mouthrinsing programs have become standard for organized school-based programs in the USA.

Many children younger than school age are not able to control their tendency to swallow, and may ingest some or all of the fluoride solution when rinsing for 1 minute.[47] Although 10 mL of 0.2% NaF solution contains only about 9 mg fluoride, that is more than desirable for routine ingestion, particularly for young children whose teeth are still forming and who may be susceptible to developing fluorosis. Consequently, fluoride mouthrinsing is not recommended for preschool age children in the USA. Often, only 5 mL of solution is used for children in kindergarten.

Several products that contain 0.05% sodium fluoride are sold as mouthrinses in retail outlets without prescriptions. The 10 mL of these rinses recommended for use contain 2.3 mg fluoride. These products have child-proof caps and are labeled as contraindicated for use by children 5 years of age or younger. Unfortunately, nearly all of these products contain alcohol for what the manufacturers consider desirable organoleptic properties.

Weekly rinsing with 0.2% NaF remains the most popular school-based caries preventive program in the United States and several other

Table 17-5

Attributes of school-based programs of weekly fluoride mouthrinsing

- Safe and effective
- Relatively inexpensive
- Easy to learn and do
- Non-dental personnel can supervise
- Well accepted by participants – good compliance
- Little time is required – 5 minutes/week

countries. Table 17-5 contains a list of some of the advantages of fluoride mouthrinsing programs accounting for their popularity compared with other organized fluoride preventive programs. It is difficult to obtain a good estimate of how many children take part in such programs. Some programs have been discontinued in recent years in several countries because of concern that they may no longer be cost-effective due to the dramatic decline in caries prevalence in some areas. Nevertheless, segments of the population remain that are at risk to high caries-attack. Organized fluoride mouthrinsing programs should be implemented or continued for these groups, who may not have access to other caries-preventive regimens or who do not sufficiently employ other caries-preventive products or practices.

Two-part fluoride rinses are marketed as self-applied caries-preventive agents for use in dental offices. These rinses are APF and SnF_2 solutions used sequentially or in combination. Their use is inherently appealing because of their perceived convenience and simplicity. They have not been tested, however, in large-scale clinical trials. The aggressive commercial promotion of these products is based largely on laboratory findings[43] and the results of small-scale studies in orthodontic and post-radiation patients. The concentrations of these rinses deviate from tested and approved products.

There also are safety concerns because these two-part rinses, when used as directed, contain 11-13 times as much fluoride as a 0.2% sodium fluoride solution used as a supervised weekly mouthrinse in schools. Products that contain APF and SnF_2 have not been recognized or approved by the American Dental Association or the US Food and Drug Administration.

Self-applied fluoride for adults with xerostomia

Adults with xerostomia, a dryness of the mouth from the lack of salivary secretions, are particularly prone to developing dental caries. Adults who have received head and neck radiation, have Sjögren's Syndrome, a chronic, autoimmune, inflammatory connective tissue disease or take medications that reduce salivary production, e.g. antidepressants, histamine antagonists or antihypertensives, are particularly prone to xerostomia and consequent rampant development of dental decay.[13]

The use of topical fluorides is essential in persons who have chronic xerostomia. Aside from professional applications of fluorides for these persons, they should also use home regimens of self-applied fluorides daily for at least 5 minutes.[33] Fluoride may be applied in mouth guards, by toothbrush or as a mouthrinse. Mouthguards containing concentrated fluorides offer the advantage of providing undiluted fluoride in close contact with the teeth, but may be painful and cumbersome for some persons. Brushing offers the advantages of being a routine procedure and easily applied, but some patients' mouths may be too sensitive to tolerate effective brushing. Mouthrinsing does not require contact with trays or toothbrushes and usually offers a pleasant relief from dryness, but provides a limited contact time between teeth and the rinse.[33]

Slow-release systems

A number of investigators have evaluated various ways to provide prolonged, sustained levels of fluoride in oral fluids in attempts to provide a ready source of fluoride for remineralization.[32] These methods include devices applied to teeth, usually molars, that release low levels of fluoride for prolonged periods, slow-release lozenges and bioadhesive tablets.

Fluoride has also been added to amalgam in an attempt to reduce the risk of recurrent caries at the margins of restorations.[44] Glass-ionomer cements release fluoride and may also inhibit secondary caries. One difficulty with these materials is controlling the rate of fluoride release.[44]

Combinations of fluoride

In texts and review articles, caries-preventive agents and methods are invariably evaluated and discussed individually. In reality, however, these agents and methods are applied and used collectively in various combinations and permutations. This is especially true for fluoride because of the multiplicity of methods, products and agents available today that contain this caries-preventive agent.

The mechanisms by which a fluoride agent prevents dental decay vary according to what agent is used, whether it is ingested in addition to being applied topically, its concentration, the vehicle used for its delivery and its frequency of use. Several mechanisms of action may operate simultaneously. Many studies have shown that fluoride toothpastes, professionally applied fluoride agents and fluoride mouthrinses, among others, provide added caries protection to children born and reared in communities with fluoridated drinking water.

There is also a logic to combining use of various topically applied fluoride agents to achieve maximal caries prevention. For example, there may be a particular rationale for combining infrequently applied concentrated fluorides, such as gels, solutions or vanishes, which are bactericidal and deposit fluoride on the outer enamel of teeth, with various dilute fluorides, like fluoride toothpastes or mouthrinses, which are applied frequently and foster the remineralization of demineralized enamel.

Some studies have shown dramatic reductions in caries prevalence or increment from the combined use of multiple fluoride agents. For example, a study in a rural setting in the USA showed that the caries prevalence of an entire school population of children in grades kindergarten through 12 was reduced by 65% after 11 years of a program of daily 1 mg fluoride tablet use in school, weekly mouthrinsing in school with a 0.2% NaF solution and home use of a toothpaste with 1000 ppm fluoride. Caries in approximal tooth surfaces declined by 90% from the combined regimen.[25] In another study, children who used both a fluoride tablet daily and a fluoride mouthrinse weekly in school developed 15% less dental decay after 8 years than children who used only the fluoride tablet and 33% less dental caries than children who used only the mouthrinse.[9]

Recommendations for use of topical fluorides

Regular use of fluoride has been a cornerstone of preventive dentistry for many years. Biannual applications have been tested in the majority of the studies involving professionally applied fluorides reviewed in this chapter. This frequency of application is not surprising given that dental practices have traditionally adopted as a standard a 6-month recall visit. Today, however, not all children or adults seem to be at risk for developing dental caries. Recent epidemiologic studies in North America and Europe have shown a major decline in dental caries prevalence and a sizable increase in children who are "caries-free". There are many reasons for this decline, but, without a doubt, the use of fluoride has played a major and predominant role. In addition, in North America, dental caries now clusters in individuals from low socioeconomic segments of society and caries-free status is a privilege that accompanies wealth and high educational status. The current skewed distribution in which 25% of children have 75% of dental decay, in addition to the widespread exposure to fluoride from other sources, challenge the practice of applying topical fluorides for all patients during recall visits.

Although fluorides should remain as one of the cornerstones for caries prevention, there is a need to determine the magnitude of their benefits under conditions that prevail today. In recent years, there has been a switch from using mass caries-preventive methods designed for all children in a community or school system to techniques that target the specific needs of individual children.[1] Diagnosis of dental caries, including an assessment of the intraoral distribution and the presence of incipient smooth surface caries and early non-cavitated carious pits and fissures, should be a prerequisite for clinical caries prevention. Based upon the caries status of a patient, sealants, fluorides, chlorhexidine, and other preventive modalities may be appropriate for use. Individuals who are most likely to benefit from fluoride applications, both professionally or self-applied, are the following:

- Caries-active individuals defined as those with past caries experience or those who develop new carious lesions on smooth tooth surfaces.

- Children shortly after periods of tooth eruption, especially those who are not caries-free.

- Individuals who are on salivary flow-reducing medications, have diseases that decrease salivary flow or have received radiation to the head and neck.

- Patients after periodontal surgery, especially when the roots of teeth have been exposed.

- Patients with fixed or removable prostheses and after placement or replacement of restorations.

- Individuals with an eating disorder or who are undergoing a change in lifestyle which may affect eating and oral hygiene habits conducive to good oral health.

- Mentally and physically challenged individuals.

The choice of topical fluoride(s) for each patient should depend on age, education, oral health habits and physical dexterity. Practitioners should concentrate on recommending for their patients agents or methods that provide frequent exposure to fluoride rather than rely on infrequently applied high concentrations of fluoride.

For public health programs, the clinical effectiveness of a universal fluoride rinse or tablet program applied to all children, many of whom may have low caries prevalence, is minimal and such a program will have low cost-effectiveness.[9] Fluoride mouthrinse programs should be recommended only after an assessment of the caries status of the targeted children. Although not widely accepted and logistically difficult, targeting of preventive services has been suggested. Based upon our current understanding of the epidemiology of dental caries in developed countries, schools located in low socioeconomic neighborhoods or in areas known to have high caries prevalence should be targeted for comprehensive caries-preventive programs with fluorides. The exact program for selection depends on severity of the caries problem, what types of tooth surfaces are predominantly affected by caries, what other fluoride sources are already available and used by the population, feasibility of implementation, the availability of personnel and sociodemographic factors that may affect acceptance and compliance.

Background Literature

Crall JJ, Novak AJ. Clinical uses of fluoride for the special patient. In: Wei SHY, ed. Clinical uses of fluorides. Philadelphia: Lea & Febiger 1985: 193-201.

Curzon MEJ, ten Cate JM, eds. Efficacy of caries preventive strategies – Proceedings of the Scientific Conference of the European Academy of Paediatric Dentistry. Caries Res 1993; 27 (Suppl 1): 29-46.

Ekstrand J. Pharmacokinetic aspects of topical fluorides. J Dent Res 1987; 162: 1061-5.

Ekstrand J. Enhancing effects of fluoride. In: Bowen WH, Tabak LA, eds. Cariology for the nineties. Rochester, NY: University of Rochester Press 1993: 409-20.

Heifetz SB, Horowitz HS. The amounts of fluoride in current fluoride therapies: safety considerations for children. J Dent Child 1984; 51: 257-69.

Horowitz HS, Heifetz SB. Methods for assessing the cost-effectiveness of caries preventive agents and procedures. Int Dent J 1979; 29: 108-17.

Horowitz HS, Heifetz SB. Topically applied fluorides. In Newbrun E, ed. Fluorides and dental caries – contemporary concepts for practitioners and students. 3rd edn. Springfield, IL: Charles C Thomas 1986: 71-114.

Kalsbeek H. Verrips GHW. Dental caries prevalence and the use of fluorides in different European countries. J Dent Res 1990; 69: 728-32.

LeCompte EJ. Clinical application of topical fluoride products – risks, benefits and recommendations. J Dent Res 1987; 65: 1066-71.

Leverett DH. Effectiveness of mouthrinsing with fluoride solutions in preventing coronal and root caries. J Public Health Dent 1989; 49: 310-6.

Manji F, Fejerskov O. Dental caries in developing countries in relation to the appropriate use of fluoride. J Dent Res 1990; 69: 733-41.

Murray JJ, Rugg-Gunn AJ. Fluoride mouthrinsing and dental caries. In Fluorides in caries prevention. Dental Practitioner Handbook No. 20. 2nd edn. Boston: Wright PSG 1982: 173-89.

Proceedings of a joint IADR/ORCA international symposium on fluorides: mechanisms of action and recommendations for use. J Dent Res 1990; 69: 771-823.

Mellberg JR, Ripa LW, eds. Professionally applied topical fluoride. In : Fluoride in preventive dentistry. Theory and clinical applications. Chicago: Quintessence Publishing Co. 1983: 181-213.

Ripa LW. Topical fluorides: a discussion of risks and benefits. J Dent Res 1987; 66: 1079-83.

Ripa LW. Review of the anticaries effectiveness of professionally applied and self-applied topical fluoride gels. J Public Health Dent 1989; 49: 297-309.

Ripa LW. A critique of topical fluoride methods (dentifrices, mouthrinses, operator- and self-applied gels) in an era of decreased caries and increased fluorosis prevalence. J Public Health Dent 1991; 51: 23-41.

Ripa LW, DePaola P, Horowitz HS, Nowak A, Schrotenboer G, Stookey GK, Volpe AR, Whall C. A guide to the use of fluorides for the prevention of dental caries. 2nd edn. J Am Dent Assoc 1986; 113: 503-65.

Rølla G, Ögaard B, Cruz R de A. Topical application of fluorides on teeth. New concepts of mechanisms of interaction. J Clin Periodontol 1993; 20: 105-8.

Stookey GK. Critical evaluation of the composition and use of topical fluorides. J Dent Res 1990; 69: 805-12.

Swango PA. The use of topical fluorides to prevent dental caries in adults: a review of the literature. J Am Dent Assoc 1983; 107: 447-50.

Whitford GM. Fluoride in dental products: safety considerations. J Dent Res 1987; 66: 1056-60.

Literature Cited

1. Arnbjerg D. Use of professionally administered fluoride among Danish children. Acta Odontol Scand 1992; 50: 289-93.

2. Banoczy J, Szoke J, Kertesz P, Toth Z, Zimmermann P, Gintner Z. Effect of amine fluoride/stannous fluoride-containing toothpaste and mouthrinsings on gingivitis, plaque and enamel F-accumulation. Caries Res 1989; 23: 284-8.

3. Berggren H, Welander E. The caries-inhibiting effect of sodium, ferric, and zirconium fluorides. A comparative study on school children using supervised brushing as the mode of application. Acta Odontol Scand 1964; 22: 401-13.

4. Bibby BG. The use of fluorine in the prevention of dental caries. II. Effect of sodium fluoride applications. J Am Dent Assoc 1944; 31: 317-21.

5. Bixler D, Muhler JC. Effect on dental caries in children in a non-fluoride area of combined use of three agents containing stannous fluoride: a prophylactic paste, a solution, and a dentifrice. II. Results at the end of 24 and 36 months. J Am Dent Assoc 1966; 72: 393-6.

6. Conchie JM, McCombie F, Hole LW. Three years of supervised toothbrushing with a fluoride-phosphate solution. J Public Health Dent 1969; 29: 11-8.

7. Council on Dental Materials, Instruments, and Equipment/Council on Dental Therapeutics, American Dental Association. Status report: effect of acidulated phosphate fluoride on porcelain and composite restorations. J Am Dent Assoc 1988; 116: 115.

8. DePaola PF. Caries in our aging population: what are we learning. In: Bowen WH, Tabak LA, eds. Cariology for the nineties. Rochester: University of Rochester Press 1993: 25-35.

9. Driscoll WS, Nowjack-Raymer R, Selwitz RH, Li S-H, Heifetz SB. A comparison of the caries-preventive effects of fluoride mouthrinsing, fluoride tablets and both procedures combined. Final results after 8 years. J Public Health Dent 1992; 52: 111-6.

10. Driscoll WS, Swango PA, Horowitz AM, Kingman A. Caries-preventive effects of daily and weekly fluoride mouthrinsing in a fluoridated community: final results after 30 months. J Am Dent Assoc 1982; 105: 1010-3.

11. Dudding NJ, Muhler JC. Technique of application of stannous fluoride in a compatible prophylactic paste and as a topical agent. J Dent Child 1962; 29: 219-24.

12. Ekstrand J, Koch G, Lindgren LE, Petersson LG. Pharmacokinetics of fluoride gels in children and adults. Caries Res 1981; 15: 213-20.

13. Engelmeir RL, King GE. Complications of head and neck radiation therapy and their management. J Prosthet Dent 1983; 49: 514-22.

14. Englander HR, Carlos JP, Senning RS, Mellberg JR. Residual anti-caries effect of repeated topical sodium fluoride applications by mouthpieces. J Am Dent Assoc 1969; 78: 783-7.

15. Englander HR, Keyes PH, Gestwicki M, Sultz HA. Clinical anti-caries effect of repeated topical sodium fluoride applications by mouthpieces. J Am Dent Assoc 1967; 75: 638-44.

16. Englander HR, Sherrill LT, Miller BG, Carlos JP, Mellberg JR, Senning RS. Incremental rates of dental caries after repeated topical sodium fluoride applications in children with lifelong consumption of fluoridated water. J Am Dent Assoc 1971; 82: 354-8.

17. Gish CW, Mercer VH, Stookey GH, Dahl LO. Self-application of fluoride as a community preventive measure: rationale, procedures, and three-year results. J Am Dent Assoc 1975; 90: 388-97.

18. Gunz GM. The effect of self-applied fluoride paste. J Public Health Dent 1971; 31: 177-81.

19. Hattab FN. The effect of air-drying on the uptake of fluoride in demineralized or abraded human enamel in vitro. J Pedod 1987; 11: 151-7.

20. Haugejorden O, Nord A. Caries incidence after topical application of varnishes containing different concentrations of sodium fluoride: 3-year results. Scand J Dent Res 1991; 99: 295-300.

21. Heifetz SB, Meyers RJ, Kingman A. A comparison of the anticaries effectiveness of daily and weekly rinsing with sodium fluoride: final results after three years. Pediatr Dent 1982; 4: 300-3.

22. Horowitz HS, Creighton WE, McClendon BJ. The effect on human dental caries of weekly oral rinsing with a sodium fluoride mouthwash: a final report. Arch Oral Biol 1971; 16: 609-16.

23. Horowitz HS, Doyle J. The effect on dental caries of topically applied acidulated phosphate-fluoride: results after three years. J Am Dent Assoc 1971; 82: 359-65.

24. Horowitz HS, Heifetz SB, McClendon BJ, Viegas AR, Guimaraes LOC, Lopes ES. Evaluation of self-administered prophylaxis and supervised toothbrushing with acidulated phosphate-fluoride. Caries Res 1974; 8: 39-51.

25. Horowitz HS, Meyers RJ, Heifetz SB, Driscoll WS, Li S-H. Combined fluoride, school-based program in a fluoride-deficient area: results of an 11-year study. J Am Dent Assoc 1986; 112: 621-5.

26. Knutson JW. Sodium fluoride solution: technique for applications to the teeth. J Am Dent Assoc 1948; 36: 37-9.

27. Knutson JW, Armstrong WD. The effect of topically applied sodium fluoride on dental caries experience. Public Health Rep 1943; 58: 1701-15.

28. LeCompte EJ, Doyle TE. Oral fluoride retention following varirous topical application techniques in children. J Dent Res 1982; 61: 1397-400.

29. Luscher B, Regolati B, Mühlemann HR. Effect of amine fluorides on plaque and caries (in vitro and animal investigations). Helv Odont Acta 1974; 18: 71-8.

30. Marthaler TM, König KG, Mühlemann HR. The effect of a fluoride gel for supervised toothbrushing 15 or 30 times per year. Helv Odont Acta 1970; 14: 67-77.

31. Miller AJ, Brunelle JA. A summary of the NIDR community caries prevention demonstration program. J Am Dent Assoc 1983; 107: 265-9.

32. Mirth DB, Shern RJ, Emilson CG, Adderly DD, Li S-H, Gomez IM, Bowen WH. Clinical evaluation of an intraoral device for the controlled release of fluoride. J Am Dent Assoc 1982; 105: 791-7.

33. Myers RE, Mitchell DL. Fluoride for the head and neck radiation patient. Milit Med 1988; 153: 411-3.

34. O'Mullane DM. Efficiency in clinical trials of caries-preventive agents and methods. Community Dent Oral Epidemiol 1976; 4: 190-4.

35. Peterson JK, Jordan WA, Snyder JR. Effectiveness of stannous fluoride-silex-silicone prophylaxis paste. Two-year report. Moorhead, Minnesota. Northwest Dent 1963; 42: 276-8.

36. Primosch RE. A report on the efficacy of fluoridated varnishes in dental caries prevention. Clin Prev Dent 1985; 7: 11-22.

37. Richardson B. Fixation of topically applied fluoride in enamel. J Dent Res 1967; 46: 87-91.

38. Ripa LW. Need for prior toothcleaning when performing a professional topical fluoride application: review and recommendations for change. J Am Dent Assoc 1984; 109: 281-5.

39. Ripa LW. An evaluation of the use of professional (operator-applied) topical fluorides. J Dent Res 1990; 69: 786-96.

40. Rølla G, Saxegaard D. Critical evaluation of the composition and use of topical fluorides, with emphasis on the role of calcium fluoride in caries inhibition. J Dent Res 1990; 69: 780-5.

41. Rugg-Gunn AJ, Holloway PJ, Davies TGH. Caries prevention by daily fluoride mouthrinsing. Report of a three-year clinical trial. Br Dent J 1973; 135: 353-60.

42. Seppa L. Studies of fluoride varnishes in Finland. Proc Finn Dent Soc 1991; 87: 541-7.

43. Shannon IL. In vitro enamel solubility reduction through sequential application of acidulated phosphofluoride and stannous fluoride. Canad Dent Assoc J 1970; 36: 308-10.

44. Skartviet L, Wefel JS, Ekstrand J. Inhibition of artificial recurrent caries by F- containing amalgam. Scand J Dent Res 1991; 99: 287-94.

45. Stookey GK, Drook CA. The effect of rinsing with water immediately after a professional fluoride gel application on fluoride uptake in demineralized enamel: an in vivo study. Pediatr Dent 1986; 8: 153-7.

46. Torell P, Siberg A. Mouthwash with sodium fluoride and potassium fluoride. Odont Revy 1962; 13: 62-72.

47. Wei SHY, Kanellis MJ. Fluoride retention after sodium fluoride mouthrinsing by preschool children. J Am Dent Assoc 1983; 106: 626-9.

48. Wei SHY, Lau EWS, Hattab FN. Time dependence of enamel fluoride acquisition from APF gels. II. In vivo study. Pediatr Dent 1988; 10: 173-7.

49. Wellock WD, Brudevold F. A study of acidulated fluoride solutions. II. The caries inhibiting effect of single annual topical applications of an acidic fluoride and phosphate solution. A two-year experience. Arch Oral Biol 1963; 8: 179-82.

50. Zero DT, Raubertas RF, Pedersen AM, Fu J, Hayes AL, Featherstone JD. Studies of fluoride retention by oral soft tissues after the application of home-use topical fluorides. J Dent Res 1992; 71: 1546-52.

FLUORIDE TOOTHPASTES

A. Richards • D.W. Banting

Introduction – Toothpastes containing 1000 ppm fluoride – Fluoride - abrasive compatibility
High fluoride (> 1000 ppm) toothpastes – Low fluoride (< 1000 ppm) toothpastes
Fluoride toothpaste and root caries – Limitations of clinical trials – Behavioral aspects
Summary and conclusions – Recommendations

Introduction

Toothbrushing with a fluoride toothpaste is by far the most common form of caries control in use today. This method of using fluoride is the simplest and most rational way of combatting caries in individuals of all ages. From a theoretical perspective the method is ideal, as it combines the mechanical effect of toothbrushing on cariogenic plaque with delivery of fluoride to the plaque-tooth interface. Thus the mechanisms whereby fluoride in a toothpaste affects the caries process are no different from the mechanisms involved when other relatively low fluoride concentration vehicles, like fluoride mouthrinses containing 0.1% fluoride, are used.

The ultimate proof of the effect of using a fluoride toothpaste is achieved by testing the product in the human clinic, and more than a hundred clinical trials, conducted over the past 50 years, have demonstrated the caries-reducing effect of using fluoride toothpastes.

Up until about 1980 most of these trials were concerned with testing various toothpaste formulations, all of which contained fluoride at a concentration of about 0.1% (1000 ppm). A summary of the results of these trials is given here as well as a description of the fluoride salts and abrasives that are considered compatible in toothpaste formulations.

The pre-1980 clinical trials tested the effects of 1000 ppm F toothpastes by comparing them with a placebo paste of the same formulation but without fluoride. As the results of the vast majority of these trials showed a positive effect, the use of fluoride toothpastes became universal (over 90% of the market in most industrialized countries). After this it was considered unethical to use non-fluoride toothpastes in clinical trials, as this would prevent trial participants from using what had become their customary fluoride toothpaste, the benefits of which were considered proven. Acceptance of the success of toothpastes containing 1000 ppm fluoride prompted manufacturers to test the possible effect of increasing the fluoride content of toothpastes to 1500-2800 ppm. The results of these trials as well as trials of toothpastes containing less than 1000 ppm fluoride are given below. Another section deals with the effects of fluoride toothpaste on root caries.

Table 18-1
Summary of clinical trials published between 1945 and 1985 which have compared toothpastes
containing 1000-1100 ppm of fluoride with a placebo toothpaste without fluoride

Fluoride source	Number of trials	Sign (p < 0.05)	% reduction DMFS increment[a]	Tooth surfaces saved per year
NaF	18	14	32[b] (11-52)[c]	0.81[b] (0.35-3.70)[c]
SnF_2	38	28	25[b] (14-64)[c]	0.76[b] (0.23-1.55)[c]
Na_2PO_3F	25	21	23[b] (15-34)[c]	0.66[b] (0.21-1.24)[c]
amine-F	5	4	25[b] (7-30)[c]	0.99[b] (0.25-1.37)[c]

a % reduction of DMFS throughout the period of the trials
b median
c range

The problems of interpreting the results of clinical trials will be described because, although clinical trials form an essential part of the evaluation of fluoride toothpastes, there are many pitfalls associated with their use. For example, statistically significant benefits may not be clinically relevant.

Concurrent with an improved understanding of how fluoride affects the caries process, the fate of fluoride in the oral environment, e.g. accumulation in plaque (see Chapter 12) has received more attention. Using toothpaste as the vehicle to introduce fluoride into the oral environment is a less precise method than, for example, supervised mouthrinsing for a fixed period of time with a measured volume of solution containing a specified amount of fluoride. Therefore, when considering how much fluoride a toothpaste should contain it is necessary to have information on how much toothpaste is normally used. Recently, it has also become obvious that it is important to consider the possible effects of how any given amount of toothpaste is used. The results of recent studies of clearance of fluoride from the mouth after use of fluoride toothpaste are given, with evidence of how different ways of using fluoride toothpastes may affect their cariostatic effect.

Finally, general conclusions are drawn about what is known about fluoride toothpastes today and a list of recommendations for use of fluoride toothpastes is given.

Toothpastes containing 1000 ppm fluoride

In clinical trials of fluoride toothpastes reported during 1945-1985 nearly all tested products contained about 1000 ppm fluoride (0.1% F = 1 mg F/g paste). This concentration of fluoride has been achieved by adding one of the following four fluoride salts: sodium fluoride (0.2% NaF), sodium monofluorophosphate (0.76% Na_2PO_3F), stannous fluoride (0.4% SnF_2), or amine fluoride (*bis*-hydroxyethyl-aminopropyl-N-hydroxyethyl-octadecylaminedi hydrofluoride).

Table 18-2
Distribution among countries of clinical trials, shown in Table 18-1, which have
compared conventional (1000-1100 ppm F) fluoride toothpastes against placebo pastes

Country	NaF	SnF$_2$	Na$_2$PO$_3$F	amine-F
USA	11	25	9	1
UK		9	11	
Sweden	4	1	2	
Denmark			1	
Holland	1			
Switzerland				3
Germany				1
Australia		2	1	
Canada	1	1	1	
Taiwan	1			

The typical clinical trial for all of these products consisted of two groups of children who were aged 11-13 years at the start of the trial. After recording caries and fillings, the children were supplied with a placebo toothpaste or a fluoride toothpaste and after a 2- or 3-year period, the means of the numbers of new tooth surfaces which had become carious or had been restored (DF-S) since the first examination were compared and the results expressed as a percent reduction in the caries increment. The results of these studies are summarized in Table 18-1, and the countries in which the trials were conducted are shown in Table 18-2. The main conclusions which may be drawn from the studies are described below.

Sodium fluoride

Toothpastes containing sodium fluoride have been compared with placebo pastes during 1945-1985. The first four studies (1945-1961) used toothpastes in which the abrasive component of the toothpaste was calcium carbonate or calcium orthophosphate, or sodium metaphosphate and none of these studies showed a caries reducing effect of the products tested. In 1961, Ericsson produced evidence which showed that in products containing calcium salts the fluoride from the highly soluble sodium fluoride reacts to produce insoluble calcium fluoride.[15] Torrild & Ericsson (1965) subsequently tested a new toothpaste formulation where the conventional calcium-based abrasive was replaced by an inert abrasive (sodium bicarbonate). This study[47] demonstrated, for the first time, a statistically significant reduction in caries increment over a 2-year period as a result of using a sodium fluoride toothpaste. In all subsequent trials, abrasives compatible with sodium fluoride were used and statistically significant benefits were found. The concept of ensuring that abrasive systems used in toothpastes are compatible with the fluoride salts used still applies today and is discussed in more detail later in this chapter.

Stannous fluoride toothpastes

As can be seen from Table 18-1, there are more reported trials of stannous fluoride toothpastes than of any of the other fluoride salts. Use and promotion of these toothpastes preceded sodium fluoride by some 10 years as the first trial reported in 1955 found a sensational 49% reduction in caries increment. Results of this and subsequent trials led for the first time to recognition of "Crest" toothpaste as a therapeutic dentifrice (Council of Dental Therapeutics of the American Dental Association 1964).[11] However, the results of later clinical trials have not consistently demonstrated statistical significance. The explanation for this may lie in the instability of the stannous fluoride salt which is subject to hydrolysis with time, resulting in formation of a variety of complex ions. The research group in Indiana, USA, who were responsible for the first trial, experimented with various pastes *in vitro* to try to overcome this problem but apparently with mixed success because, although they reported benefits in 12 different trials, other workers were not always as successful even though they used the same products. Stannous fluoride toothpastes have now more or less been abandoned not only because of the inconsistency of trial results but also because a marked disadvantage was that these toothpastes caused brown staining of the teeth.

Sodium monofluorophosphate toothpastes
Twenty-one trials (Table 18-1), reported during the period 1963-1983, have shown the benefits of using a monofluorophosphate toothpaste compared with a placebo. The background for using this compound was twofold. First of all, monofluorophosphate had been successfully used in topical fluoride solutions. These topical fluoride solutions were developed with the intention of incorporating fluoride into sound enamel and the phosphate ion was considered important for this purpose. Secondly, and of great importance for toothpaste manufacturers, were the results of *in vitro* studies which showed that this salt could be used with calcium carbonate and other abrasives not compatible with sodium fluoride.

Amine-fluoride toothpastes
The philosophy behind using an organic fluoride compound in a toothpaste was based on studies which suggested that uptake of fluoride in enamel could be enhanced by using a substance with affinity for the enamel surface. Also, *in vitro* studies had demonstrated that amine fluorides could reduce enamel solubility and retard enzyme activity in plaque. Only a few trials have been reported. The results were encouraging but the last trial which was conducted in the USA gave negative results and the possible toxicity of the compound has been questioned.

Fluoride – abrasive compatibility

Today the market is dominated by toothpastes containing either sodium fluoride or sodium monofluorophosphate. As described above, the success of these salts as the source of fluoride has been dependent on producing formulations in which the concentration of soluble fluoride is not affected by the abrasive in the product. The most commonly used abrasives are presented in Table 18-3. Only the first five abrasives on the list (Table 18-3) are generally considered to be compatible with sodium fluoride, whereas all are considered to be compatible with sodium monofluorophosphate. It would, however, be wrong to assume that all toothpastes contain soluble fluoride concentrations equal to their stated total fluoride content. This is because with storage of the products a gradual reduction in soluble fluoride content may occur, as shown in Fig. 18-1. For this reason regulatory bodies such as the US Food and Drug Administration, Standards Association of Australia and the European Community have produced rules for the minimum amount of soluble fluoride which must be present in a fluoride toothpaste throughout its shelf life. These rules typically require that at least 60% of the total fluoride content is present as a soluble

Table 18-3

Commonly used toothpaste abrasives which are considered suitable for maintaining concentrations of soluble fluoride during the shelflife of toothpastes containing sodium fluoride or sodium monofluorophosphate

Toothpaste abrasives	
calcium pyrophosphate – $Ca_2P_2O_7$	
hydrated silica – SiO_2	
sodium bicarbonate – $NaHCO_3$	**NaF and MFP**
insoluble sodium metaphosphate - $(NaPO_3)_x$	
acrylic polymer	
alumina trihydrate – $Al_2O_3.3H_2O$	
anhydrous dicalcium phosphate – $CaHPO_4$	**MFP only**
dicalcium phosphate dihydrate – $CaHPO_4.2H_2O$	
calcium carbonate – $CaCO_3$	

ion. This means F^- or, in the case of monofluorophosphate, F^- and $PO_3F_2^-$. The latter ion is now known to be rapidly hydrolyzed in the mouth to provide F^-. However, some hydrolysis does occur slowly from the time of manufacture and combine with abrasives or other toothpaste constituents to form insoluble compounds so that the total soluble fluoride concentration falls with time, as illustrated in Fig 18-1.

The crucial factor for the caries-inhibiting effect of a toothpaste or any other fluoride vehicle is the available fluoride ion concentration and it would appear that far too little attention has been paid to the question of compatible abrasives. Thus, although various regulations may ensure that major manufacturers use so-called compatible abrasive/fluoride combinations, they have been given considerable leeway concerning shelf life and minimum concentrations of soluble fluoride. Unfortunately, very few independent workers have published data on reduction in soluble fluoride concentration with time and commercial interests have

probably prohibited manufacturers from publishing such data. In view of the fact that there is now considerable evidence from clinical trials that even small changes in fluoride concentration can produce measurable differences in caries increments, it seems that this problem warrants attention in the future.

The percent caries reductions and surfaces saved per year shown in Table 18-1 suggest that sodium fluoride toothpastes are marginally more effective than monofluorophosphate toothpastes. Attempts have been made in recent years, for example using meta-analysis of selected trials,[24,45] to provide some measure of the superiority of sodium fluoride dentifrices. Theoretically, such superiority, if it exists, could be explained by possible differences in concentrations of soluble fluoride available in the mouth during and after toothbrushing. Concentrations are lower for monofluorophosphate as they are dependent upon hydrolysis of monofluorophosphate ion in the oral environment.

However, differences in ages of subjects, lo-

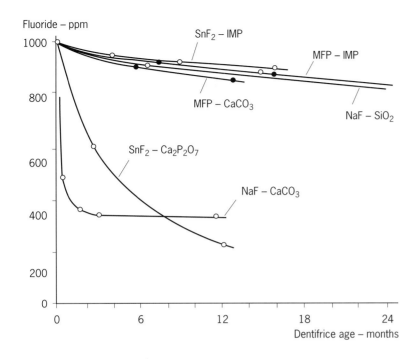

Fig. 18-1. Total soluble fluoride in dentifrices prepared with various fluoride salts and abrasives. (By courtesy of Quintessence Publishing Co., Inc[30,35]).

cation of trials, caries prevalences, fluoride exposure from other sources, etc., between the trials summarized in Table 18-1 prohibit true comparisons between sodium fluoride and monofluorophosphate with these and similar data.[50] Only a few studies have addressed this problem in a scientifically appropriate manner by making direct comparisons in the same trial and these studies have not provided sound evidence of the superiority of sodium fluoride toothpastes. Similarly, in recent years, trials have been carried out to test the possible benefit of using products containing a combination of sodium fluoride and monofluorophosphate. The conclusion from these studies is that – provided the total fluoride concentration is the same – there is no additional benefit to be gained from using a combination of the two salts instead of one salt alone.

High fluoride (> 1000 ppm) toothpastes

The possible benefit of using toothpastes containing more than 1000 ppm fluoride has been tested in clinical trials which have compared conventional 1000 ppm products with test pastes containing concentrations of 1500-2800 ppm. The results of 12 reports from these trials are summarized in Table 18-4. Use of toothpaste containing 1500 ppm resulted in statistically significantly lower caries increments in eight out of nine comparisons. In three out of three trials, 2000 ppm was found to be better than 1000 ppm but not significantly better than 1450 or 1500 ppm. Of seven trials of toothpastes with more than 2000 ppm, two failed to find a significant difference from 1000 ppm. Finally, two trials have tested pastes with 1500 ppm F against those with 2000 ppm F or more and in

Table 18-4

Summary of clinical trials which have compared fluoride dentifrices containing 1450 ppm F or more with products containing 1000 or 1100 ppm

Study	Subject's age	No.	F conc.	DMFS increment	Stat. sign.
Hodge et al., England (1980)[22]	11-12	194	1000[a]	7.31[d]	...
		200	1450[b]	6.08[d]	S
		203	1450[b]	5.94[d]	S
Barnaud & Finidori, Polynesia (1984)[2]	6-11	206	1250[b]	2.74	...
		152	2500[b]	1.61	S
Buhe et al., Germany (1984)[8]	12	438	1000[a]	14.1	...
		421	1500[a]	12.6	S
Bogopolsky et al., France (1984)[4]	7-13	–	1000[b]	1.2	...
		–	2500[b]	0.3	S
Diodati et al., USA (1986)[12]	10.5	602	1000[a]	3.08	...
		590	1450[b]	2.73	S
		592	2000[b]	2.71	S[e]
Triol et al., USA, (1987)[48]	10	–	1000[a]	3.21	...
		–	1450[a]	2.95	S
		–	2000[a]	2.79	S[e]
Stephen et al., Scotland (1988)[46]	12	469	1000[a]	6.83	...
		464	1500[a]	6.27	S
		239	2500[a]	5.56	S[f]
Lu et al., USA (1987)[28]	10	703	1100[c]	4.40	...
		673	2800[a]	4.37	ns
		679	2800[c]	3.88	S
Conti et al., USA (1988)[10]	11	1228	1000[a]	2.39	...
		1187	1500[a]	1.87	S
Fogels et al., USA (1988)[17]	9	950	1000[a]	2.36	...
		963	1500[a]	2.02	S
Ripa et al., USA (1988)[42]	11.7	827	1000[a]	3.74	...
		824	1000[b]	3.63	...
		858	2500[b]	3.67	ns
Marks et al., USA (1992)[29]	6-13	1120	1000[a]	4.23	...
	6-13	1116	1500[a]	4.23	ns
	6-13	1076	2000[a]	4.08	ns
	6-13	1112	2500[a]	3.77	S[g]

S $p < 0.05$

a MFP; **b** mixed-fluoride containing both NaF and MFP; **c** NaF; **d** DFS; **e** not significantly different from 1450 ppm; **f** significantly different from 1500 ppm; **g** not significantly different from 2000 ppm

Table 18-5

Summary of clinical trials which have compared fluoride dentifrices containing less
than 1000 ppm F with products containing 1000 ppm

Study	Subject's age	No.	F conc.	DMFS increment	Stat. sign.
Reed, USA (1973)[40]	5-14	397	0	4.00	...
		379	250[a]	3.70	ns
		387	500[a]	3.66	ns
		362	1000[a]	3.22	S
Forsman, Sweden (1974)[18]	10-11 (boys)[f]	75	0	3.05	
		77	250[b]	2.83	
		73	250[a]	2.53	
		79	1000[b]	3.10	...
	10-12R(boys)[f]	73	0	5.73	
		71	250[b]	5.08	ns
		66	1000[b]	5.13	...
Gerdin, Sweden (1974)[19]	3.5	108	250[c]	1.58[e]	S
		105	1000[a]	1.84[e]	
Koch et al., Sweden (1982)[26]	12	96	250[a]	7.5	ns
		96	1000[a]	7.2	
		96	1000[b]	6.7	
Mitropoulos et al., England (1984)[31]	12	365	250[b]	4.29	S
		360	1000[b]	3.61	
Petersson et al., Sweden (1989)[38]	12	74	136[a]		ns
		75	136[a]		ns
		67	1000[a]		
		68	1000[a]		
Winter et al., England (1989)[51]	2	1104	550[d]	2.52[e]	ns
		1073	1055[b]	2.29[e]	
Koch et al., Iceland (1990)[25]	12	203	250[a]	12.7	S
		209	700[b]	10.9	
		211	980[b]	8.8	
		209	950[a]	10.1	
		203	930[a]	10.1	

S $p < 0.05$
a NaF ; **b** MFP; **c** $KMnO_4F$; **d** MFP and NaF; **e** dfs; **f** similar results were found for girls

one of these there was a significant improvement with the highest fluoride concentration but not in the other. Overall, the results of these studies show that there is a dose-response relationship in favor of using fluoride concentrations above 1000 ppm. As can be seen from Table 4, large numbers of subjects were used in many of these trials in order to achieve statistical significance for relatively small improvements in efficacy which may not be considered of clinical significance in populations with low caries prevalences.

Low fluoride (< 1000 ppm) toothpastes

Results of studies which have tested toothpastes containing less than 1000 ppm of fluoride are summarized in Table 18-5. Three of these studies failed to demonstrate statistically significant differences between products containing 250 or 136 ppm and those containing 1000 ppm. Although there was a general trend for the low fluoride pastes to provide poorer caries inhibition in these studies, it has been argued on the basis of these studies that low fluoride toothpastes may be just as good as conventional pastes with 1000 ppm. However, the numbers of subjects in these studies were small (less than 100 per group) and statistically significant differences in favor of the higher fluoride concentrations were found in three other studies with larger numbers of subjects. Overall, the results of low fluoride studies in 12-year-olds, in keeping with high fluoride studies, support the hypothesis that there is an inverse relationship between fluoride concentration in a toothpaste and caries increments.

The main argument for lowering the fluoride content of toothpastes is to reduce total fluoride exposure in pre-school children in order to reduce the risk of development of dental fluorosis. Although fluoride toothpastes are in-

tended for topical application, it is estimated that almost 50% of the fluoride from a dentifrice is ingested by 2-3-year-olds. Fortunately, the amount decreases with age, reaching 25% in 6-7-year-olds. Assuming that the average amount of dentifrice used per brushing is 0.5 g and that children brush on average twice daily with a dentifrice containing 1000 ppm fluoride, fluoride ingestion through toothpaste can be substantial (Tables 18-6 and 18-7). Ingestion of fluoride from toothpaste alone can exceed recommended daily dosage for young children and represents a major contribution to their total fluoride intake. Recommendations regarding total daily intake for Canadians have recently been developed.[27]

The widespread use of fluoride products, including fluoride toothpaste, in North America raises legitimate concerns about the degree of fluoride exposure in pre-school children when the drinking water is also fluoridated at around 1 ppm. Fig. 18-2 represents the estimated daily fluoride intake for a 4-year-old child weighing 20 kg and living in areas with low, optimal and high levels of fluoride in the drinking water. The minimum estimated daily intake from all sources approaches 1 mg/ day in communities with low and optimal levels of fluoride but can easily surpass the recommended daily intake depending on the amount of water and other beverages consumed, foods eaten, fluoride supplements received and the quantity of toothpaste swallowed. This illustrates dramatically the vast variability in total fluoride ingestion that may occur from many sources, one of which is toothpaste, among young children (compare with dose-response considerations in Chapter 9).

Because of the widespread community benefits and favorable cost/effective ratio of community water fluoridation, it has been recommended that twice daily toothbrushing using a fluoride toothpaste be promoted for the prevention of dental caries but that, for children under 6 years of age, toothbrushing be

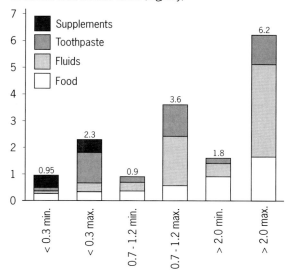

Estimated total fluoride intake (mg/day)

Fluoride in drinking water (mg/L)

Fig. 18-2. Estimated daily fluoride intake for a 4-year-old child weighing 20 kg according to fluoride content of drinking water. Minimum and maximum intakes have been estimated by assuming low or high estimates of amounts of water and other beverages consumed and quantities of toothpaste swallowed.[1]

supervised by an adult, the amount of toothpaste kept to the minimal amount needed and that swallowing of the fluoride toothpaste be discouraged.[39] Additional recommendations have addressed product labeling or package instructions relating to these guidelines, studies to investigate the efficacy of lower dose fluoride dentifrices and the marketing of toothpastes.

In this context therefore it may be relevant to consider the results of the two studies on 2-3-year-old children. The first of these[19] found that a 250 ppm F paste was significantly better than a 1000 ppm F paste. The numbers of subjects was small but the fluoride source used in the test paste was potassium manganese fluoride salt, which has never been tested before or since, whereas the positive control paste contained sodium fluoride. The only other study in this age group[51] used over a thousand children in each group and failed to demonstrate a statistically significant difference between 500 ppm and 1000 ppm after 3 years. This study sup-

ports the hypothesis that 500 ppm is just as good as 1000 ppm for this age group. However, the results of one study alone do not justify general recommendation of low fluoride dentifrices for everyone. Furthermore, the scientific value of this study is marred by the fact that the authors did not consider it necessary to carry out a baseline examination of their subjects at the outset of the trial.

Fluoride toothpaste and root caries

The etiology and pathogenesis of root and coronal caries are similar,[36] and therefore parallel approaches can be rationally entertained to avoid their consequences. Thus fluoride should be considered fundamental to the control of root caries as well as enamel caries.[37]

Only one clinical study has been conducted on the effectiveness of sodium fluoride toothpaste to prevent root caries initiation but it is limited in its utility because it was of only 1

Table 18-6
Amount of dentifrice used per brushing (g) or fluoride per brushing (mg)[a] by age

Study	2-3	4	5	6-7	8-10	11-13	16-35
Ericsson & Forsman[16] (1969)[b]		0.45		0.45			
Hargreaves et al.[21] (1972)[c]			0.33			1.10	
Barnhart et al.[3] (1974)[b]	0.86			0.94			1.39
Glass et al.[20] (1975)[b]					1.04[d]		
Dowell[13] (1981)[c]	0.55						
Bruun & Thylstrup[7] (1988)[c]	0.55[d]			0.75[d]	1.10[d]		1.55[d]
Simard et al.[44] (1989)[b]	0.46	0.78	0.65				
Naccache et al.[33] (1990)[b]	0.50		0.47				
Naccache et al.[32] (1992)[b]	0.55	0.45	0.52	0.50			
Mean value	**0.58**	**0.56**	**0.50**	**0.66**	**1.07**	**1.10**	**1.5**
(no. of studies)	(6)	(3)	(4)	(4)	(3)	(1)	(2)

a If one assumes that the dentifrice contains 0.1% (1000 ppm), then the ingestion of x grams of dentifrice results in the ingestion of x mg of fluoride; b Supervised dentifrice use study; c Home use study; d No attempt was made to control for spillage of dentifrice

year's duration and because it has not been replicated.[23] Nevertheless, a clinically and statistically significant reduction (67%) in the rate of new root caries development favoring the test group was observed. In addition, other studies have shown that toothbrushing with a fluoride dentifrice can convert active lesions to inactive lesions,[34,37] and the histopathology of arrested root caries lesions has been described.[43]

Limitations of clinical trials

When they are considered as a group, the results of all the clinical trials summarized in Table 18-1 provide overwhelming evidence of the caries-reducing effect of using a fluoride toothpaste. Likewise, it is clear from the trials summarized in Tables 18-4 and Table 18-5 that when large populations have been used, the reductions in caries incidence are dose-dependent. However, it is important to appreciate that

Table 18-7
Percent ingestion of dentifrice fluoride by age

Study	Age range (year)						
	2-3	4	5	6-7	8-10	11-13	16-35
Ericsson & Forsman[16] (1969)[a]		30		26			
Hargreaves et al.[21] (1972)[b]			28				
Barnhart et al.[3] (1974)[a]	35			14		6	3
Glass et al.[20] (1975)[a]					12[c]		
Simard et al.[44] (1989)[a]	59	48	34				
Naccache et al.[33] (1990)[a]	41		30				
Naccache et al.[32] (1992)[a]	57	49	42	34			
Mean value	**48**	**42**	**34**	**25**	**12**	**6**	**3**
(no. of studies)	(4)	(3)	(4)	(3)	(1)	(1)	(1)

a Supervised dentifrice use study; b Home use study; c No attempt was made to control for spillage of dentifrice

clinical trials vary greatly in design and methodology. Results of individual trials are therefore not comparable, which means that they cannot be used to evaluate the relative efficacy of the various formulations tested.

Many of the early trials did not live up to the general requirements of a double-blind, randomized trial. Subjects were not stratified according to age, numbers of teeth present, caries prevalence at the start of the study, etc. Diagnostic criteria were poorly described and no details of examiner calibration or measurements of inter- and intraexaminer reliability were stated.

Although later studies have fulfilled such basic requirements, there are many other factors which should be considered when faced with the results of a single study. Reporting results as percentage reductions of DMFS increments (as shown in Table 18-1) can be misleading as the actual numbers of tooth surfaces "saved" over a given period is the relevant factor to be used when considering the clinical rather than the statistical significance of the results of a trial. Thus, in some cases, the results of trials in some populations have recorded mean DMFS increments of less than one over a 3-year period, while in other populations 3-year increments of 12 or more have been reported.

Expressing results of 2- or 3-year clinical trials as percentages have led some workers to consider the 20-40% reductions found to be rather modest when compared to the more than 50% reductions consistently shown to occur as a result of water fluoridation (see

Chapter 15). However, such comparisons may not be justifiable as most clinical trials normally only run for 2 or 3 years, whereas results of effects of drinking fluoridated drinking water represent the effect of lifelong exposure. In fact, fluoride toothpastes may be more effective than fluoridated drinking water, and in populations with widespread and frequent use of fluoride toothpastes the efficacy of these products may also be superior to that of fluoridated drinking water.

DMFS measurements provide a rather crude indication of the disease situation in a population and the missing and filled components are highly dependent upon the diagnostic threshold for treatment used by the clinicians treating the trial subjects both before and during a trial.

In some populations, a continuing decline in the prevalence and incidence of caries has led to a situation where use of conventional DMFS measurements means that more than half of the subjects recruited to a clinical trial are recorded as caries free at the outset and remain so throughout the period of the study. As a consequence, it has become common to conduct trials with thousands of subjects in order to be certain of attaining statistically significant differences between means of DMFS increments. It should be remembered that the level of statistical significance normally chosen ($p < 0.05$) means there is always a one in 20 risk that the results may have occurred by chance.

It may seem reasonable to require the sales promotion claims of superior efficacy of new formulations made by toothpaste manufacturers to be adequately supported by properly conducted clinical trials. On the other hand, as far as fluoride is concerned, provided that a new product has been shown to contain a given amount of fluoride in, soluble form, throughout its shelf life, it seems reasonable to expect that it will provide benefits in keeping with the results found in previous studies.

Clinical trials are time-consuming and expensive and have nearly always been funded by the few major multinational companies in the cosmetics industry. This is a highly competitive market and clinical trials are likely to continue to play an important role in sales promotion. The more recent clinical trials have aimed at producing evidence for an effect of a wide variety of other therapeutic agents which may further enhance the effect of fluoride. Market forces will ensure that this practice continues even though the limitations of clinical trials described above means that the results are too variable and imprecise for optimizing different toothpaste formulations. Even if clinical trials were more precise, "head on" comparisons of products from different manufacturers would not be given financial support for commercial reasons. Also, trials which fail to produce evidence of superiority of a new formula are less likely to be published than "successful" trials. These factors should be borne in mind when evaluating the results of a single and otherwise scientifically sound clinical trial.

Behavioral aspects

Benefits of using a toothpaste containing fluoride have been apparent and widely accepted for more than three decades without much attention having been paid to how they should be used. In recent years, however, a number of studies have focused on the possible effects of various oral care habits on the efficacy of fluoride toothpastes.

Not surprisingly, perhaps, it has been shown that frequency of toothbrushing is directly related to the degree of benefit achieved. As early as 1982, a review of controlled clinical trials showed that there was a tendency for the largest caries reductions to occur in studies where toothbrushing was supervised (Fig. 18-3), suggesting that there was an increased frequency of toothpaste use in the supervised trials.[6] The obtaining of reliable data on toothbrushing fre-

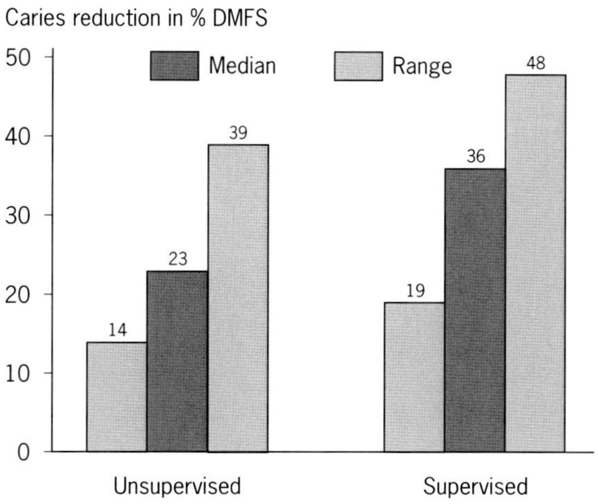

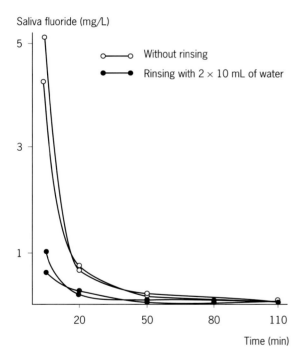

Caries reduction in % DMFS

Fig. 18-3. Percentage caries reductions recorded in supervised and unsupervised clinical trials of conventional (1000-1100 ppm F) fluoride toothpastes. (Modified from Bruun et al.[6]).

Fig. 18-4. Changes in salivary fluoride concentrations with time after application of 1 g sodium fluoride toothpaste (1000 ppm F) for 1 min. Chewing the toothpaste for 1 minute followed by swallowing without rinsing the mouth with water, resulted in higher concentrations of fluoride in saliva up to 110 minutes after than were achieved by toothbrushing with the same amount of the toothpaste for 1 minute followed by rinsing the mouth with 2 × 10 mL of water.[41]

quency is dependent on accurate reporting by children, who may not always be willing to disclose how seldom they brush their teeth. In some studies with large numbers of subjects, statistically significantly lower caries increments have been found in trial participants who claimed they had brushed twice daily or more compared with those who stated they had brushed once daily or less.[9,49]

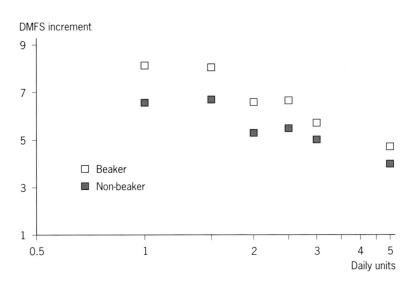

DMFS increment

Daily units

Fig. 18-5. Differences in caries increments in relation to reported rinsing of the mouth after toothbrushing, frequency of toothbrushing and concentration of fluoride in toothpaste. Data are from a 3-year clinical trial with toothpastes containing 1000, 1500, and 2500 ppm fluoride. The subjects were also divided according to whether they brushed their teeth once or twice daily and also according to whether they used a beaker of water or not to rinse their mouth after toothbrushing. Assuming brushing 1 × daily with 1000 ppm is equivalent to 1 arbitrary unit of fluoride exposure, then 1.5 units = 1 × daily using 1500 ppm, 2 units = 2 × daily using 1000 ppm, 2.5 units = 1 × daily using 2500 ppm, 3 units = 2 × daily using 1500 ppm, and 5 units = 2 × daily using 2500 ppm.[9]

Factors affecting fluoride elimination

As the whole purpose of adding fluoride to a toothpaste is to increase the concentration of fluoride at the plaque–enamel interface (in plaque fluid and, if possible, in liquid within pores of caries lesions) it may be expected that the efficacy of a fluoride toothpaste depends upon the extent to which it is capable of producing increased levels of fluoride in the oral environment for prolonged periods of time. Concentrations of fluoride in plaque have been shown to be related directly to concentrations of fluoride in toothpaste,[14] and initial saliva concentrations after toothbrushing and the length of time saliva fluoride levels are elevated after fluoride dentifrice use have also been

shown to be directly related to the fluoride concentration.[5] However, as shown in Fig. 18-4, rinsing the mouth with water after toothbrushing may cause profound reductions in the amount of fluoride available in the oral environment after toothbrushing.

In a recent study[9] of toothpastes containing 1000, 1500 and 2500 ppm fluoride, the subjects were asked about frequency of toothbrushing and how they rinsed their mouths after toothbrushing. Fig. 18-5 summarizes the results of this study; mean DMFS increments were higher for subjects who used a beaker of water when they rinsed their mouths. The Figure also demonstrates the effects of fluoride concentration and toothbrushing frequency and it is tempting to speculate from these results that oral care habits such as frequent brushing and limited rinsing after toothbrushing with a 1000 ppm fluoride toothpaste may be just as effective as infrequent brushing and thorough rinsing with a toothpaste with a fluoride concentration greater than 1000 ppm.

Amount of paste used

Another aspect of oral care habits is the question of how much toothpaste is used at each toothbrushing session. Table 18-6 shows the mean amount of toothpaste used per brushing by age. The data indicate reasonable consistency of use by age, with increasing amounts used with increasing age. The mean value of 0.5-0.58 g paste for 2-5-year-olds approximates the "pea-size" amount which has been recommended for young children, a recommendation which is printed on toothpaste packages in some countries. The increasing amount of toothpaste used with age probably reflects the size of the toothbrush head – junior and adult toothbrushes being larger than children's toothbrushes taken together with the habit of dispensing enough toothpaste to cover all the bristles. The reason for this practice is open to conjecture but it may reflect what is taught by dental health personnel and/or mimic what the commercial product advertisements portray.

Summary and conclusions

In developed countries worldwide, fluoride dentifrices most likely have made the greatest single contribution to the decline in the prevalence of dental caries. The evidence from countless clinical trials conducted to test a variety of fluoride preparations applied in a toothpaste vehicle on a wide spectrum of populations of diverse age from all parts of the world falls clearly on the side of fluoride toothpastes being universally accepted as the primary preventive strategy for coronal caries because of their ease of use, ability to produce significant reductions in dental decay and low cost. The commonly repeated figure of a 50% reduction in dental caries prevalence as a direct consequence of fluoridated toothpaste is probably an underestimate of its global impact. The parallel use of fluoride toothpaste for root caries lacks the intensity of study applied to coronal caries but the results are expected to be similar.

An observed increase in the milder forms of dental fluorosis, in areas both with and without community water fluoridation, have raised concerns about the total daily intake of fluoride of young children and have prompted recommendations to use less dentifrice, supervise the toothbrushing activity and discourage swallowing of the toothpaste by children under the age of 6 years. However, taking the dose-response considerations presented in Chapter 9 into account, it is obvious that, rather than restricting the use of toothpaste containing fluoride, efforts should be focused on minimizing systemic exposure to fluoride from sources such as tablets and drops.

Recommendations

There is good scientific evidence in the dental literature to support the following recommendations regarding the use of fluoride dentifrices:

- Fluoride dentifrice should be used daily for toothcleaning by persons of all ages to control development and progression of dental caries lesions.

- With young children, the amount of fluoride dentifrice should be reduced and the toothbrushing activity should be supervised to minimize the ingestion of fluoride (which can add significantly to the total daily fluoride intake leading to an increased risk of mild dental fluorosis).

- Although there is a dose-response relationship between fluoride concentration in a dentifrice and dental caries reduction, the clinical significance of fluoride concentrations in toothpastes containing more than 1100 ppm has not been proven, and the risk of developing milder forms of dental fluorosis increases with dosage.

- Lower concentrations (< 1100 ppm) of fluoride in toothpastes may be as effective as higher (1100 ppm) concentrations but sufficient evidence is not yet available to recommend the routine use of lower fluoride concentrations.

- Sodium fluoride and sodium monofluorophosphate are equally efficacious anticaries agents when used in dentifrices at 1100 ppm concentration and are preferred to stannous fluoride and amine fluoride at this time.

Literature cited

1. Banting DW. The future of fluoride. J Am Dent Assoc 1991; 123: 86-91.

2. Barnaud J, Finidori C. Étude de l'efficacité preventive d'une pâte à haute teneur en fluorures. J Int Assoc Dent Child 1974; 15: 21-31.

3. Barnhart WE, Hiller LK, Leonard GJ, Michaels SE. Dentifrice usage and ingestion among four age groups. J Dent Res 1974; 53: 1312-7.

4. Bogopolsky S, Albertini H, Goldberg W. Étude clinique d'une pâte (dentifrice) à haute teneur en fluorures à Marseilles. In: Vaillant JM, Barmes D, eds. Le Point Sur Le Fluor, Symposium, Institut de Stomatologie et de Chirurgie Maxillo-Faciale, La Salpetriere, Paris 1984.

5. Bruun C, Givskov H, Thylstrup A. Whole saliva fluoride concentrations after toothbrushing with NaF and MFP dentifrices with different F concentrations. Caries Res 1984; 18: 282-8.

6. Bruun C, Lambrou D, Larsen MJ, Fejerskov O, Thylstrup A. Fluoride in mixed human saliva after different topical treatments and possible relation to caries inhibition. Community Dent Oral Epidemiol 1982; 10: 75-9.

7. Bruun C, Thylstrup A. Dentifrice usage among Danish schoolchildren. J Dent Res 1988; 67: 1114-7.

8. Buhe H, Buttner W, Barlage B. Uber einen dreijahrigen klinischen Zahncremetest mit Zahnpasten unterscheidlicher Fluoridkonzentration: 0.8% und 1.2% Natriumfluorophosphat. Quintessenz 1984; 35: 1-9.

9. Chesters RK, Huntington E, Burchell CK, Stephen KW. Effect of oral habits on caries in adolescents. Caries Res 1992; 26: 299-304.

10. Conti AJ, Lotzkar S, Daley R, Cancro L, Marks RG, McNeal RG. A 3-year clinical trial to compare efficacy of dentifrices containing 1.14% and 0.76% sodium monofluorophosphate. Community Dent Oral Epidemiol 1988; 16: 135-8.

11. Council on Dental Therapeutics. Reclassification of Crest toothpaste. J Am Dent Assoc 1964; 69: 195-6.

12. Diodati RR, Triol CW, Kranz SM, Korn LR, Volpe AR. Clinical anticaries effect of various dentifrices. J Dent Res 1986; 65: 198.

13. Dowell TB. The use of toothpaste in infancy. Br Dent J 1981; 150: 247-9.

14. Duckworth RM, Morgan SN, Burchell CK. Fluoride in plaque following use of dentifrices containing sodium monofluorophosphate. J Dent Res 1989; 68: 130-3.

15. Ericsson Y. Fluorides in dentifrices. Investigations using radioactive fluorine. Acta Odontol Scand 1961; 19: 41-77.

16. Ericsson Y, Forsman B. Fluoride retained from mouthrinses and dentifrices in pre-school children. Caries Res 1969; 3: 290-9.

17. Fogels HR, Meade JJ, Griffith J, Miragliuolo R, Cancro LP. A clinical investigation of a high-level fluoride dentifrice. J Dent Child 1988; 55: 210-5.

18. Forsman B. Studies on the effect of dentifrices with low fluoride content. Community Dent Oral Epidemiol 1974; 2: 166-75.

19. Gerdin PO. Studies on dentifrices, VIII. Clinical testing of an acidulated non-grinding dentifrice with reduced fluoride content. Swed Dent J 1974; 67: 283-97.

20. Glass RL, Peterson JK, Zuckerberg DA, Naylor MN. Fluoride ingestion resulting from the use of a monofluorophosphate dentifrice by children. Br Dent J 1975; 138: 423-6.

21. Hargreaves JA, Ingram GS, Wagg BG. A gravimetric study of the ingestion of toothpaste by children. Caries Res 1972; 6: 237-43.

22. Hodge HC, Holloway PJ, Davies TGH, Worthington HV. Caries prevention by a dentifrice containing a combination of sodium monofluorophosphate and sodium fluoride. Br Dent J 1980; 149: 201-4.

23. Jensen ME, Kohout F. The effect of a fluoridated dentifrice on root and coronal caries in an older adult population J Am Dent Assoc 1988; 117: 829-32.

24. Johnson MF. Comparitive efficacy of NaF and SMFP dentifrices in caries prevention. A meta-analytic overview. Caries Res 1993; 27: 328-36.

25. Koch G, Bergmann-Arnadottir I, Bjarnason S, Finnbogason S, Hoskuldsson O, Karlsson R. Caries preventive effect of fluoride dentifrices with and without anticalculus agents: a 3-year controlled clinical trial. Caries Res 1990; 24: 72-9.

26. Koch G, Petersson LG, Kling E, Kling L. Effect of 250 and 1000 ppm fluoride dentifrice on caries. Swed Dent J 1982; 6: 233-8.

27. Lewis DW, Banting DW, Burgess RC, Ismail A, Clark DC, Leake JL. Recommendations regarding total daily fluoride intake for Canadians. J Can Dent Assoc 1994; 60: 1050-60.

28. Lu KH, Ruhlman CD, Chung KL, Sturzenburger OP, Lehnoff RW. A three-year clinical comparison of a sodium monofluorophosphate dentifrice with sodium fluoride dentifrices on dental caries in children. J Dent Child 1987; 54: 241-4.

29. Marks RG, D'Agostino R, Moorehead JE, Conti AJ, Cancro L. A fluoride dose response evaluation in an anticaries clinical trial. J Dent Res 1992; 71: 1286-91.

30. Mellberg JR. Fluoride dentifrices. In Mellberg JR, Ripa LW, Leske GS, eds. Fluoride in preventive dentistry. Theory and clinical applications. Chicago: Quintessence, 1983: 215-33.

31. Mitropoulos CM, Holloway PJ, Davies TGH, Worthington HV. Relative efficacy of dentifrices containing 250 or 1000 ppm F- in preventing dental caries – report of a 32 month clinical trial. Community Dent Health 1984; 1: 193-200.

32. Naccache H, Simard PL, Trahan L, Brodeur JM, Demers M, Lachapelle D, Bernhard PM. Factors affecting the ingestion of fluoride dentifrice by children. J Public Health Dent 1992; 52: 222-6.

33. Naccache H, Simard PL, Trahan L, Demers M, Lapointe C, Brodeur JM. Variability in the ingestion of toothpaste by preschool children. Caries Res 1990; 24: 359-63.

34. Nemes J, Banoczy J, Wierzbicka M. Clinical study on the effect of amine fluoride/stannous fluoride on exposed root surfaces. J Clin Dent 1992; 3: 51-3.

35. Noren B, Harse C. The stability of the monofluorophosphate and fluoride ions in dentifrice containing calcium carbonate. J Soc Cosmet Chem 1974; 18: 3-11.

36. Nyvad B. Microbial colonization of human tooth surfaces (Thesis). APMIS 1993; 101: Suppl. 32.

37. Nyvad B, Fejerskov O. Active root surface caries converted into inactive caries as a response to oral hygiene. Scand J Dent Res 1986; 94: 281-4.

38. Petersson LG, Johansson M, Jonsson G, Birkhed D, Gleerup A. Caries preventive effect of toothpastes containing different concentration and mixture of fluorides and sugar alcohols. Caries Res 1989; 23: 120.

39. Recommendations from report of the 1992 Canadian Conference on the Evaluation of Current Recommendations concerning Fluorides. J Can Dent Assoc 1993; 59: 330-6.

40. Reed MV. Clinical evaluation of three concentrations of sodium fluoride in dentifrices. J Am Dent Assoc 1973; 87: 1401-3.

41. Richards A, Larsen MJ, Hovgaard O, Fejerskov O. Fluoride toothpastes and fluoride concentrations in saliva. Dan Dent J 1988; 92: 146-50.

42. Ripa LW, Leske GS, Forte F, Varma A. Caries inhibition of mixed NaF-Na$_2$PO$_3$F dentifrices containing 1,000 and 2,500 ppm F: 3-year results. J Am Dent Assoc 1988; 116: 69-73.

43. Schupbach P, Lutz F, Guggenheim B. Human root caries: Histopathology of arrested lesions. Caries Res 1992; 26: 153-64.

44. Simard PL, Lachapelle D, Trahan L, Naccache H, Demers M, Brodeur JM. The ingestion of fluoride dentifrice by young children. J Dent Child 1989; 56: 177-81.

45. Stamm JW. Clinical studies of neutral sodium fluoride and sodium monofluorophosphate dentifrices. In: Bowen WH, ed. Relative efficacy of sodium fluoride and sodium monofluorophosphate as anti-caries agents in dentifrices. London: The Royal Society of Medicine Press Limited, 1995: 43-58.

46. Stephen KW, Creanor SL, Russell JI, Burchell CK, Huntington E, Downie CFA. A 3-year dose-response study of sodium monofluorophosphate dentifrices with and without zinc citrate: anticaries results. Community Dent Oral Epidemiol 1988; 16: 321-5.

47. Torell P, Ericsson Y. Two year clinical tests with different methods of local caries-preventive fluoride in Swedish schoolchildren. Acta Odontol Scand 1965; 23: 287-322.

48. Triol CW, Mandanas BY, Juliano GF, Yraolo B, Cano-Arevalo M, Volpe AR. A clinical study in children comparing anticaries effect of two fluoride dentifrices. Clin Prev Dent 1987; 9: 22-4.

49. Tucker GJ, Andlaw RJ, Burchell CK. The relationship between oral hygiene and dental caries incidence in 11-year old children. A 3-year study. Br Dent J 1976; 141: 75-9.

50. Volpe AR, Petrone ME, Davies RM. A critical review of the 10 pivotal caries clinical studies used in a recent meta-analysis comparing the anticaries efficacy of sodium fluoride and sodium monofluorophosphate dentifrices. Am J Dent 1993; 6: 13-42.

51. Winter GB, Holt RD, Williams BF. Clinical trial of a low-fluoride toothpaste for young children. Int Dent J 1989; 39: 227-35.

CHAPTER 19

Rational use of fluorides in caries control

B.H. Clarkson • O. Fejerskov • J. Ekstrand • B.A. Burt

Introduction – cariostatic mechanisms in historical perspective
Enamel fluoride and caries experience
Caries experience related to fluoride in plaque and oral fluids
Fluoride: A therapeutic agent – Clinical implications – Recommendations

Introduction

This final chapter presents a rationale for the uses of fluoride from the personal, professional and public health standpoint. Since the publication of the first edition of this book, scientific developments in the field of fluoride have included: (i) subtle advances in our knowledge of the dynamics of caries lesion formation; (ii) a more precise understanding of the mechanism of action of fluoride; (iii) an expansion of our knowledge of the pharmacokinetics of fluoride; (iv) a reevaluation of the toxicologic effects of fluoride, especially its link at relatively low concentrations with fluorosis; and (v) a reassessment of fluoride's effects on skeletal tissues during development and disease. The purpose of this chapter is to synthesize these advances in knowledge, all of which have been described in detail throughout this book. The end result is a science-based rationale for the use of fluorides in dental practice and in public health.

Our understanding of the mechanism of the action of fluoride, added to the documented increase in fluorosis in North America, dictates how fluoride should be used both in dental practice and in public health. In essence, however, it does not change the argument underlying the biologic rationalism of fluoride usage, [rationalism being defined in the American Heritage dictionary as the theory that "...the exercise of reason, rather than the acceptance of empiricism, authority or spiritual revelation, provides the only valid basis for action"].

Basically, we are dealing with fluoride's direct and indirect effects on two very different structures, teeth and plaque. In simple terms, one can view fluoride as having an effect on caries by reducing the dissolution of teeth, and/or by accelerating the remineralization of initial lesions, and/or by preventing plaque bacteria from producing sufficient organic acids to demineralize tooth surfaces. If one can now use the facts available today to identify the predominant mechanism of action, the most beneficial and cost-effective way of using fluoride to combat dental caries can be chosen without the risk of physiologically "saturating

347

the environment" with fluoride. By using fluoride in precise amounts, and at the most appropriate times in terms of dental development, the benefits of fluoride will be maximized and the detrimental side effect of dental fluorosis will be minimized.

Cariostatic mechanisms in historical perspective

Theories of the mechanism of action of fluoride, and how they developed, are best viewed in a historical perspective. The fact that the cariostatic effect of fluoride was first discovered in relation to the natural fluoride content of drinking water was logically interpreted as meaning that fluoride's cariostatic effect was due to the systemic, preeruptive incorporation of fluoride into the tooth. Having established a theory, scientists attempted to find a plausible explanation as to how fluoride "worked" once it was incorporated into enamel. It had already been discovered that acids initiated dental decay; therefore, fluoride's effect was expected to be related to reducing the solubility of tooth enamel. Laboratory experiments were performed which seemed to suggest that the solubility of enamel was reduced by incorporating fluoride, but closer scrutiny revealed that it only affected the enamel solubility significantly when incorporated at a relatively high concentration. Despite that, a hypothesis evolved which suggested that fluoride helped to make the enamel crystal "more perfect," and therefore less acid soluble. Sophisticated analysis of both fluoridated and non-fluoridated bone mineral supported this hypothesis, so the "void and substitution theorem" became the means by which a theory to explain how fluoride reduces dental caries evolved into dogma.

Consequently, a corollary to having "established" that the best method for obtaining maximum cariostatic effect of fluoride was by a systemic route was that topical application, while second best, was still useful. It could also be inferred from the above dogma that increasing the amount of fluoride in enamel would make more crystals more perfect and, therefore, such enamel would be more acid resistant. Much time and effort have been spent on trying to develop topical formulations or regimens which would significantly increase the fluoride content of sound enamel. To this end, many different fluoride concentrations were used, a variety of vehicles were developed, the pH of the vehicle was lowered, the frequency and mode of application were altered, and various fluoride compounds were tested. Many methods were studied extensively both in the laboratory and in clinical trials. Virtually all of these developments, however, were based on the philosophy that in order for fluoride to evoke its cariostatic effect it should be incorporated into the tooth surface, and in as high a concentration as possible.

It should also be remembered that the efficacy yardstick by which these different topical modalities have been measured was the 50-60% caries reduction obtained from water fluoridation. However, most clinical trials of topical fluoride agents ran for approximately 1-3 years and produced caries reductions of approximately 25-30% when compared with control groups. These reductions were taken as support for the concept that no topical fluoride use was as effective as systemic use, despite the fact that the populations examined in water fluoridation studies had been exposed for some 10-15 years as opposed to the 1-3 years in clinical trials for topical fluorides. The comparisons were therefore hardly valid.

More recently, other observations have had an effect on our thinking with respect to the cariostatic mechanism of fluoride. One involves the realization of the consequences of enamel apatite being impure, while others concern the role which the reaction products calcium fluoride and "free" fluoride, absorbed onto the enamel crystal surface, might play in the dissolution and remineralization chemistry of dental hard tissues.

Enamel apatites contain a number of foreign ions, including carbonate at approximately 2-5% wet weight. The carbonated apatites are more reactive and therefore more soluble, and fluoride has been shown to reduce the dissolution rate of this apatite.[2,8] Thus the elimination of the carbonated apatite crystals and reprecipitation of fluoridated hydroxyapatite could be valuable in preventing caries lesion progression. Such activity may also be part of the early, so-called "secondary maturation" process, which includes subclinical levels of demineralization and remineralization and thus helps to prevent the development of clinically detectable lesions.

The undesirable reaction product of earlier attempts to incorporate fluoride into enamel in a permanently bound state, calcium fluoride, has become a celebrated cariostatic moiety. The formation of calcium fluoride after topical fluoride applications is thought to act as a fluoride reservoir, from which fluoride dissolves at the site of caries formation under appropriate chemical conditions and then promotes the reprecipitation of mineral. It has even been speculated that calcium fluoride may act as a more effective blocker of acid diffusion through enamel than fluoridated hydroxyapatite, and can therefore help limit both the penetration and progression of the carious lesion.

The presence of "free" or intercrystalline fluid fluoride in enamel has been recognized for some time. In fact, it is suggested that it contributes approximately 25% of the fluoride present in developing rat enamel.[1] More recently, it has been shown that a relatively high percentage of the fluoride in mature human surface enamel can be extracted with urea.[7] If this is true this would indicate that such fluoride is "free" in the intercrystalline fluid, and/or easily dissociated from the enamel

crystals, and/or associated with the organic matrix of enamel. This fluoride may be more readily available to interact chemically at the inception of lesion formation, providing conditions which both limit demineralization and promote remineralization of the dental tissue.

Mechanistically, these recent observations argue against the need to use a systemic route to incorporate fluoride into enamel. This is because the elimination of carbonated apatite, the production of calcium fluoride, and the presence and "topping-up" of the free fluoride can all be achieved by topical applications of fluoride.

Enamel fluoride and caries experience

In addition to the above considerations it has become evident during the last two decades that the fluoride concentration in enamel does not reflect the relative susceptibility of the tooth to decay *in vivo*. The fluoride concentration in whole enamel is relatively low and mainly reflects fluoride incorporated during preeruptive formation and mineralization of the tissue. In spite of the difference in caries experience between those born and raised in high- rather than low-fluoride areas, there is little difference in enamel fluoride concentration between these two populations. However, when individuals move from a low-fluoride water supply to one where the water contains 1.0 mg F/L, their subsequent caries experience is improved when compared to that in comparable populations in the low-fluoride community they left. Similarly, in regions where fluoridation of water supplies was discontinued for one reason or another, the population returned to caries levels comparable to those existing prior to the introduction of fluoridation. These observations demonstrate that caries resistance depends more upon day-to-day exposure to fluoride than on the presence of "permanently" bound fluoride in the enamel.

In addition, lesions formed *in vitro* in tooth enamel from non-fluoridated and fluoridated areas show little difference with respect to lesion depth, degree of demineralization, and histologic features. The same finding has been observed when the fluoride-rich outer enamel surface was removed in both groups.[10] Thus it is not surprising that a clear-cut inverse relationship between caries experience and the fluoride content of surface enamel cannot be demonstrated.

In research over the years, much cariostatic importance has been attached to the conversion of hydroxyapatite to fluoridated hydroxyapatite. Complete substitution of hydroxyl ions in human enamel corresponds to a fluoride content of 3.7%, but even in severely fluorosed enamel such complete substitution is never achieved because less than one-quarter of the hydroxyl ions in the outer enamel have been replaced by fluoride. In human enamel formed in areas with 1.0-1.5 mg F/L in the water there are significantly smaller fluoride concentrations as the substitution amounts to only 10%, corresponding to about 3,000 ppm of fluoride in the outer enamel.[6] As a consequence, it has been shown that carious lesions can be produced *in situ* in shark enamel, which is virtually pure fluorapatite, under plaque subjected to appropriate cariogenic conditions.[9] Thus the need to convert hydroxyapatite to fluoridated hydroxyapatite via systemic or topical means should not, in itself, be a goal for inhibiting carious lesion progression. The therapeutic goal should be to have fluoride available in the oral fluids when conditions exist which favor either demineralization or remineralization of the hard tissue. The source of this fluoride is not important *per se*.

Caries experience related to fluoride in plaque and oral fluids

Plaque contains 5-10 mg F/kg wet weight in low fluoride areas and some 10-20 mg F/kg wet weight in areas with fluoridated water. Most of it, up to 95%, is bound in some form. These levels of fluoride do not appear to affect the bacterial composition of plaque, and they do not encourage the selection of stable fluoride-resistant strains. But if mobilized they may inhibit acid production at any pH range. The combination of fluoride with a metallic ion, e.g. stannous fluoride, can cause plaque disruption, while very high concentrations of fluoride, such as those in professional gels, may have a transitory effect on plaque bacterial metabolism. Therefore, although there is some evidence that fluoride may affect plaque metabolism when combined at high concentrations with other ions, it is difficult to envisage fluoride's effect on plaque bacteria as a major cariostatic mechanism. Much more evidence exists to suggest that the primary cariostatic mechanism comes from the effects of fluoride concentrations in both plaque fluid and saliva on the mineral dynamics of the caries process.

Plaque fluid fluoride concentrations are relatively low (0.04-0.1 ppm), although there is probably variation from site to site in the same mouth.[11] The analysis of plaque fluid from individuals who exhibit either caries resistance or caries susceptibility has been revealing.[4,5] A positive relationship between higher plaque fluid pH and low caries susceptibility in "starved" individuals, and a similar positive relationship between low caries susceptibility and the degree of supersaturation with all calcium and phosphorus phases of biologic interest, has been shown.[3] Thus, relatively small increases in pH and fluoride concentration will help cause the precipitation of apatitic phases into the demineralized dental hard tissue.

The fluoride concentrations in mixed saliva, although two to three times higher in individuals in a 1.0-1.5 mg F/L area than in a 0.2 mg F/L area, are still relatively low. For a long time this was thought to be of no significance in relation to caries. However, the improved understanding of fluoride kinetics in oral fluids in combination with what is known today about the effect of very low concentrations of fluoride on the physicochemical behavior of enamel has initiated an entirely new concept of how fluoride exerts its cariostatic effect.

We must conclude therefore that the predominant cariostatic effect of fluoride is that of a direct effect on the de- and remineralizing processes in the dental hard tissues. This concept explains why significant caries reductions are achieved after various topical treatments with high fluoride concentrations, and, equally importantly, why fluoride at very low levels (1.0 mg F/L and below) in the oral fluids affects the rate of mineral dissolution and enhances redeposition of calcium and phosphate.

From the foregoing discussion and from previous chapters in this book, certain important facts emerge:

- Available evidence suggests that fluoride's effect is predominantly one which involves an interaction with the hard tissue during caries lesion development and progression.

- It is apparent that there is no relationship between *in vitro* acid solubility of enamel and clinical caries reduction.

- The difference in fluoride content in enamel, whether surface or subsurface, either from areas of low water-fluoride concentration (< 0.2 mg F/L) or from areas of higher concentration (approximately 1.0 mg F/L), is not of sufficient magnitude even to theoretically explain a 50% difference in caries experience.

- It is apparent that there is no relationship between the fluoride content of enamel, as

such, and the caries experience of the individual. This is evident in both the primary and permanent dentitions and when the fluoride levels of more caries-prone sites, i.e. approximal surfaces, are compared with less caries-prone sites such as free smooth surfaces.

- People born and reared with drinking water at 1.0 mg F/L develop caries to the same degree as those in a low fluoride area if, after tooth eruption, they move into these low fluoride areas (assuming they are exposed to a comparable cariogenic challenge).

- Topical fluorides achieve levels of caries reduction unrelated to how much fluoride is incorporated into the enamel.

- Although both laboratory and clinical evidence exists that fluoride can affect bacterial metabolism and plaque colonization, there is no convincing, consistent evidence which directly links this effect with caries reductions in humans.

- Evidence is accruing which suggests that the prevalence of fluorosis is increasing in some populations where there is extensive exposure to fluorides.

- Fluoride in plaque fluid and saliva at relatively low concentrations can inhibit the progression of a carious lesion.

In reviewing these statements, and combining them with discussions from earlier chapters, certain observations can be made which indicate that caries reduction in humans is *not* dependent upon (a) fluoride being administered via a systemic route; (b) having high levels of fluoride in sound enamel; or (c) having fluoride affect either the bacterial metabolism or bacterial colonization of enamel. The inhibition of caries, however, is predominantly effected by fluoride being present during active caries development at the plaque/enamel interface, where it will directly alter the dynamics of mineral dissolution and reprecipitation. This is not to say that fluoride incorporated into enamel apatite does not reduce its rate of dissolution to some extent, but this factor alone cannot explain the caries reductions observed. These considerations should govern the use of fluoride in caries prevention and treatment.

Fluoride: A therapeutic agent

Acceptance of these arguments pinpoints an anachronism in our present thinking, which is that fluoride is a primary preventive agent for caries. To illustrate, caries reductions in clinical trials are usually measured by gross clinical observations pertaining to the absence or presence of cavitated carious lesions. This approach ignores the fact that before a lesion develops to a level where it is clinically obvious, actual lesion formation may have been going on for months or even years. Rather than concluding that fluoride "prevents lesion formation" because the test group developed fewer cavitated lesions during the test period, it would be more correct to state that fluoride has interfered with lesion development to the extent that lesion progression rate has been slowed down, or even stopped, in the test subjects. In this light, fluoride should be thought of as an active treatment for carious lesions rather than a preventive measure in the strict sense.

This viewpoint may seem to be of only theoretical interest, but it is a crucial issue when a clinician or public health administrator is determining how to use fluoride. When it is understood that fluoride acts by interfering with the disease process at all stages, it can then be used appropriately as a therapeutic agent which reduces the demineralization rate and enhances mineral uptake.

What conclusions can now be drawn from the preceding arguments and how can they be applied by the clinician, the public health official or the general public at large? The guiding principle is that the fluoride ion has to be active at the site of the developing lesion. A topical mode of delivery is appropriate for patients in a dental practice, and fluoride toothpaste is a fundamental vehicle in societies where toothbrushing is a cultural norm. However, public health delivery often has to rely on modes where systemic absorption is inevitable, such as drinking water and salt fluoridation. These modes of delivery are easily the most cost-effective means of providing fluoride to large populations, and in many instances are the only feasible way of achieving large-scale fluoride availability. The trade-off to their effectiveness is that some dental fluorosis will be observed. So long as the fluorosis is within acceptable limits, their public health benefits will be widespread and obvious.

In order to optimize fluoride's preventive effect as a topical agent, a regimen using low fluoride concentrations is desirable, and as demineralization occurs at every cariogenic challenge, high frequency of fluoride application is recommended (e.g. fluoride in the water supply and/or regular toothbrushing with fluoride toothpaste) to maintain appropriate therapeutic intraoral fluoride levels.

Finally, it must be recognized that fluoride therapy alone will not arrest caries development and progression at every site in every individual. To do that, microbial deposits have to be removed and the patients made to understand the importance of proper oral hygiene; dietary management and sealants may also need to be employed. If excellent oral hygiene is combined with selective fluoride therapy, however, a substantial reduction in disease incidence can be achieved in most, otherwise healthy, individuals.

Clinical implications

The caries-reducing effect of fluoride was first identified from epidemiologic surveys associating water fluoride concentrations and caries experience in large populations. Ever since, we have by tradition looked upon fluoride use as a mass prophylactic measure in public health. This is reflected in the way that topical fluorides have been used in programs aiming at large groups of schoolchildren, where the assumption is that all these children would benefit, irrespective of their actual caries experience. This approach was understandable when fluoride was thought to prevent caries on a lifelong basis by being incorporated into sound enamel, and when virtually all children had a high caries experience. However, with our present knowledge of how caries develops and how fluoride affects it, public health programs targeted at whole populations may not always be an automatic choice. A rational use of fluoride as a therapeutic agent has to be based on caries-fluoride interactions as well as the pharmacokinetic and toxicologic behavior of the fluoride agents. In addition, cost-effectiveness, meaning whether the amount of disease prevented justifies the cost of the program, is always an issue in today's low-caries populations.

Having brought the argument to this point, it can be seen that *it is not possible to recommend a "one and only" or "best" fluoride program.* Decisions on the most appropriate type of public health program to implement should also take into account these factors:

- The economic development of the community

- Educational levels

- Caries prevalence, incidence and distribution in the population

- Oral hygiene status

- Access to dental services

- Special living conditions or dietary habits of a population or individual

- Other fluoride exposures, e.g. water fluoride concentration, and use of fluoride toothpastes.

A good example of why there can not be a "one and only" fluoride program is given when one compares the different Scandinavian countries, which have all shown similar reductions in dental caries in recent years though they have used different fluoride measures and programs to achieve it. Moreover, present day caries experience in the USA and the Nordic countries is similar, although fluorides are used in very different ways in those countries.

The clinician faces an even greater dilemma when trying to individualize his or her fluoride recommendations for a patient, and some general guidelines would seem appropriate.

In patients with little caries or in whom caries activity is controlled, the clinician will not need to use new fluoride regimens as the patient will most probably be receiving high-frequency, low-concentration fluoride via toothpaste or drinking water, or both. There may be cases, in fact, where the clinician recommends a reduction in the number of fluoride modalities being used; e.g. if a patient clinically has no active caries and is living in a community with fluoridated water and is using a fluoride rinse as well as a fluoride toothpaste, the patient may be advised to stop using the rinse. If, by contrast, the clinician decides to prescribe the use of a professionally applied topical fluoride gel for a patient with high caries activity, which one should the dentist use? There is little evidence to suggest that any one high-concentration topical fluoride agent is significantly more effective than another.

The ultimate aim of all clinicians should be to achieve and then maintain a high-frequency, low-fluoride concentration regimen for their patients because low levels of fluoride in the oral fluids significantly affect ongoing de- and remineralization. Patients would benefit if dental personnel would instruct them, when necessary, about the benefits of such a simple regimen as the regular use of fluoride toothpastes. Many patients, as well as some dental health personnel, consider toothpaste only as a vehicle for removing food debris, dental plaque and for improving mouth odors. However, from current knowledge it is evident that fluoride toothpaste should be applied specifically at sites which may be at particular caries risk. This should be done after the regular brushing procedure is finished, particularly at bedtime because salivary secretion is reduced during the night. Therefore, the toothpaste thus applied will act as an excellent fluoride reservoir. This regimen has proven effective in the arrest of active root-surface caries lesions in elderly patients.

In this context, we stress that fluoride toothpastes probably constitute the most rational and simple way of providing fluoride therapy to everybody, at least in the economically developed countries where such toothpaste is inexpensive and widely available. Although difficult to prove, it is reasonable to assume that a good part of the decline in dental caries over recent years in most industrialized countries, notably those Northern European countries without water fluoridation, can be explained by the widespread use of fluoride toothpastes. This reduction in caries has not been paralleled by a reduction in sugar intake, but it does follow a significant increase in the use of fluoride toothpastes by the public. Fluoride toothpastes now account for over 90% of toothpaste sales in most economically developed countries. A major challenge to manufacturers and public health agencies is how to bring the benefits of fluoride toothpaste to Third World countries, where products that are standard in the developed world are too expensive for the local economies. The challenge is, technologically, to produce an effective but inexpensive product; logistically, to distribute it widely; and educationally, to promote its use among people who may not have toothbrushing as part of their culture.

Returning to patients in a private practice, for those who are highly caries susceptible and have shown little progress with standard fluoride therapy, a controlled release fluoride delivery system would probably be beneficial. Unfortunately, there is at present no effective slow-release vehicle available. These patients are those in whom caries develops and progresses rapidly, and where the background factors which cause this high activity are difficult to alter. Such patients may include individuals with poor salivary secretion as a result of certain diseases or radiation therapy to the head and the neck region, or those taking psychosedative drugs or other drugs that affect salivary gland function. These patients need frequent professional oral hygiene intervention and frequent professional application of topical fluorides (i.e. gels, varnishes). Furthermore, daily use of fluoride lozenges or chewing tablets or chewing gum for these patients may be prescribed in order to achieve an elevated fluoride concentration in the oral environment throughout the day. In very severe cases it may even be necessary to recommend daily home treatment with a fluoride gel.

The foregoing considerations are naturally applicable only in countries with a well-developed dental care delivery system. Recommendations for fluoride use in developing countries are complicated by the many logistical problems in those countries. While water fluoridation, for example, is a highly effective method for reaching large populations, it can only be used when there is a well-controlled public water system, a water treatment facility and a trained staff. The majority of the world's population live in rural areas with no organized drinking water system, and as mentioned earlier they usually have no access to fluoride toothpaste either. Dental services are also scarce to non-existent in such situations.

In view of these problems, a number of developing countries have chosen to implement salt fluoridation as a method of bringing fluoride to their populations (though as noted in Chapter 16 it also has been adopted by some European countries). Salt fluoridation has been evaluated in field trials (Chapter 16), and while it appears to be effective there are a number of questions that still surround its use. One concerns its cariostatic action. As this book has made clear, fluoride is a therapeutic agent whose predominant cariostatic action involves interaction with the dental hard tissues during lesion development and progression. Following that principle, it has not yet been demonstrated how fluoridated salt increases the fluoride levels in oral fluids to the extent that they interfere with the carious process. A second issue is that the appropriate concentration of fluoride in salt needs to be established for each country adopting the measure; what is appropriate for Switzerland does not necessarily apply to Costa Rica.

Recommendations

- Water fluoridation is a highly effective and cost-effective method for reducing the prevalence and severity of caries in large populations, especially among those people who rarely visit a dentist. Fluoridation does bring with it some risk of mild fluorosis. The prevalence and severity of fluorosis related to water fluoride concentrations is well established, and in such areas other ingestible fluoride agents should not be used.

- If water fluoridation is not an option, for whatever reason, we do not recommend the use of fluoride supplements in young children because of the problems they incur. Compliance in their use is frequently poor, and supplements are known to be a risk factor for dental fluorosis when ingested during the early years of life. Supplements are effective in children when chewed or sucked prior to swallowing, but should not be used before the age of 6 years in order to avoid the risk of fluorosis. They might be effective and practical therapy for caries-susceptible adults, although this approach has not yet been clinically tested. From all the evidence given on fluoride's mode of action, supplements cannot be recommended for pregnant women as a means of providing cariostatic benefits for the offspring.

- Salt fluoridation is a practical method, and sometimes the only method, of bringing fluoride to large populations where water fluoridation cannot be used. But because there are still outstanding questions on the mechanism of action of the fluoride in salt, and because the amounts of salt ingested can vary considerably among individuals, salt fluoridation should be the methed of last resort for fluoride administration in public health. Over-consumption of salt has been associated with hypertension, and it should never be assumed that because salt is fluoridated people should eat more of it. Where salt fluoridation is used, the concentration should be established so that normal consumption provides dental benefits.

- The topical use of fluorides which are not intended for ingestion is recommended where possible. Certainly, fluoride in toothpaste is the method of choice because it can be used by everybody irrespective of age, it is a cultural norm in many societies and it is an efficient way of maintaining appropriate intraoral fluoride levels. Fluoride toothpaste is a risk factor for fluorosis when swallowed by young children, so careful supervision and use of small amounts of toothpaste are called for when youngsters are learning to brush their teeth.

- Fluoride rinsing can be recommended as a school-based prophylactic measure where caries prevalence is high, though it is not cost-effective in child populations with low caries incidence. Rinsing can also be recommended as a daily routine for individual patients who are more than usually susceptible to caries.

- Professionally applied fluoride gel treatment may be very useful in high risk patients. Because such treatment is necessarily expensive, it should be seen as an individual treatment for problem patients only.

To conclude the theme we have promoted throughout this book, fluorides are used in caries treatment to interfere with the ongoing caries process. This happens most efficiently when a low level of fluoride is constantly present in the mouth, and this status requires high-frequency exposure to low-concentration fluoride. Fluoride should be specifically used to slow down the caries progression rate by altering the mineral dynamics at sites where there is active lesion formation, and it should also be combined with oral hygiene measures to obtain the maximum caries-reducing effect. If fluorides are used in this way, it is not only possible to arrest caries lesion development and progression in virtually everybody, but to do so with little concern for dental fluorosis.

Background literature

Bowden GH, Milnes AR, Boyar R. Streptococcus mutans and caries: State of the art 1983. In: Guggenheim B, ed. Cariology today. Basel: Karger, 1984: 173-91.

Brudevold F, McCann HG, Gron P. Caries resistance as related to the chemistry of the enamel. In: Wolstenholme GEW, O'Connor M, eds. Caries resistant teeth, Ciba Foundation Symposium. London: Churchill 1965: 121-48.

Burt BA, ed. Proceedings for the Workshop: Cost effectiveness of caries prevention in dental public health. J Public Health Dent 1989; 49 (Spec Iss): 251-352.

Clarkson BH. Caries prevention – fluoride. Adv Dent Res 1991; 5: 41-5.

Driessen FMC. Mineral aspects of dentistry. Monographs in Oral Science, Vol. 10. Basel: Karger 1982.

Ekstrand J, Spark C-J, Vogel G. Pharmacokinetics of fluorid in man and its clinical relevance. J Dent Res 1990; 69: 550-5.

Fejerskov O, Manji F, Baelum V, Moller IJ. Dental fluorosis – a handbook for health workers. Copenhagen: Munksgaard, 1988.

Fejerskov O, Thylstrup A, Larsen MJ. Rational use of fluorides in caries prevention – a concept based on possible mechanisms. Acta Odontol Scand 1981; 39: 241-7.

Fomon S, Ekstrand J. Fluoride, Chapter 18. In: Fomon SJ, ed. Infant Nutrition. S. Louis: C.V. Mosby, 1993: 299-310.

Guggenheim B, ed. Cariology today. Basel: Karger, 1984: 223-78.

Johansen E, Olsen TO. Topical fluorides in the prevention and arrest of dental caries. In: Johansen E, Taves DR, Olsen TO, eds. Continuing evaluation of the use of fluorides. (AAS selected symposium). Colorado: Westview Press, 1979: 66-110.

Konig K, Brown W, eds. Cariostatic mechanisms of fluoride. Caries Res 1977; 11: Suppl. 1.

Larsen MJ, Bruun C. Enamel/saliva – inorganic chemical reactions. In: Thylstrup A, Fejerskov O, eds. Textbook of cariology. Copenhagen: Munksgaard, 1986: 181-203.

Loesche WJ. Dental caries: A treatable infection. Springfield: Thomas, 1984.

Luoma H, Fejerskov O, Thylstrup A. The effect of fluoride on dental plaque, tooth structure and dental caries. In: Thylstrup A, Fejerskov O, eds. Textbook of cariology. Copenhagen: Munksgaard, 1986: 199-334.

Szpunar SM, Burt BA. Evaluation of appropriate use of dietary fluoride supplements in the U.S. Community Dent Oral Epidemiol 1992; 20: 148-54.

Tatevossian A. The chemistry of plaque fluid. Frontiers of oral physiology, Vol 3. Basel: Karger, 1981: 66-77.

World Health Organization. Fluorides and oral health; Report of an Expert Committee. Technical Report Series no. 846. Geneva: WHO 1994.

Literature cited

1. Aoba T, Collins J, Moreno EC. Possible function of matrix proteins in fluoride incorporation into enamel mineral during porcine amelogenesis. J Dent Res 1989; 68: 1162-68.

2. Featherstone JDB, Shields CP, Khademazad B, Olderstraw MD. Acid reactivity of carbonated apatite with strontium and fluoride substitutions. J Dent Res 1983; 62: 1049-53.

3. Margolis HC. Enamel-plaque fluid interactions. In: Bowen WH, Tabak LA, eds. Cariology for the nineties, Rochester, NY: University of Rochester Press 1993: 173-86.

4. Margolis HC, Duckworth JH, Moreno, EC. Composition of pooled resting plaque fluid from caries-free and caries-susceptible individuals. J Dent Res 1988; 67: 1468-75.

5. Margolis HC, Duckworth, JH, Moreno, EC. Composition and buffer capacity of pooled starved plaque fluid from caries-free and caries susceptible individuals. J Dent Res 1988; 67: 1476-82.

6. Margolis HC, Moreno EC. Physicochemical perspectives on the cariostatic mechanisms of systemic and topical fluoride. J Dent Res 1990; 66 (Spec Iss): 606-13.

7. Nainar HSM, Clarkson BH. Fluoride profile in mature unerupted enamel following removal of surface organic material. Caries Res 1993; 28: 83-8.

8. Nelson DGA, Featherstone JDB. Preparation analysis and characterization of carbonated-apatite. Calcif Tissue Int 1982; 34: 569-81.

9. Ogaard B, Rolla G, Ruben J, Dijkman T, Arends J. Microradiographic study of demineralization of shark enamel in a human caries model. Scand J Dent Res 1988; 96: 209-11.

10. Silverstone LM. The surface zone in caries and in caries-like lesions produced *in vitro*. Br Dent J 1968; 125: 145-57.

11. Vogel GL, Ekstrand J. Fluoride in saliva and plaque fluid a 0.2% NaF rinse: Short term kinetics ond distribution. J Dent Res 1992; 71: 1553-7.

Index

Index

Toothpastes 163, 328
Topical agents 268
Topical fluorides 311, 323
Total fluorine 33
Toxic dose 170
Toxic substance 167
Toxicity considerations 317
Treatment of acute fluoride toxicity 180
Treatment modalities 102

V
Vitamin D 102

W
Water fluoridation 275
Water fluoridation as social policy 285
Water fluoride concentrations 286
Water fluoride studies 156
"White spot" lesion 192
Whole plaque 34
World status of fluoridation 281

X
Xerostomia 322

Z
Zinc ion 227